Pathology of Sinonasal Tumors and Tumor-Like Lesions

Alessandro Franchi
Editor

Pathology of Sinonasal Tumors and Tumor-Like Lesions

Springer

Editor
Alessandro Franchi
Department of Translational Research
and of New Technologies in Medicine and Surgery
University of Pisa
Pisa
Italy

ISBN 978-3-030-29850-0 ISBN 978-3-030-29848-7 (eBook)
https://doi.org/10.1007/978-3-030-29848-7

This Springer imprint is published by the registered company Springer Nature Switzerland AG
The registered company address is: Gewerbestrasse 11, 6330 Cham, Switzerland

Contents

Part I

General Features

Epidemiology of Sinonasal Cancer

Lucia Miligi, Carlotta Buzzoni, and Sara. Piro

Introduction

Sinonasal cancers (SNCs) represent less than the 0.2% of all malignant cancers yearly diagnosed in the world [1] and about 3.6% of all malignancies arising in the head and neck area [2]. Despite this low frequency, a great variety of histological types may be found, and the most frequent are keratinising squamous cell carcinoma (SCC), adenocarcinomas (AD), cylindrical cell (non-keratinising) carcinoma, undifferentiated carcinoma, lymphoma, melanoma and olfactory neuroblastoma.

SNCs may be classified as *rare cancer*, but the low absolute risk in the general population effectively contrasts with the high relative risks for specific chemical exposures and occupational settings. SNCs are indeed considered rare cancers with high occupational attributable fraction (AF: 20–43%) [3, 4]. In this chapter, we review the current knowledge on epidemiological aspects of SNC.

L. Miligi (✉) · S. Piro
Unit of Environmental and Occupational Epidemiology, Institute for Cancer Research, Prevention and Clinical Network (ISPRO), Florence, Italy
e-mail: l.miligi@ispro.toscana.it; s.piro@ispro.toscana.it

C. Buzzoni
Tuscany Cancer Registry, Clinical and Descriptive Epidemiology Unit, Institute for Cancer Research, Prevention and Clinical Network (ISPRO), Florence, Italy

Incidence, Mortality and Survival

Incidence

SNCs represent less than the 0.2% of all malignant cancers yearly diagnosed in the world. The incidence rates are around 1/100,000 inhabitants, as reported in the publication *Cancer Incidence in Five Continents-Volume XI,* a report published approximately every 5 years by the *International Agency for Research on Cancer* and *the International Association of Cancer Registries,* which provides comparable high-quality statistics on the incidence of cancer from cancer registries around the world [1]; in volume XI, the period 2008–2012 is analysed.

The annual number of new cases is available where population-based cancer registries exist, with some approximation, because current statistics are by site and the three-digit ICD-O-3 codes C30–C31 (cancers of the nasal cavity, middle ear and paranasal sinuses) encompass middle ear cancers too [5]. The percentage distribution of cancers across subsites of the sinonasal region is different in different geographic areas. Generally, the subsite 'middle ear' is the less represented (e.g. in males it accounts for less than 3% of cases in the USA). Nevertheless, when descriptive epidemiology of cancers of the SNC are presented, current statistics must be interpreted considering that the ICD-O-3 codes for SNC take into account also middle ear.

A. Franchi (ed.), *Pathology of Sinonasal Tumors and Tumor-Like Lesions*,
https://doi.org/10.1007/978-3-030-29848-7_1

SNCs may be classified as *rare cancer*: according to the European Parliament and Council of the European communities, rare diseases are defined as those with a prevalence of <50 per 100,000 [6], while, in line with the Orphan Drug Act, in the USA rare diseases are those affecting <200,000 persons [http://www.fda.gov/orphan/oda.htm]. However, a published analysis of rare cancers in the USA employed the definition of <15 incident cases per 100,000 per year [7]. In 2010, the EU funded RARECARE—Surveillance of rare cancers in Europe project [8] and proposed a new definition of rarity for cancers and a list of rare cancers in Europe.

The low frequencies of rare cancers, and the consequent limited medical expertise on the matter, create specific problems in clinical decision making, clinical research and healthcare organisation. In addition, patients and their families are confronted with a wide range of difficulties arising directly from the rarity of the pathologies. Such difficulties may include wrong diagnosis leading to inaccurate treatments, delays in the period between the onset of the first symptoms and the diagnosis, insufficient scientific knowledge and lack of appropriate quality healthcare.

Geographic Differences

In North America, crude incidence rates are about 1.1/100,000 inhabitant among men and 0.6/100,000 among women, with similar values in Asia (about 1.0/100,000 men and 0.6/100,000 women). Rates are slightly higher in Europe (about 1.2/100,000 men and 0.7/100,000 women) and Oceania (about 1.1/100,000 men and 0.6/100,000 women) and lower in Central/South America (about 0.5/100,000 men and 0.3/100,000 women) and Africa (about 0.4/100,000 men and 0.3/100,000 [1].

In the period 2008–2012, the highest incidence age-standardised rates (ASR) per 100,000 inhabitants (standard: world population) have been reported among men in some small registries in Australia (Tasmania: 1.7), Spain (Asturias: 1.7), South America (French Guiana: 1.7), Africa (Zimbabwe, Harare: 1.3), France (Lille, Limousin and Vendee: 1.2), Switzerland (Neuchatel: 1.2) and Thailand (Lopburi: 1.2) [1], but these rates are unstable because it is based on small populations. In selected major registries (or groups of registries), ASR per 100,000 inhabitants (standard: world population) in males present a smaller statistical variability, and the highest incidence rates have been reported in Belgium (Flanders) as shown in Table 1.

Table 1 Cancers of the nasal cavity, middle ear and paranasal sinuses (codes ICD-O-3: C30–C31)

Nord America	Cases	Crude rate	ASR (W)
Population			
USA, NPCR	6261	0.9	0.6
USA, NPCR: White	5375	0.9	0.6
USA, NPCR: Black	595	0.6	0.6
Asia			
China, Hong Kong	171	1.0	0.6
India, Mumbai	150	0.4	0.5
Japan, Osaka	371	1.7	0.8
Korea	1035	0.8	0.7
Europa			
Belgium	480	1.8	1.1
Denmark	217	1.6	0.9
Germany, North Rhine-Westphalia	627	1.4	0.8
The Netherlands	475	1.2	0.6
Norway	119	1.0	0.8
Ukraine	1263	1.2	0.7
United Kingdom	1442	0.9	0.6
Oceania			
Australia, New South Wales	182	1.0	0.7

Number of new cases in 5 years, crude rates (per 100,000 inhabitants) and age-standardised rates (per 100,000 inhabitants) by selected Registries. Males, years 2008–2010 (Modified from Bray [1]). *NPCR* National Program of Cancer Registries, *ASR* age standardized rate, *W Standard* world population

Table 2 Cancers of the nasal cavity, middle ear and paranasal sinuses (codes ICD-O-3: C30–C31), period 2008–2012

	Male			Female		
Population	Cases	Crude rate	ASR (W)	Cases	Crude rate	ASR (W)
Africa	82	0.30	0.60	60	0.20	0.40
Peru	72	0.50	0.60	52	0.40	0.30
Puerto Rico	67	0.70	0.50	44	0.40	0.30
Canada	504	0.80	0.50	385	0.60	0.30
USA	6608	0.90	0.60	4366	0.60	0.30
China	1087	0.70	0.50	604	0.40	0.20
India	523	0.40	0.50	339	0.30	0.30
Israel	104	0.60	0.50	76	0.40	0.30
Japan	1195	1.70	0.80	648	0.90	0.40
Korea	433	0.70	0.60	240	0.40	0.30
Philippines	180	0.50	0.80	116	0.30	0.40
Thailand	171	0.60	0.50	128	0.40	0.30
Turkey	158	0.50	0.50	86	0.30	0.20
Austria	230	1.10	0.70	119	0.60	0.30
Belarus	220	1.00	0.70	132	0.50	0.30
Belgium	480	1.80	1.10	169	0.60	0.30
Bulgaria	206	1.10	0.70	91	0.50	0.20
Croatia	135	1.30	0.80	67	0.60	0.30
Czech Republic	225	0.90	0.50	300	1.10	0.60
Denmark	217	1.60	0.90	165	1.20	0.60
France	404	1.50	0.90	169	0.60	0.30
Germany	1837	1.40	0.80	1100	0.80	0.40
Ireland	72	0.60	0.50	52	0.50	0.30
Italy	715	1.20	0.60	398	0.60	0.30
Lithuania	96	1.30	0.90	54	0.60	0.30
The Netherlands	475	1.20	0.70	340	0.80	0.50
Norway	119	1.00	0.60	83	0.70	0.40
Poland	211	0.70	0.50	135	0.40	0.20
Russian Federation	176	0.90	0.70	113	0.50	0.30
Spain	264	1.00	0.60	133	0.50	0.30
Switzerland	136	1.30	0.70	65	0.60	0.30
Ukraine	1263	1.20	0.90	797	0.60	0.40
United Kingdom	1442	0.90	0.60	975	0.60	0.30
Australia	572	1.00	0.70	311	0.60	0.30
New Zealand	85	0.80	0.50	41	0.40	0.30

Number of new cases in 5 years, crude rates (per 100,000 inhabitants) and age-standardized rates (per 100,000 inhabitants) by sex and country with total number of diagnosed cases >100 (Modified from Bray [1]); *ASR* Age Standardized Rate, *W Standard* World population

Table 2 compares incidence data from different countries in the world, including only countries with 100 or more diagnosis during the considered period, 2008–2012. Differences are more pronounced in crude rates than age-standardised rates: part of the observed heterogeneity is related to the distribution across countries. Among males, crude rates vary from 0.3 (Africa) to 1.8 per 100,000 (Belgium), and ASR varies from 0.5 (India) to 1.1 (Belgium). Among female, crude rates vary from 0.2 (Africa) to 1.2 per 100,000 (Denmark), and ASR varies from 0.2 (Turkey) to 0.6 (Denmark). The male/female ratio in ASR varies from 0.8 in Czech Republic to 3.7 in Belgium.

Fig. 1 Cancers of the nasal cavity, middle ear and paranasal sinuses (codes ICD-O-3: C30–C31). Incidence age-specific rates per 100,000 inhabitants. Italian areas covered by a general cancer registry, males and females, years 2008–2012 (Source: Bray [1])

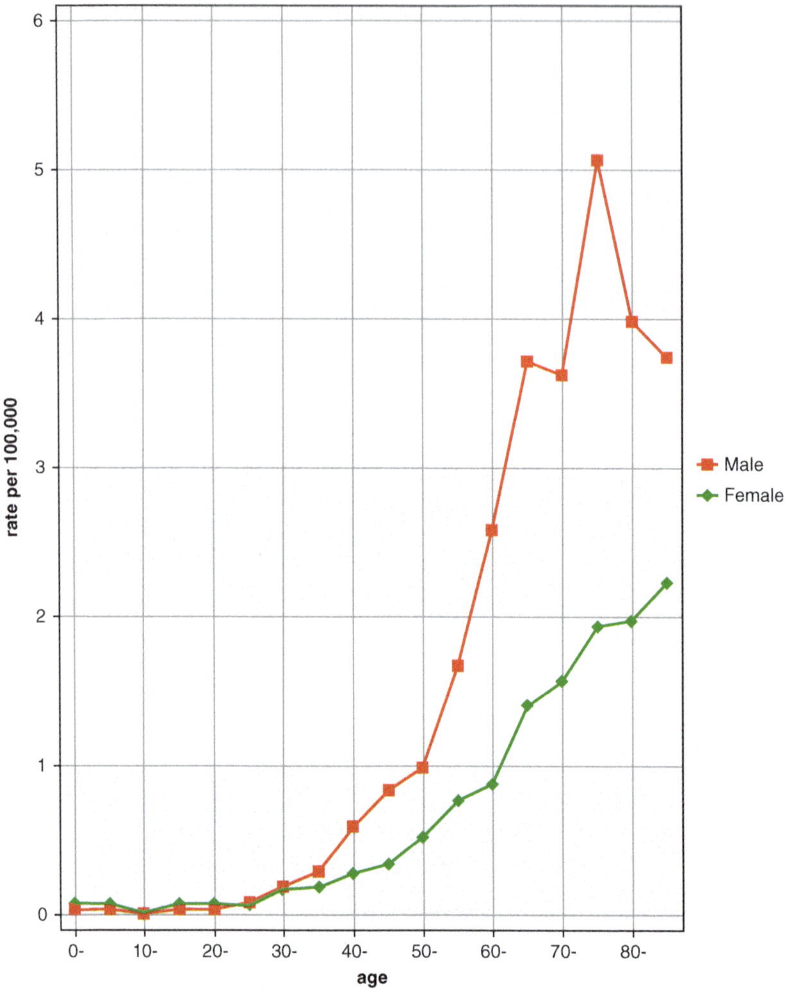

Age-Specific Rates

Age-specific incidence rates for cancers of the nasal cavity, middle ear and paranasal sinuses (ICD-O-3: C30–C31) increase with age. As an example, data from Italy, an area with high SNC incidence, are shown in Fig. 1. The median age at diagnosis was 65 years in men and 67 years in women.

Time Trends

Trend analysis on the SEER data base suggests a slight decrease in the incidence of the SNC over time although this difference is not statistically significant [9], and considering histological subtypes, the incidence of SCC decreases substantially in the study period considered. Denmark shows incidence rates higher than other countries and continuing to trend upwards [10] with AD subtypes more common than SCC suggesting the role of occupational risk factors. Occupational risk factors, in particular wood dust exposure, may influence disparities in the risk of developing SNC in different countries. Difference in the proportion of workers exposed to wood dust, in exposure levels, in processing methods, control measures developed and the presence of concomitant carcinogens in the workplaces may be important factors that may influence differences between countries [10].

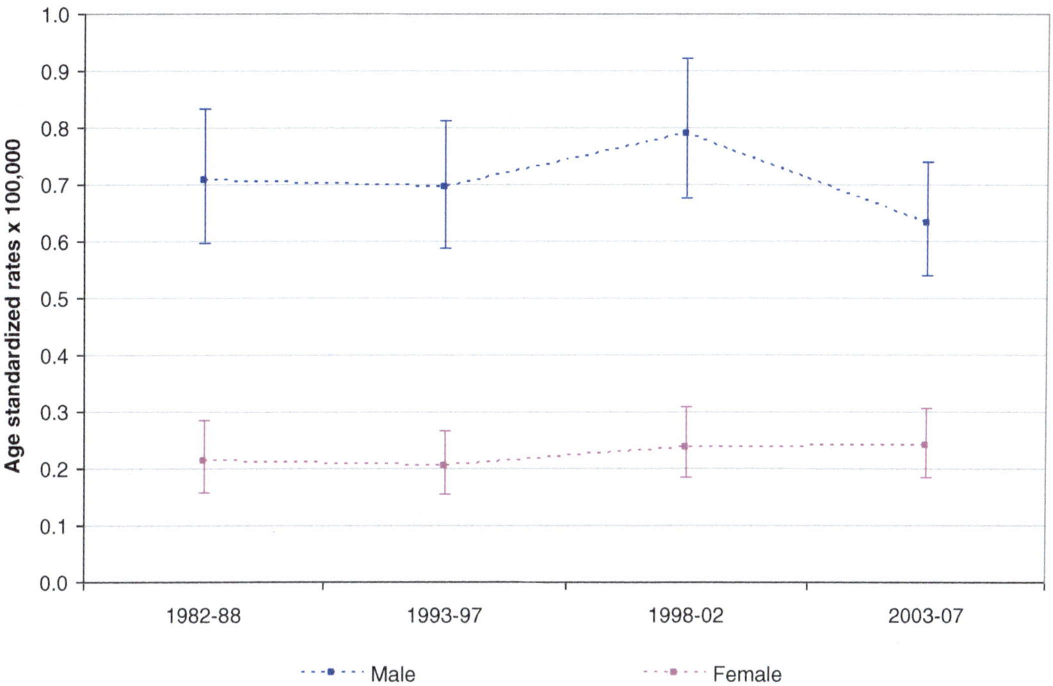

Fig. 2 Cancers of the nasal cavity, middle ear and paranasal sinuses (codes ICD-O-3: C30–C31). Incidence age-standardised rates (standard: world population) per 100,000 inhabitants and confidence intervals 95% per time periods. Italian areas covered by a general cancer registry, males and females, years 1982–2012 (http://ci5.iarc.fr/CI5plus/Pages/table3_sel.aspx)

However, the decreasing rates observed for SCC that is mainly associated with smoking may be consistent with the decreasing smoking rates in many developed countries in the last decades [9].

In Italian areas covered by a general cancer registry, the incidence age-standardised rates for cancers of the nasal cavity, middle ear and paranasal sinuses (ICD-O-3: C30–C31) in subsequent 5-year periods from the 1980s to 2000s is shown in Fig. 2. Only cancer registry with data available in all periods are included: a small increase in females in the two more recent periods was observed; among males, instead, an increase in the late 1990s, followed by a reduction in 2000s, was observed.

Data by Subsite and Morphology

The US analysis on SNC incidence and survival [9] found that almost half of SNCs are localised in the nasal cavity, followed by maxillary and ethmoid sinus. These lesions were represented mostly by cancers of epithelial origin including SCC (51%), AD (13%), esthesioneuroblastoma (6%) and adenoid cystic carcinoma (6%).

In Italy, based on AIRTUM data, cancers originate more often in nasal cavity in both genders, as shown in Table 3 (almost 60% of all SNCs in both sexes). Maxillary and ethmoidal sinuses are the next most common subsites. On the basis of the morphologic ICD-O-3 codes, malignant epithelial neoplasms are the most frequent subtypes in both genders (77% of all malignant cancers of this site among males, 68% among females) (Table 4); SCC outnumbered all other carcinomas. Intestinal- type adenocarcinomas represent 6% of all SNCs among males and 2% among females (Table 4). However, distribution by morphology may be affected by the bias due to the presence of unspecified neoplasms; nevertheless unspecified morphologies represent a small amount (<10%) of all diagnosis. For the same reason, data on intestinal-type adenocarcinoma

Table 3 Cancers of the nasal cavity, middle ear and paranasal sinuses (codes ICD-O-3: C30–C31)

Subsite	Males		Females	
	n.	%	n.	%
C30.0 nasal cavity	393	57%	230	59%
C30.1 middle ear	29	4%	18	5%
C31.0 maxillary sinus	116	17%	79	20%
C31.1 ethmoidal sinus	87	13%	25	6%
C31.2 frontal sinus	6	1%	1	0%
C31.3 sphenoidal sinus	14	2%	5	1%
C31.8 overlapping lesion	10	1%	12	3%
C31.9 unspecified sinus	33	5%	23	6%
All	688	100%	393	100%

Number of new cases in 5 years by subsite (four-digit codes ICD-O-3), by gender and by Registries Association: AIRTUM. Males and females, years 2008–2012 (http://ci5.iarc.fr/CI5plus/Pages/table3_sel.aspx)

Table 4 Cancers of the nasal cavity, middle ear and paranasal sinuses (codes ICD-O-3: C30–C31)

	Males		Females	
Morphology	n.	%	n.	%
Epithelial neoplasms	532	77%	267	68%
Epithelial NOS	66	10%	33	8%
Squamous cell	278	40%	166	42%
Adenocarcinomas, of which	177	26%	61	16%
Adenocarcinoma, intestinal type	40	6%	6	2%
Others epithelial	11	2%	7	2%
Non-epithelial neoplasms	110	16%	89	23%
Malignant neoplasm unspecified	46	7%	37	9%
All	688	100%	393	100%

Number of new cases in 5 years by morphology, by gender and by Registries Association: AIRTUM. Males and females, years 2008–2012 (http://ci5.iarc.fr/CI5plus/Pages/table3_sel.aspx)

Table 5 Cancers of the nasal cavity (C30.0), maxillary sinus (C31.0) and ethmoidal sinus (C31.1)

	Male						Female					
	C30.0 nasal cavity		C31.0 maxillary sinus		C31.1 ethmoidal sinus		C30.0 nasal cavity		C31.0 maxillary sinus		C31.1 ethmoidal sinus	
Morphology	n.	%	n.	%	n.	%	n.	%	n.	%	n.	%
Epithelial neoplasms	293	75%	96	83%	70	80%	156	68%	57	72%	18	72%
Epithelial NOS	25	6%	10	9%	15	17%	19	8%	5	6%	5	20%
Squamous cell	174	44%	58	50%	14	16%	107	47%	33	42%	8	32%
Adenocarcinomas, of which	89	23%	25	22%	40	46%	28	12%	16	20%	3	12%
Adenocarcinoma, intestinal type	24	6%	0	0%	11	13%	3	1%	0	0%	1	4%
Others epithelial	5	1%	3	3%	1	1%	2	1%	3	4%	2	8%
Non-epithelial neoplasms	84	21%	10	9%	9	10%	64	28%	13	16%	4	16%
Malignant neoplasm unspecified	16	4%	10	9%	8	9%	10	4%	9	11%	3	12%
All	393	100%	116	100%	87	100%	230	100%	79	100%	25	100%

Number of new cases in 5 years by morphology and by gender. AIRTUM: Italian Cancer Registries Association, data from the pool of Italian Cancer Registries, males and females, years 2008–2012 (http://ci5.iarc.fr/CI5plus/Pages/table3_sel.aspx)

might be underestimated, and we cannot exclude that some cancers of this specific histotype could have been classified as simple 'adenocarcinomas not otherwise specified'. Intestinal-type adenocarcinomas are 6% of all nasal cavity cancers and 13% of all ethmoidal sinus cancers among males (Table 5).

Survival and Mortality

The prognosis of patients with sinonasal cancer is generally poor and has not changed substantially over the last three decades [9]. Turner extracted survival data from SEER database for the most common sinonasal malignancies and evaluated the trend for the period 1973–2001. Five-year relative survival was 54.5 ± 0.9%. The author observed a nonstatistical significant trend toward an improved survival over time, and no differences were noted between men and women or by histological subtype, but considering the site of origin, cancers originating in the nasal cavity had substantially improved survival compared with cancer of the accessory sinuses [9, 11]. It is therefore conceivable that the improved survival noted for sinonasal adenocarcinoma in the USA may be secondary to a decline in the rate of high-grade intestinal variants of the disease often attributed to exposure to wood dust and other industrial contaminants [9].

Based on the Italian report on rare cancer published in 2016 [12], the 5-year survival for epithelial tumours of the nasal cavity and sinuses diagnosed during 2000s is 47% (95% CI: 43%; 52%), male and female together. For SCC the 5-year survival is 52% (95% CI: 47%; 57%), for undifferentiated carcinoma it is 33% (95% CI: 22%; 50%), for intestinal-type adenocarcinoma it is 65% (95% CI: 45%; 93%), and the last estimate is based only on 26 cases. Five-year survival estimates in Italy are similar to those observed in Europe in the other European areas [13]. The estimate proportion of prevalent cases of SNC in Italy is 3.7 × 100,000 inhabitants, for SCC the proportion is 3.0 × 100,000 and for intestinal-type adenocarcinoma it is 0.1 × 100,000 [12].

Similar to incidence, mortality rates were higher for males than females: the rates between 2004 and 2008 varied from 1.3 per million in Sweden to 3.3 in Denmark in men and from 0.5 per million in the Netherlands to 1.5 per million in Denmark [10]. Significant ongoing decreases in mortality rate dating back to 1970s were observed in both males and females in Australia, Canada, Greece, Hong Kong, Ireland, the Netherlands, the United Kingdom and the USA.

Risk Factors

Malignant tumours of the nose and paranasal sinuses are uncommon neoplasms. This low absolute risk in the general population has been accompanied by a high relative risk, in particular of epithelial tumours, for specific chemical exposures and occupational settings [14].

SNC has been investigated in several epidemiological studies, but few have examined the risks by histological types such as AD and SCC. Here a review on possible risk factors is presented focusing above all on occupational risks.

Woodworking and Wood Dust Exposure

Considering exposure to wood dust, it has been estimated that in 25 member states of the European Union, in 2000–2003 about 3.6 million workers were occupationally exposed to inhalable wood dust. Among these 1.5 million workers were exposed to low levels <0.5 mg/m^3 and 0.2 million to high levels above 5 mg/m^3 of wood dust [15]. At the end of the 1960s, a cluster of patients with sinonasal AD was reported in the furniture industry in Great Britain [16, 17]. Since then reports of sinonasal cancer among woodworkers were published in several other countries, and a number of descriptive studies, based on occupational title and considering cancer mortality or incidence among woodworkers, corroborated the indication of an increased risk for nasal cancer in woodworkers [18, 19].

A number of cohort studies have been conducted among workers with a job entailing potential wood exposure. In a cohort of about 40,000 members of Danish carpenters and cabinet makers union and a cohort of more than 5000 British furniture workers, a significant increase in mortality from nasal cancer was observed, with all the nasal cancer among UK cohort being AD [20, 21]. A pooled reanalysis of cancer mortality among five cohorts of 28,704 workers (furniture workers, plywood workers and wood model makers) in wood-related industries observed a significant excess of nasal cancer [22]. An excess of SNC was observed among the British furniture workers with the highest wood dust exposure but not among US furniture workers [22].

In a review of North American cohort studies published in 1997, rates of nasal cancer were not reported to be significantly elevated [23]. A geographic discrepancy was suggested between European and American furniture industry with more elevated rates of nasal cancers among Europeans in the furniture industry.

Some other cohort studies assessed cancer risks in woodworkers in Estonia [24] and in Finland [25] and Sweden [26].

Given the rarity of nasal cancers, the number of cases in the cohort studies is small so that the association with woodworking jobs could not to be adequately investigated with the cohort approach.

The case-control approach is more suitable to study the association between rare cancers and exposure. Several case-control studies were conducted in different countries to investigate the association between occupational exposures and SNC, and some of these studies considered also the different subtypes of SNC. Case-control studies with high risks of nasal cancer were reported in Germany, the Netherlands, Italy and France [18]. In the case-control studies conducted in North America, the association between nasal cancer and woodworking occupations has been less strong than in Europe [18]. Possible explanations for the different epidemiological findings between North America and Europe include differences in concentration or types of wood dust, wood processing methods, and/or presence of other carcinogenic exposures in the European workplaces [18].

A pooled analysis of 12 case-control studies conducted in seven countries (China, France, Germany, Italy, Netherlands, Sweden and the USA) was performed with the aim to examine the relationship between wood dust and SNC [27]. Seven categories of jobs with potential exposure to wood dust were defined combining occupation and industry title: forestry workers, loggers, pulp and paper workers, sawmill workers, furniture makers, other wood product workers and carpenters. Furthermore, the jobs were classified with regard to the wood dust level of exposure on the basis of an ad hoc job exposure matrix. The combined data set consisted of 680 male cases, 2349 male controls, 250 female cases and 787 female controls. Overall, men employed in any wood-related job had a statistically significant OR of 2.0 for all histologies combined, the highest risk being for furniture workers, sawmill workers, wood product workers and carpenters. No excess risk was observed in forestry workers, logging and pulp and paper workers. Considering SNC subtypes, a high risk for AD was associated with employment in wood-related jobs, and the risk was highest for furniture workers. No association was observed among men between SCC and employment in all wood-related occupations. The odds ratio (OR) for all sinonasal cancer and AD among women were elevated but lower than those observed in men; the risk for SCC was similar in men and women. The results for men by high level of wood exposure showed a statistically significant OR of 5.8 for all histologies considered and 45.5 for AD. Considering women, very few were classified in the high level of wood exposure, and increased non-significant risk for any exposure level was 1.5; the analysis by subtype showed an OR of 2.5 for AD and 2.1 for SCC, but this analysis was not statistically significant.

For the AD subtypes, the relative risk increased also with duration of exposure, but also men employed in the shortest category of exposure (less than 5 years) appeared to be at elevated risk. The authors of the pooled analysis observed the highest risk in the European studies, while a lower risk was observed in the American and Shanghai studies. France, Italy and the Netherlands had both the highest proportion of cases that were AD and the highest relative risk, and 77% of the European AD cases had worked in wood dust exposed jobs, as compared with the 20% of non-European studies. Furthermore, the authors pointed out that the evidence regarding SCC was ambiguous, and there was a great deal of heterogeneity observed in individual study results. This may be due to differences in risk associated with exposure to hardwood and softwoods or with other aspects related to the exposures [27].

As pointed out by the International Agency for Research on Cancer (IARC) in the monograph Vol. n 62, the excess appears to be attributable to wood dust per se rather than to other exposures in the workplaces, because the excess was observed in various countries during different periods and among different occupational groups and because direct exposures to other chemicals do not produce RR of the magnitude associated with exposure to wood dust [18].

Considering wood type, AD of the nasal cavity and paranasal sinuses is clearly associated with exposures to hardwood dust. In several series of AD from different countries, a high proportion of cases was exposed to hard wood, and these findings were confirmed in several case-control studies [18]. There are too few studies to evaluate cancer risks attributable to softwood exposure alone. In these studies, SNC risk was elevated but lower than that in studies with exposure to hard wood or mixed [18]. The overall evaluation of the IARC working group was that wood dust is carcinogenic to humans (Group 1) considering that there is sufficient evidence in humans for the carcinogenicity of wood dust and inadequate evidence in experimental animals for the carcinogenicity of wood dust [18].

A case-control study among men in four Nordic countries [28] conducted with the aims to provide stronger evidence to aid the role of cumulative exposure to mixed wood dust in aetiology of nasal cancer found that wood workers had elevated risk in nasal cancer particularly for AD subtype. Because wood workers in the study population are primarily exposed to softwood dust, the study results imply that softwood could also be carcinogenic.

In 1998, results of a meta-analysis of 14 studies on SNC (but usable results were available for 12 studies) showed a summary OR of all SNCs of 2.6 (95% CI 2.1–3.3) among male wood workers, whereas OR was 18 (95% CI 12–28) for AD and 0.8 (95% CI 0.6–1.2) for SCC [29]. ORs for AD were higher for furniture workers than for carpenters. Results for selected characteristics of the study design for all histologic subtypes presented higher pooled ORs for studies conducted in countries with a prevalent use of hard wood [29]. A pooled analysis of the European studies published in 1999 confirmed that exposure to wood dust was strongly associated with SNC risk in men [30]. The excess risk observed for wood dust was particularly high for AD (OR 12.20, 95% CI 7.43–20.0). Among men, analysis by exposure level showed that excess risk was almost exclusively found among workers in the highest wood dust exposure category of levels higher than 5 mg/m^3 (OR = 6.69), while there was no association between wood dust at any level of exposure for SCCs. In women the situation is different due to the fact that only few women were exposed to wood dust (OR 1.17 95% CI 0.31–4.47) [30].

In 2012 on the basis of the new available data, IARC in the monograph Vol. 100C revaluated the carcinogenicity of wood dust and confirmed the previous evaluation: wood dust causes cancer of nasal cavity and paranasal sinuses. The evidence in humans was also sufficient for nasopharynx [19].

An industry-based case-control study on AD of the nasal cavity and paranasal sinuses in the Germany wood industry reported data also on cumulative and average exposure to wood dust, quantified with a job exposure matrix, based on wood dust measurements at recent and historical workplaces [31]. AD occurred more frequently among workers that had ever worked as cabinet makers or joiners. Average exposure to inhalable wood dust ≥5 mg/m^3 was associated with a high significant risk (OR 48.47, 95% CI 13.30–176.63) compared with levels below 3.5 mg/m^3. Exposure between 3.5 and 5 mg/m^3 was also found to pose a risk [31]. Furthermore, in an Italian case-control study conducted in Piedmont on incident cases occurred between 1996 and 2000, a very high risk was observed for AD and exposure to wood dust (OR 58.6, 95% CI 23.74–144.8), among subjects exposed to high level of wood dust the OR for AD was of 179.9 (95% CI 55.37–584.4) [32].

A recent meta-analysis of published studies after 1985 with a case-control and cohort design (11 cohort and 17 case-control studies) found a RR pooled of 5.91 (95% CI 4.31–8.11) for case-control studies and a RR 1.61 (95% CI 1.10–2.37) for the cohort studies in the wood dust exposed subjects [33]. The strongest associations are with AD 29.43 (95% CI 16.46–52.61), but a slight increased risk was also observed for SCC (RR pooled 1.46 95% CI 1.01–2.1). Analysis by duration of wood dust exposure suggests a possible exposure response relationship (RR pooled <15 years 2.40, RR pooled >15 years 9.19 *p* 0.001) [33].

Shoe and Leather Industry and Leather Dust Exposure

In 1981, and again in 1987, IARC concluded that there is an excess risk of cancer among people employed in the boot and shoe manufacture and repair industry. The strongest evidence cited was for excess risks of nasal cancer and leukaemia [34, 35]. AD has been caused by employment in boot and shoe manufacture and repair industry. Elevated risks in excess of tenfold have been reported from studies in the boot and shoe manufacturing industry in England and in Italy [35]. A far higher risk of nasal cancer was found for subjects who worked in the dustiest operations and for those classified into the category of 'heavy' exposure to leather dust. A similar pattern was noted when only AD was considered.

Furthermore, exposure to leather dust may occur in the production of leather clothes and other leather goods. In 1987, IARC concluded that there was inadequate evidence for carcinogenicity to humans for leather goods manufacture and classified these industries in Group 3, and the IARC working group observed that the number of cases of nasal cancer reported is insufficient to make an association with employment in the manufacture of leather goods [35]. Also, leather tanning and processing was classified in Group 3 in 1987, with an inadequate evidence for carcinogenicity to humans [35]. Considering nasal cancer, the IARC working group concluded that there was no evidence suggesting an association between leather tanning and nasal cancer [35]. Furthermore, exposure to leather dust, which had caused increased risks for sinonasal cancer in the shoe and boot-making industry, might be substantial in the tanning industry. There have also been indications of an association for tannery workers [36–40], but in some cases, results were non-significant and based on very few cases. AD was the most frequent type observed, and exposure other than leather dust was suggested such as chromium salts and natural tannins [40]. However, it has been observed that there are 10 times fewer articles published on leather goods compared with wood dust which also induces SNC [41].

The pooled analysis of European case-control studies found an excess risk for SNC for leather dust exposure of 1.92 (95% CI 1.10–3.35) among men and an OR of 2.71 (95% CI 0.78–9.43) among women [30]. Leather dust exposure was principally associated with AD (OR 2.99 95% CI 1.33–6.73), and lower and non-significant excess risk was seen for SCC (OR 1.45 95% CI 0.70–2.99).

In a recent review on SNC and exposure to leather dust, papers published in English or Italian since 1980–2006 were included [41]. Fourteen studies were considered, including one meta-analysis. Four out of five of the case-control studies found an excess risk associated with exposure to leather dust, and of five cohort mortality studies, an excess risk was found in all studies conducted in shoe trades. The four studies of the incidence of SNC confirm the excess risk in shoemaking. The excess was observed especially among those working in shining, finishing and shoe repair in which exposure levels to leather dust were particularly high. A significant dose-response effect (all histological subtypes) in the profession was also observed [36]. Histological classification was provided in several studies focusing on the shoe trades: AD accounted for 80% of cases according to Battista

[40], 88% according to Acheson [42] and 75% according to Cecchi [43]. The Italian study conducted in Piedmont observed an OR of 14.4 (95% CI 3.03–68.87) considering all histological subtypes with the AD subtypes particularly associated with leather dust (OR 26. 6 95% CI 5.09–139.0) [32].

A series of cases of SNC have been observed among shoemakers (11 cases) and tannery workers (8 cases) in the leather production area in Tuscany (Italy) in the period 1990–2002 [44]. The possible etiologic role of tannins both in leather and in wood industry was stressed [44].

In the pooled analysis of Binazzi and coauthors, the RR [33] pooled for exposure to leather dust was 11.89 (95% CI 7.69–18.36) with higher risk observed for AD (RR pooled 35.26; 95% CI 20.62–60.28), and the pooled risk for SCC was 2.09 (95% IC 1.12–3.9).

Other Occupational Exposures

Formaldehyde

In the monograph Vol. 100F (2012) confirming previous evaluation, IARC concluded that there is sufficient evidence in humans for the carcinogenicity of formaldehyde that causes cancer of nasopharynx and leukaemia, and a positive association has been also observed between exposure to formaldehyde and sinonasal cancer [45]. IARC evaluated six case-control studies, and four of these reported an increased risk [45]. An analysis of proportionate cancer incidence among industrial workers in Denmark showed in increasing risk for SCC. No excess of mortality from SNC cancer was observed in three recent updates of industrial garment in the USA and chemical workers in the United Kingdom [45].

The IARC working group noted that case-control studies that observed positive associations might reflect problems of residual confounding by wood dust exposure which is strongly associated with SNC. Due to these observations, IARC working group concluded that there is only limited epidemiological evidence that formaldehyde causes SNC in humans [45].

The RR pooled for exposure to formaldehyde found in the recent analysis pooled of Binazzi was 1.68 (95% CI 1.37–2.06), for AD the RR pooled was 3.81 (95% 1.39–10.41) and 2.37 (95% CI 1.69–3.33) for SCC [33].

Nickel and Chromium

Also nickel exposure was associated with nasal cancer, and nickel compounds were evaluated as carcinogenic to human by IARC in 2012 [19]. These agents cause cancer of the lung and nasal cavity and paranasal sinuses.

Increasing risks for SNC were found to be associated with exposures during high temperature oxidation of nickel matte and nickel copper matte in cohort studies in Canada, Norway and United Kingdom, in the electrolytic refining in Norway. In the Norwegian study, a dose–response relationship was also observed. An update of nasal cancer in Finnish refinery workers after 20 years from the first exposure to nickel reported an elevated SIR. One study on Ni-Cd battery workers exposed to nickel hydroxide and cadmium oxide demonstrated a significant risk of SNC, and in a cohort of Swedish battery workers, a strong risk was also found in men [19].

IARC in 2012 evaluated the carcinogenicity of chromium VI compounds on the bases of the results of nine cohort studies, some case reports and three case-control studies. In aggregate the epidemiological evidence remains suggestive but inconclusive regarding the effect of chromium VI on nasal cancers, and in the overall evaluation, IARC concluded that there is sufficient evidence in humans for the carcinogenicity of these compounds that cause cancer of the lung and limited evidence for SNC. In the pooled study of Binazzi, the pooled RR on the basis of the six studies that considered nickel/chromium exposure was 18.0 (95% CI 14.55–22.27) [33].

Radiation

IARC in the monograph volume 100D concluded there is sufficient evidence in humans for the carcinogenicity of radium-226 that causes bone sarcomas and carcinomas of paranasal sinuses and mastoid process [46].

Other Exposures

Increased risks of SNC have also been observed with some inconsistencies for many occupations including farm workers [47], textile [48–50] and construction [47].

A pooled analysis showed that exposure to textile dust was associated with non-significantly elevated risk of AD, among women only, with an OR for the high level of cumulative exposure of 2.5 (95% CI 0.7–9.0) [50]. In the IARC Monograph Vol. 48, the working group concluded there is limited evidence that working in the textile manufacturing industry entails a carcinogenic risk. This evaluation is based mainly on findings of bladder cancer among dyers (possibly due to exposure to dyes) and among weavers (possibly due to exposure to dusts from fibres and yarns) and of cancer of the nasal cavity among weavers (possibly due to exposure to dusts from fibres and yarns) and among other textile workers. Working in the textile manufacturing industry entails exposures that are possibly carcinogenic to humans (Group 2B) [51].

Recently, Binazzi and co-authors found a RR pooled in the textile industry of 2.03 (95% CI 1.47–2.8) which increased risk particularly for AD (RR pooled 3.5 95% CI 1.88–6.54), and considering the construction sector, a significant pooled risk has been observed (RR pooled, 1.62 95% CI 1.11–2.36), while farming resulted non-significantly associated with the risk of SNC (RR pooled, 1.01 95% CI 0.75–1.38) [33].

Also, chemical workers and welders were suggested to be associated with SNC [52]. An OR of 4.1 (95% CI 1.66–10.13) for SCC subtype was found among those exposed to welding fumes in an Italian study [32].

Other Risk Factors

Although occupational agents are the most important etiological agents for SNC, an excess risk was also observed in some studies in association with cigarette smoking. In the Monograph 100 E IARC concluded that the evidence of an association between tobacco smoking and SNC is based on the results of case-control studies each of which may be subjects to different source of bias. However, the presence of a dose–response relationship in most studies, the decrease in risk associated with time since quitting, the consistently higher risk for SCC than for AD and the lack of potential confounding support the existence of a casual association [53].

Benign nasal conditions, such as recurrent nasal polyps, sinusitis and nosebleed, have been suspected to be risk factors for SNC [54].

Attributable Risk

The pooled analysis of the European case-control studies has produced attributable risk estimates for occupations, exposures and smoking [30]. The attributable risk for SNC associated with occupations was 33% (95% CI 12–89%), but considerable differences were observed between men and women. In men, up to 39% (95% CI 18–92%) of all SNC cases could be attributed to occupational exposure, while in women occupation explained 11% (95% CI 0.1–100%). Considering histological subtypes, for AD occupational exposures were related to 77% (95% CI 60–100%) of all cancers, while a lower attributable risk of 22 (95% CI 3–100%) was observed for SCC, mainly due to exposures in other than wood- or leather-related occupations. Fifteen percent of all SNCs could be attributed to smoking, this proportion being higher for SCC (23%).

A recent French study produced a range of AF of sinonasal cancer attributable to specific occupational risk, the estimate of AF for wood dust ranges from 0.15 (low value %) to 1.85 (high value %) for women and for men from 9.75 to 23.85, and considering exposure to leather dust, the AF is 7.15 for women and 1.98 for men (only low value %) [55].

Italian Sinonasal Cancer Registry

In Italy, a SNC incidence has been under compulsory surveillance since 2008, through the 'Sinonasal cancer national registry' (Registro Nazionale dei Tumori Naso Sinusali—ReNaTuNS), a national cancer registry coordinated by National Institute for Insurance Against Accident at Work (INAIL). Currently, the registry covers a proportion of Italian territory through regional structures (COR), and the cases recorded in ReNaTuNS in the period 2000–2016 were 1529. The age-standardised incidence rates per 100,000 person-years were 0.64 in men and 0.26 in women. Occupational exposures were predominant among the attribute exposure setting primarily to wood and leather dust. Other putative agents were chrome, solvents, tannins, formaldehyde, textile dust and pesticides [56].

Sinonasal Inverted Papilloma

Sinonasal inverted papilloma (SIP) also known as Schneiderian papilloma is an infrequent benign tumour that constitutes 70% of all sinonasal papillomas. About 10% of cases may evolve into sinonasal malignancies, mainly SCC. The aetiology of SIP is not fully understood; the presence of human papillomavirus, smoking habit and presence of nasal polyposis are suggested to be risk factors for SIP [57–59]. The role of occupational exposure has also been suggested [58, 59].

A recent case-control study conducted in Piedmont, Italy, found a significant association and a significant dose–response relationship with occupational exposure to organic solvents. Also, exposure to welding fumes was found to be associated, but a dose–response relationship was not observed. Even exposure to nickel compounds was found to be associated with SIP, but based on few exposed cases. The authors concluded that these associations should be further investigated in future case-control studies [60].

Conclusion

In conclusion, SNC is a rare cancer with predominant occupational aetiology associated with exposures to specific carcinogens such as wood and leather dust and other agents. Occupational exposure to carcinogens contributes greatly to the aetiology of SNC, primarily for intestinal-type adenocarcinoma. Other occupational exposures are also suggested to be associated with SNC (formaldehyde, nickel and chromium compounds, textile industry, farming and construction). Furthermore, tobacco smoking is a well-known carcinogenic agent also for SNC. Monitoring trends in the burden of disease attributable to work is very important in the control of occupational health hazards. Epidemiological surveillance of SNC cases and their occupational history is fundamental for monitoring the occurrence of the disease in exposed workers in industrial sectors. Implementation of risk reduction strategies and the prevention of disease caused by workplace exposures is an important public health objective.

References

1. Bray F, Colombet M, Mery L, et al., editors. Cancer incidence in five continents, Vol. XI (electronic version). Lyon: International Agency for Research on Cancer; 2017. http://ci5.iarc.fr. Accessed 16 Jan 2018.
2. Muir C, Weilard L. Upper aerodigestive tract cancers. Cancer. 1995;75:147–53.
3. Slack R, Young C, Rushton L, British Occupational Cancer Burden Study Group. Occupational cancer in Britain. Nasopharynx and sinonasal cancers. Br J Cancer. 2012;107(Suppl 1):S49–55.
4. Rushton L, Hutchings SJ, Fortunato L, et al. Occupational cancer burden in Great Britain. Br J Cancer. 2012;107(Suppl 1):S3–7.
5. Fritz A, Percy C, Jack A, editors. International classification of diseases for oncology. 3rd ed. Geneva: World Health Organization; 2000.
6. European Parliament and Council of the European Communities. Decision no. 1295/1999/EC of the European parliament and of the council of 29 April 1999 adopting a programme of Community action on rare diseases within the framework for action in the field of public health (1999 to 2003). Off J Eur Community. 1999;42:22.
7. Greenlee RT, Goodman MT, Lynch CF, et al. The occurrence of rare cancers in US adults, 1995-2004. Public Health Rep. 2010;125(1):28–43.
8. Gatta G, Van der Zwan JM, Casali PG, et al. Rare cancers are not so rare: the rare cancer burden in Europe. Eur J Cancer. 2011;47(17):2493–511.
9. Turner JH, Reh DD. Incidence and survival in patients with sinonasal cancer: a historical analysis of population-based data. Head Neck. 2012;34(6):877–85.
10. Youlden DR, Cramb SM, Peters S, et al. International comparisons of the incidence and mortality of sinonasal cancer. Cancer Epidemiol. 2013;37:770.
11. Dutta R, Dubal PM, Svider PF, et al. Sinonasal malignancies: a population-based analysis of site-

specific incidence and survival. Laryngoscope. 2015;125(11):2491–7.
12. AIRTUM Working Group. The burden of rare cancers in Italy. Epidemiol Prev. 2016;40(1 Suppl 2):1–12.
13. Van Dijk BA, Gatta G, Capocaccia R, et al. Rare cancers of the head and neck area in Europe. Eur J Cancer. 2012;48(6):783–96.
14. Comba P, Belli S. Etiological epidemiology of tumours of the nasal cavities and the paranasal sinuses. Ann Ist Super Sanita. 1992;28(1):121–32.
15. Kauppinen T, Vincent R, Liukkonen T, et al. Occupational exposure to inhalable wood dust in the member states of the European Union. Ann Occup Hyg. 2006;50:549–61.
16. Acheson ED, Hadfield EH, Macbeth RG. Carcinoma of the nasal cavity and accessory sinuses in woodworkers. Lancet. 1967;11:311–2.
17. Acheson ED, Cowdell RH, Hadfield E, et al. Nasal cancer in woodworkers in the furniture industry. Br Med J. 1968;8:587–96.
18. IARC monographs on the evaluation of carcinogenic risks to humans. Vol. 62: Wood dust and formaldehyde. Lyon: IARC; 1995.
19. IARC. Monographs on the evaluation of carcinogenic risks to humans: arsenic, metals, fibres and dusts, vol. 100C. Lyon: IARC; 2012.
20. Olsen J, Sabroe S. A follow-up study of non-retired and retired members of the Danish Carpenter/Cabinet Makers' Trade Union. Int J Epidemiol. 1979;8(4):375–82.
21. Acheson ED, Pippard EC, Winter PD. Mortality of English furniture makers. Scand J Work Environ Health. 1984;10:211–7.
22. Demers PA, Boffetta P, Kogevinas M, et al. Pooled reanalysis of cancer mortality among five cohorts of workers in wood-related industries. Scand J Work Environ Health. 1995;21:179–90.
23. Blot WJ, Chow WH, McLaughlin JK. Wood dust and nasal cancer risk. A review of the evidence from North America. J Occup Environ Med. 1997;39:148–56.
24. Innos K, Rahu M, Rahu K, et al. Wood dust exposure and cancer incidence: a retrospective cohort study of furniture workers in Estonia. Am J Ind Med. 2000;37(5):501–11.
25. Siew SS, Kauppinen T, Kyyrönen P, et al. Occupational exposure to wood dust and formaldehyde and risk of nasal, nasopharyngeal, and lung cancer among Finnish men. Cancer Manag Res. 2012;
26. Hemelt M, Granström C, Hemminki K. Occupational risks for nasal cancer in Sweden. J Occup Environ Med. 2004;46(10):1033–40.
27. Demers PA, Kogevinas M, Boffetta P, et al. Wood dust and sino-nasal cancer: pooled reanalysis of twelve case-control studies. Am J Ind Med. 1995;28(2):151–66.
28. Siew SS, Martinsen JI, Kjaerheim K, et al. Occupational exposure to wood dust and risk of nasal and nasopharyngeal cancer: a case-control study among men in four Nordic countries—with an emphasis on nasal adenocarcinoma. Int J Cancer. 2017;141(12):2430–6.
29. Gordon I, Boffetta P, Demers PA. A case study comparing a meta-analysis and a pooled analysis of studies of sinonasal cancer among wood workers. Epidemiology. 1998;9:518–24.
30. 't Mannetje A, Kogevinas M, Luce D, et al. Sinonasal cancer, occupation, and tobacco smoking in European women and men. Am J Ind Med. 1999;36:101–7.
31. Pesch B, Pierl CB, Gebel M, et al. Occupational risks for adenocarcinoma of the nasal cavity and paranasal sinuses in the German wood industry. Occup Environ Med. 2008;65:191–6.
32. D'Errico A, Pasian S, Baratti A, et al. A case-control study on occupational risk factors for sino-nasal cancer. Occup Environ Med. 2009;66(7):448–55. https://doi.org/10.1136/oem.2008.041277.
33. Binazzi A, Ferrante P, Marinaccio A. Occupational exposure and sinonasal cancer: a systematic review and meta-analysis. BMC Cancer. 2015;15:49. https://doi.org/10.1186/s12885-015-1042-2.
34. IARC monographs on the evaluation of carcinogenic risks to humans. Vol. 25: Wood, leather and some associated industries. Lyon: IARC; 1981.
35. IARC monographs on the evaluation of carcinogenic risks to humans. Supplement No. 7: Overall evaluations of carcinogenicity: an updating of IARC monographs. Vols. 1 to 42. Lyon: IARC; 1987.
36. Merler E, Baldasseroni A, Laria R, et al. On the causal association between exposure to leather dust and nasal cancer: further evidence from a case-control study. Br J Ind Med. 1986;43:91–5.
37. Comba P, Belli S. Etiological epidemiology of tumors of the nasal cavities and the paranasal sinuses. Ann Ist Super Sanita. 1992;28:121–32.
38. Mikoczy Z, Schütz A, Hagmar L. Cancer incidence and mortality among Swedish leather tanners. Occup Environ Med. 1994;51:530–5.
39. Mikoczy Z, Hagmar L. Cancer incidence in the Swedish leather tanning industry: updated findings 1958-99. Occup Environ Med. 2005;62:461–4.
40. Battista G, Comba P, Orsi D, et al. Nasal cancer in leather workers: an occupational disease. J Cancer Res Clin Oncol. 1995;121:1–6.
41. Bonneterre V, Deschamps E, Persoons R, et al. Sinonasal cancer and exposure to leather dust. Occup Med (Lond). 2007;57:438–43.
42. Acheson ED, Pippard EC, Winter PD. Nasal cancer in the Northamptonshire boot and shoe industry: is it declining? Br J Cancer. 1982;46:940–6.
43. Cecchi F, Buiatti E, Kriebel D, et al. Adenocarcinoma of the nose and paranasal sinuses in shoemakers and woodworkers in the province of Florence, Italy (1963-77). Br J Ind Med. 1980;37:222–5.
44. Iaia TE, Farina G, Ferraro MT, et al. A series of cases of sinonasal cancer among shoemakers and tannery workers. Epidemiol Prev. 2004;28:169–73.
45. IARC monographs on the evaluation of carcinogenic risks to humans. Vol. 100F: Chemical agents and related occupational exposures. Lyon: IARC; 2012.

46. IARC. Monographs on the evaluation of carcinogenic risks to humans: radiation, vol. 100D. Lyon: IARC; 2012.
47. Luce D, Leclerc A, Morcet JF, et al. Occupational risk factors for sinonasal cancer: a case-control study in France. Am J Ind Med. 1992;21:163–75.
48. Brinton LA, Blot WJ, Becker JA, et al. A case-control study of cancers of the nasal cavity and paranasal sinuses. Am J Epidemiol. 1984;119:896–906.
49. Laakkonen A, Kyyrönen P, Kauppinen T, et al. Occupational exposure to eight organic dusts and respiratory cancer among Finns. Occup Environ Med. 2006;63:726–33.
50. Luce D, Leclerc A, Bégin D, et al. Sinonasal cancer and occupational exposures: a pooled analysis of 12 case-control studies. Cancer Causes Control. 2002;13:147–57.
51. IARC. Monographs on the evaluation of carcinogenic risks to humans: some flame retardants and textile chemicals, and exposures in the textile manufacturing industry, vol. 48. Lyon: IARC; 1990.
52. Hernberg S, Westerholm P, Schultz-Larsen K, et al. Nasal and sinonasal cancer. Connection with occupational exposures in Denmark, Finland and Sweden. Scand J Work Environ Health. 1983;9:315–26.
53. IARC. Monographs on the evaluation of carcinogenic risks to humans. Vol. 100E: Tobacco smoke and involuntary smoking. Personal habits and indoor combustions. Lyon; 2012.
54. Hiyama T, Oshima A, Hanai A, et al. Chronic maxillary sinusitis and the epidemiology of cancer of the maxillary sinus. In: Reznick G, Stinson SF, editors. Nasal tumors in animal and man, Anatomy, physiology and epidemiology, vol. 1. Boca Raton: CRC Press. p. 137–49.
55. Serrier H, Sultan-Taïeb H, Luce D, et al. Respiratory cancers attributable to occupational exposures: what is the cost to society in France. Sante Publique. 2017;29(4):509.
56. Binazzi A, Corfiati M, Di Marzio D, Cacciatore AM, Zajacovà J, Mensi C, Galli P, Miligi L, Calisti R, Romeo E, Franchi A, Marinaccio A. Sinonasal cancer in the Italian national surveillance system: epidemiology, occupation, and public health implications. Am J Ind Med. 2018;61(3):239–50.
57. Lawson W, Schlecht NF, Brandwein-Gensler M. The role of the human papillomavirus in the pathogenesis of Schneiderian inverted papillomas: an analytic overview of the evidence. Head Neck Pathol. 2008;2(2):49–59.
58. Sham CL, Lee DL, van Hasselt CA, et al. A case-control study of the risk factors associated with sinonasal inverted papilloma. Am J Rhinol Allergy. 2010;24(1)
59. Barbieri PG, Tomenzoli D, Morassi L, et al. [Sinonasal inverted papillomas and occupational etiology]. G Ital Med Lav Ergon. 2005;27(4):422–6.
60. d'Errico A, Zajacova J, Cacciatore A, et al. Occupational risk factors for sinonasal inverted papilloma: a case-control study. Occup Environ Med. 2013;70(10):703–8.

Molecular Pathology of Sinonasal Tumors

Mario A. Hermsen, C. Riobello, R. García-Marín, V. N. Cabal, L. Suárez-Fernández, F. López, and J. L. Llorente

Introduction

This chapter will present an overview of what is known about the genes involved in the sinonasal cancer types described in this book. As these tumors are rare and some subtypes even rarer, the number of genetic studies is limited and often include a relatively low number of cases. Another difficulty that hampers genetic analyses is the fact that poorly differentiated tumor types are often difficult to classify correctly, possibly a cause of "diagnostic contamination" in published results. Furthermore, tumor subtypes as sinonasal undifferentiated carcinoma (SNUC) and sinonasal adenocarcinoma (SNAC) may still be considered a heterogeneous group of malignancies, representing a category with a diagnosis of exclusion [1]. These considerations will be taken into account in this chapter. Nonetheless, recent years have seen a notable increase in publications, some of which leading to the definition of a tumor subtype by its characterizing genetic abnormality.

The lionshare of the available data concerns malignant tumors, but a number of well-defined benign and precursor lesions are included as well. Genetic aberrations discussed in this section include chromosomal amplification, deletion and translocation, gene mutation and methylation and viral infection, but not changes in gene or protein expression.

Cancer can be regarded a genetic disease, and indeed all malignancies carry numerical or structural changes in the DNA sequence, either a few or a multitude of them. Not all of these alterations are necessarily important, and the concept of "driver" versus "passenger" events is widely accepted. An older categorization considered early and late events, for example, those involved in tumor initiation and tumor progression. Also, genetic changes associated with the process of metastasis or the development of resistance to specific anticancer therapy have been sought over the years. In 2000, Hanahan and Weinberg proposed six "hallmarks of cancer," which further

M. A. Hermsen (✉)
Department of Head and Neck Oncology, Instituto de Investigación Sanitaria del Principado de Asturias (ISPA), Oviedo, Spain

Instituto Universitario de Oncología del Principado de Asturias (IUOPA), Centro de Investigación Biomédica en Red (CIBER-ONC), Oviedo, Spain

Department of Otolaryngology, Hospital Universitario Central de Asturias (HUCA), Oviedo, Spain
e-mail: mhermsen@hca.es

C. Riobello · R. García-Marín · V. N. Cabal
L. Suárez-Fernández
Department of Head and Neck Oncology, Instituto de Investigación Sanitaria del Principado de Asturias (ISPA), Oviedo, Spain

F. López · J. L. Llorente
Department of Otolaryngology, Hospital Universitario Central de Asturias (HUCA), Oviedo, Spain

A. Franchi (ed.), *Pathology of Sinonasal Tumors and Tumor-Like Lesions*,
https://doi.org/10.1007/978-3-030-29848-7_2

elaborated to ten hallmarks in 2011, which can be affected by genetic abnormalities and contribute to the great variety that characterizes cancer behavior [2, 3]. The present chapter will present genetic alterations in epithelial, neuroendocrine, and mesenchymal tumor types that may define or aid diagnosis, that may be related to prognosis and resistance to therapy and that may indicate the usefulness of modern specific inhibitors in personalized therapy.

Epithelial Tumors

Squamous Cell Carcinoma (SNSCC)

Genome-wide genetic studies have shown that SNSCC generally have complex, aneuploid genomes that carry a wide variety and a large number of chromosomal aberrations [4, 5] similarly to most solid tumors. In SNSCC, DNA copy number gains are found frequently at chromosomal regions 3q, 7p, 8q, 11q13, 17q, 19p, and 20q, with losses at 3p, 8p, 9p, 13q, 17p, 17q, and 18q. Most of these aberrations are also recurrent in the head and neck SCC. A curious exception are gains at chromosome 5p and loss at 5q; these are very frequent in head and neck SCC but not so in sinonasal SCC [6]. Recurrent high-level amplifications of chromosomal loci include 7p12, 11p13, 11q13, and 17q21, which contain the suggested candidate oncogenes EGFR, CD44, CCND1/CTTN, and ERBB2, respectively [5, 7]. In addition, using fluorescence in situ hybridization, gene amplification of FGFR1 and SOX2 was demonstrated in 20% and 37% of SNSCC cases, respectively [8, 9].

Studies of the involvement of specific genes in SNSCC, particularly TP53, CDKN2A KRAS, and EGFR, have often been guided by findings from more-frequent and better-studied head and neck squamous cell carcinoma, in spite of the difference in etiology. TP53 mutation has been reported in 70% of tumors [10]. Mutations in KRAS and HRAS, which encode proteins downstream of EGFR in the EGF signalling pathway, have been found in approximately 1% in SNSCCs [11, 12], whereas BRAF mutations have not been detected [11]. However, Udager et al. reported KRAS mutations in 51/51 (100%) oncocytic papillomas (OSP) and 5/5 (100%) OSP-associated SNSCC, suggesting that OSP may be precursor to a subset of SNSCC [13]. A number of recent publications have described EGFR mutations, especially affecting exon 20 (Fig. 1), in SNSCC associated with inverted papilloma (ISP), albeit in varying frequencies, from 30% up to 91% of tumors [14–17]. Detecting the same mutation in

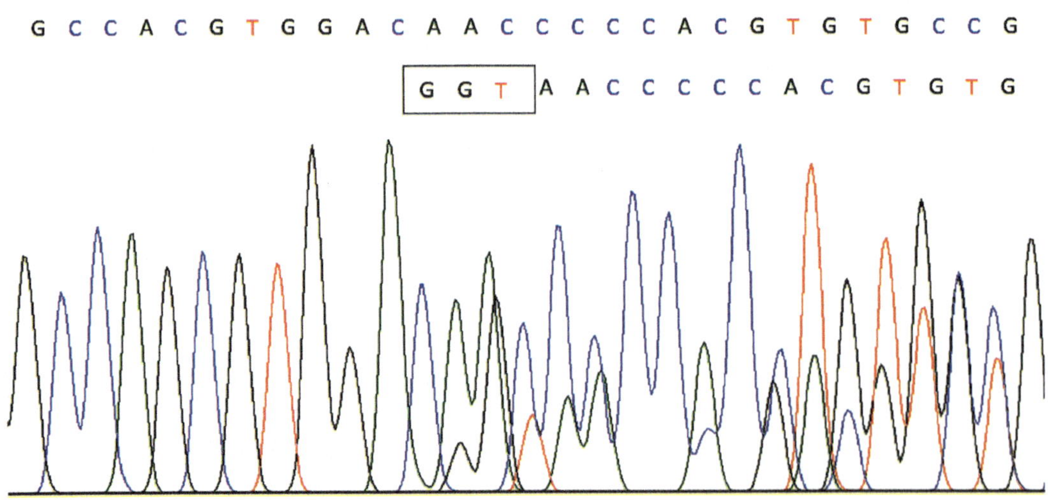

Fig. 1 EGFR exon 20 insertion mutation p.N770_N771insG c.2310_2311insGGT in a sinonasal squamous cell carcinoma associated with inverted papilloma

SNSCC and in the corresponding ISP positively demonstrated that the malignant SNSCC indeed clonally arises from the precursor ISP. These studies also indicate that EGFR-mutated cases carry a better prognosis than wild-type tumors. EGFR exon 20 mutation is also found in lung cancer patients that developed resistance to first-line EGFR inhibitors (gefitinib and erlotinib), which has led to the development of new drugs as neratinib, afatinib, and dacomitinib, now investigated in clinical trials. These drugs may also prove useful in SNSCC, and indeed preclinical studies using SNSCC cell lines have shown promising results [14]. Two SNSCCs, one HPV-positive and one HPV-negative, were included as part of a large exome-sequencing study of head and neck squamous cell carcinoma, and both were discovered to be among the tumors with the lowest number of mutations [18]. TP53 was the only mutated gene identified in the HPV-positive SNSCC, whereas the other HPV-negative tumor was found to tumor two mutated genes, SYNE1 and NOTCH3, which have both been implicated in the regulation of nuclear polarity and terminal differentiation of squamous epithelia. Microsatellite instability was observed in 21% and in 41% of SNSCC, based on mononucleotide (more reliable) and dinucleotide markers, respectively [19, 20]. This percentage is similar to head and neck SCC.

A study using methylation-sensitive MLPA has indicated up to 19% of SNSCC with possible silencing of expression through promotor hypermethylation of RASSF1, a gene similar to the RAS effector proteins, of CDH13 coding H-cadherin, and of CHFR, a mitotic checkpoint regulator. Methylation of these genes has also been reported in head and neck SCC and lung cancer [21].

HPV infection has been described in 38% of benign and 31% malignant tumors [15, 16, 22–28]. In addition, 21% of SNSCC overexpressed p16INK4A (cyclin-dependent kinase inhibitor 2A), often used as surrogate marker of HPV-positive cases [22, 23]. ISP-associated SNSCC also harbor 13–23% HPV, with 5–13% concerning oncogenic subtypes. In 10–24% of ISP, only non-oncogenic HPV types were found. Possibly EGFR mutation and HPV infection represent two different pathways of progression from ISP to SNSCC; indeed, they appear to occur in a mutually exclusive manner [15, 16].

Intestinal-Type Adenocarcinoma (ITAC)

Genome-wide genetic studies have shown that ITAC generally have complex, aneuploid genomes that carry a wide variety and a large number of chromosomal aberrations, with the exception of papillary-type ITAC, which seems to be predominantly diploid with few genetic aberrations [4, 29–33]. The major chromosomal regions showing gain or loss in more than 40% of cases were losses at 5q, 8p, 17p, and 18 and gains at 5p, 7p, 8q, and 20q. Univariate statistical analysis revealed seven specific CNAs significantly associated with worse overall survival: gains at 1q22–23, 3q28–29, 6p22, and 13q31–33 and losses at 4p15–16, 4q32–35, and 10q24 [32, 33]. These prognostic CNAs were found least frequent in papillary and most frequent in solid-type ITAC. Cluster analysis performed on 66 defined CNAs resulted in five groups of tumors with distinct CNA profiles with marked differences in overall survival. Mucinous-type ITACs may be genetically different from the other subtypes, and they have been shown to have less frequent TP53 mutation and expression, more frequent loss of membranous E-cadherin staining, and less expression of β-catenin and EGFR [34, 35]. Using fluorescence in situ hybridization, gene amplification was not found in studies on FGFR1 and cMET, while SOX2 copy number gains were demonstrated in 8% of ITACs [8, 9, 36]. Also using FISH, Pacheco et al. reported absence of chromosomal translocations of ALK in a series of 96 ITACs [37].

Studies of the involvement of specific genes in ITAC have often been guided by findings from more-frequent and better-studied tumors with similar histology, such as colorectal and lung adenocarcinoma, respectively. Mutation of the TP53 gene has been associated with exposure to wood dust, with a frequency of 40–50% [38–43].

Interestingly, the frequency of p53 overexpression, a proxy for TP53 mutation, seems to be markedly lower in mucinous-type ITAC compared with the other ITAC subtypes [38]. Being a tumor histopathologically similar to intestinal adenocarcinoma, activation of the Wnt pathway has been suspected and studied in ITAC. However, the key components of the Wnt cascade APC (encoding adenomatous polyposis coli protein) or CTNNB1 (encoding β-catenin) have not been found mutated in sinonasal carcinomas [40] Still, nuclear expression of β-catenin has been reported in 31–53% of cases [38, 44, 45], indicating that activation of the Wnt pathway probably does contribute to the development of ITAC. Mutations in KRAS and HRAS, which encode proteins downstream of EGFR in the EGF signalling pathway, have been found in approximately 15% of ITACs, whereas BRAF mutations have not been detected in these tumors. EGFR mutations were not detected [7, 12, 35, 40, 44, 46–48]. Microsatellite instability detection based on mononucleotide markers was observed in 1 of 41 ITAC, suggesting that this mechanism of genomic instability does not play an important role [19]. Methylation-sensitive MLPA on 50 cases of ITAC revealed the following recurrent methylated genes CDH13 (36%), ESR1 (26%), APC (14%), TIMP3 (10%), CASP8 (6%), and HIC1 and RASSF1 (4%). Papillary and colonic ITAC subtypes carried a mean of 1.26 gene methylations per tumor versus 0.63 in solid and mucinous subtypes. Methylation of TIMP3 was associated with a significantly worse survival in ITAC patients [21].

Sinonasal Undifferentiated Carcinoma (SNUC)

A microarray CGH study on 24 SNUC revealed chromosomal copy number gains occurred in >50% of cases at 1q, 2q, 3q, 4q, 6p, 7, 8q, 12, 17q, and 20 and losses in >35% of cases at 13q and 17p [49]. Most of these findings have been confirmed by other studies on SNUC observing gains at 1q, 3q, 8q, 17q, and 20q and losses at 3p and 17p [50–52]. Takahasi et al. created a stable SNUC tumor cell line that carried an amplification at 17q12 [53]. As ERBB2 gene is located in this region, this gene was tested and found overexpressed. Gain or amplification of ERBB2 at 17q12 was not found in the 35 cases studied by Jo et al. and López-Hernández et al. [49, 50]. Frequent gain and amplification at 3q26 and 17q23–24, respectively, may include transcription factors SOX2 and SOX9 involved in cellular differentiation processes [49, 50, 54]. Other hotspots of amplification concerned chromosomal bands 8p11 and 8q24 with possible candidate oncogenes FGFR1 and cMYC [8, 49].

Gelbard et al. analyzed mutations of 12 cancer-related genes (AKT, BRAF, CDK4, CTNNB1, EGFR, FBXW7, JAK2, c-KIT, KRAS, PDGFR, PI3K, VEGF) in 13 SNUCs, but none were found [54]. Better luck was obtained with a study sequencing all coding exons of 300 cancer-related genes and 113 introns across 35 genes for chromosomal rearrangement detection [50]. Several genes were found to harbor mutation in 2 or more of 11 analyzed SNUCs: IDH2, TP53, PIK3CA, ARID1A, CREBBP, KMT2D, SETD2, and TET2. A similar study including 10 SNUC reported recurrent mutations in SOX17, cKIT, SETD2, and IDH2 [51]. Interestingly, both studies demonstrated frequent loss-of-function alterations in genes involved in epigenetic regulation. However, the most outstanding mutation concerned IDH2 (Fig. 2), in 55% (5/11) of cases, while subsequent publications confirmed the importance of this gene, presenting 49% (26/53) up to 82% (14/17) of cases with IDH2 mutation [50, 51, 55]. It is thought that the abnormal activity of mutated IDH2 causes an accumulation of the (R)-2-hydroxygluuotarate (2-HG) oncometabolite, thus inducing global DNA hypermethylation and interruption of the differentiation of lineage-specific progenitor cells into terminally differentiated cells [56]. Capper et al. have recently claimed "sinonasal IDH2 carcinoma" as a new entity apart from IDH2 mutation characterized by high levels of methylation, which is in agreement with the above studies, and also 17q deletions and histopathologically by frequent necrosis [52]. Three of these tumors were sequenced using a panel of 560 cancer-related genes, finding no other mutation than IDH2. Whether or not IDH2 mutation is a characteriz-

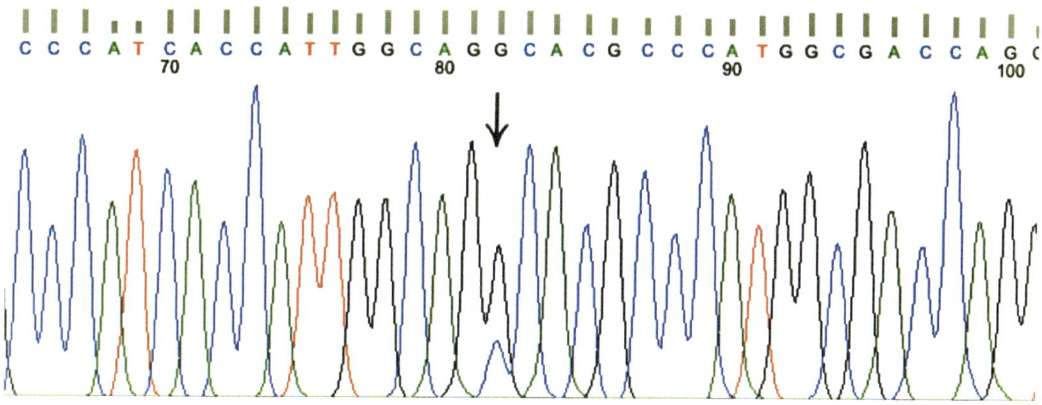

Fig. 2 IDH2 R172S point mutation (C > G, see arrow) in a sinonasal undifferentiated carcinoma

ing event for SNUC remains to be seen, because they have also been detected in sinonasal undifferentiated high-grade carcinomas and neuroendocrine carcinoma [51, 55].

Other Carcinomas

A number of other carcinomas have been classified by specific, characterizing genetic alterations, but still little more is known about additional copy number abnormalities or mutations that may be related to prognosis or response to therapy. These tumors include SMARCB1-deficient sinonasal basaloid carcinoma, nuclear protein in testis (NUT) midline carcinoma, HPV-related sinonasal adenoid-cystic-like carcinoma, non-intestinal-type adenocarcinomas, and teratocarcinosarcoma.

SMARCB1-deficient sinonasal basaloid carcinoma is defined by the absence of SMARCB1/INI1 protein expression as detected by immunohistochemical staining. López-Hernández et al. analyzed whole-genome copy number changes in two SNUC cases that showed complete absence of SMARCB1 staining [49]. Both demonstrated simple karyotypes, which is in agreement with Jackson et al. [57] who showed that SMARCB1 inactivation occurs by a variety of mechanisms, including deletions, LOH, and mutations, although in sinonasal tumors, no mutations have been reported yet [58]. Reported deletions involving the SMARCB1 gene have demonstrated great complexity of rearrangements of chromosome 22 compared with the low frequency of alterations involving the other chromosomes [57]. Four signalling pathways have been reported to be affected by SMARCB1: the p16INK4a-Rb-E2F pathway regulating chromosomal stability, the WNT signaling pathway shown by WNT/β-catenin overexpression, the Shh signaling pathway through regulation of GLI1, and repression of polycomb genes through elevated expression and recruitment of EZH2 [59].

NUT carcinoma harbors a defining chromosomal translocation alteration involving the nuclear protein in testis gene (NUT1 on 15q14), in 70% of cases, creating a fusion protein with BRD4 (19p13) and in 6% with BRD3 (9q34.2), NSD3 (8p12), ZNF532 (18q21.32), ZNF592 (15q25.3), and CIC (19q13.2) [60–65]. A diffuse NUT1 protein expression of >50% is also accepted for diagnosis [1]. NUT carcinomas typically have simple karyotypes often with the t(15;19) translocation as sole aberration, a finding supported by recent whole genome next-generation sequencing finding few if any additional oncogenic mutations [62, 66, 67].

HPV-related sinonasal adenoid-cystic-like carcinoma (also named HPV-related multiphenotypic sinonasal carcinoma) is defined by the presence of high-risk HPV in the absence of the t(6;9) MYB-NFIB rearrangement. However, variable immunohistochemical staining of cMYB has been reported [68]. Interestingly, not the well-known oncogenic HPV types 16 and 18 are involved, but in two thirds of cases HPV 33 and further HPV types 35, 56, 26, and 52 [69–72]. To date, there are no studies that have analyzed genetic abnormalities additional to HPV infection.

Non-intestinal-type adenocarcinomas concern a heterogeneous and poorly described group of tumors. Andreasen et al. first described a recurrent translocation t(12;15)(p13;q25) involving the genes ETV6 and NTRK3 in four cases and another translocation between ETV6 and RET [73, 74]. This latter translocation was previously described by Skalova et al. in mammary analog of secretory carcinoma of the salivary gland [75]. Moreover, Baneckova et al. found two cases of ETV6-NTRK3 translocation in sinonasal secretory carcinoma [76]. However, they have shown that these two tumors, although sharing the same translocations, are indeed two separate entities. Yet another translocation fusing SYN2 and PPARG genes was described by Soon et al. [77]. The t(3;3) SYN2-PPARG fusion has been reported in pulmonary small cell carcinoma. Villatoro et al. detected CTNNB1 mutations in two cases of sinonasal non-ITAC with morular metaplasia and CDX2/β-catenin nuclear expression [78]. Finally, Franchi et al. reported BRAF mutations in 2 of 12 low-grade SNAC [35]. It remains to be clarified whether or not all these cases with specific genetic characteristic also represent distinct tumor entities.

Teratocarcinosarcoma is so extremely rare that hardly any genetic studies have been published to date. Using cytogenetic analysis, Vranic et al. described a case carrying trisomy chromosome 12 with a subclone of cells also showing partial loss on chromosome arm 1p [79]. Thomas et al. have reported another case carrying an extra copy of chromosome 12 in a subpopulation of cells as detected by FISH [80]. A recent study presented two teratocarcinosarcomas, one of which analyzed by exome sequencing. They found 1209 sequence variants and after filtering focused on a pathogenic mutation in CTNNB1, coding the β-catenin gene. This mutation caused the accumulation of β-catenin protein in the nucleus, particularly in the mesenchymal component, a pattern that was also observed in the second tumor [81].

Neuroectodermal/Melanocytic Tumors

Neuroendocrine Carcinoma (SNEC)

Microarray CGH analysis of 18 SNEC cases showed a profile with frequent gains and losses. Hotspot gains occurring in >50% of cases were seen at 1q, 6p, 7, 8q, 12, 14, 17q, 18q, and 20, and >35% losses occurred at 5q, 16p, and 22q (Fig. 3). Compared to SNUC, losses appeared almost exclusively in 5q, 6q, 9q, 16p, and 22q in SNEC [49].

Very little is published on gene mutations in SNEC. One recent study evaluated mutations in TP53 in a tumor showing both SNEC and SNSCC differentiation, and they only found TP53 mutations in the SNEC phenotype [82]. The presence of TP53 mutations in SNEC was also demonstrated by Dogan et al., in addition to RB1 mutations [51]. These pathways are also frequent in pulmonary small cell carcinomas suggesting a common genetic background.

Olfactory Neuroblastoma (ONB)

In a Affymetrix array CGH study of 11 ONB, López-Hernández et al. reported a markedly low frequency of CNAs, with gains in >35% of cases at 7q, 14q, 18q and 20 and losses at 1p, 2p, 3, and 4. Losses were more frequent than gains. Eight of 11 cases carried only whole chromosome CNAs (Fig. 4), whereas gains or losses of segments of chromosomes were rare. The low level of chromosome instability of these tumors was also reflected by the absence of amplifications. Markedly, gains at 8q, perhaps the most frequent alteration in all solid tumors, was completely absent in ONB [49]. An almost identical pattern of gains and losses was found in 42 ONB studied by methylation microarray that also provided DNA information [52]. Another report with similar results on 12 ONB mentioned a striking pattern with chromosomes 3, 10 and 17q and 20 being affected almost exclusively by deletions or overrepresentations, respectively [83]. Apart from whole chromosome 5, 11, and 20 gains, Lazo de la Vega also reported focal gains involving CCDN1 at 11q13 and FGFR3 at 4p16 [84].

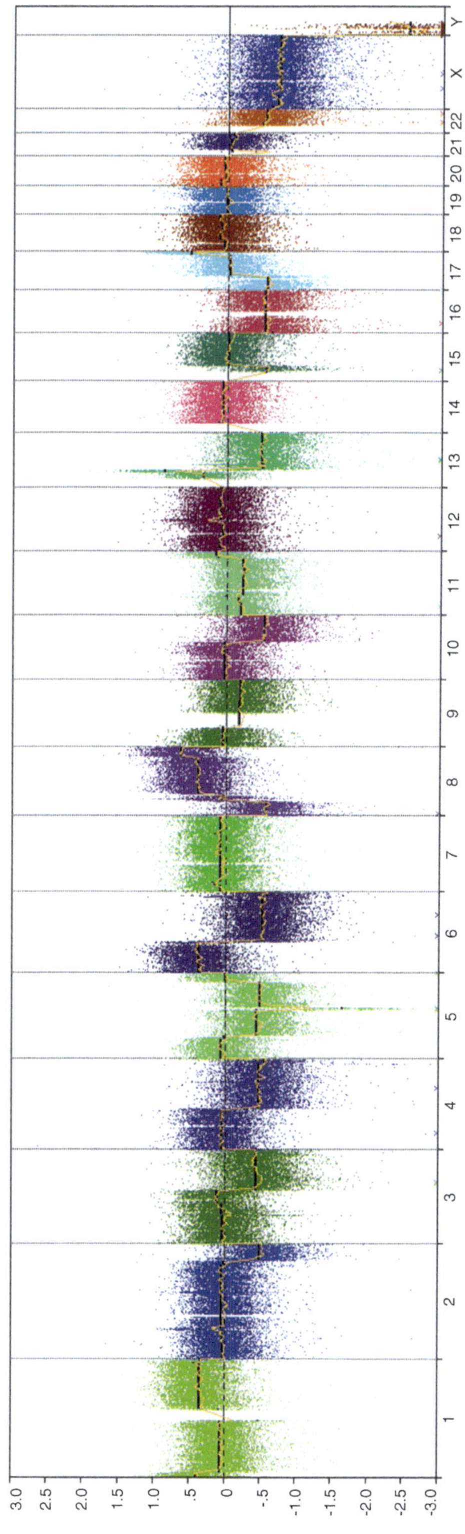

Fig. 3 Sinonasal neuroendocrine carcinoma showing a complex karyotype with copy number gains and losses affecting almost all chromosomes

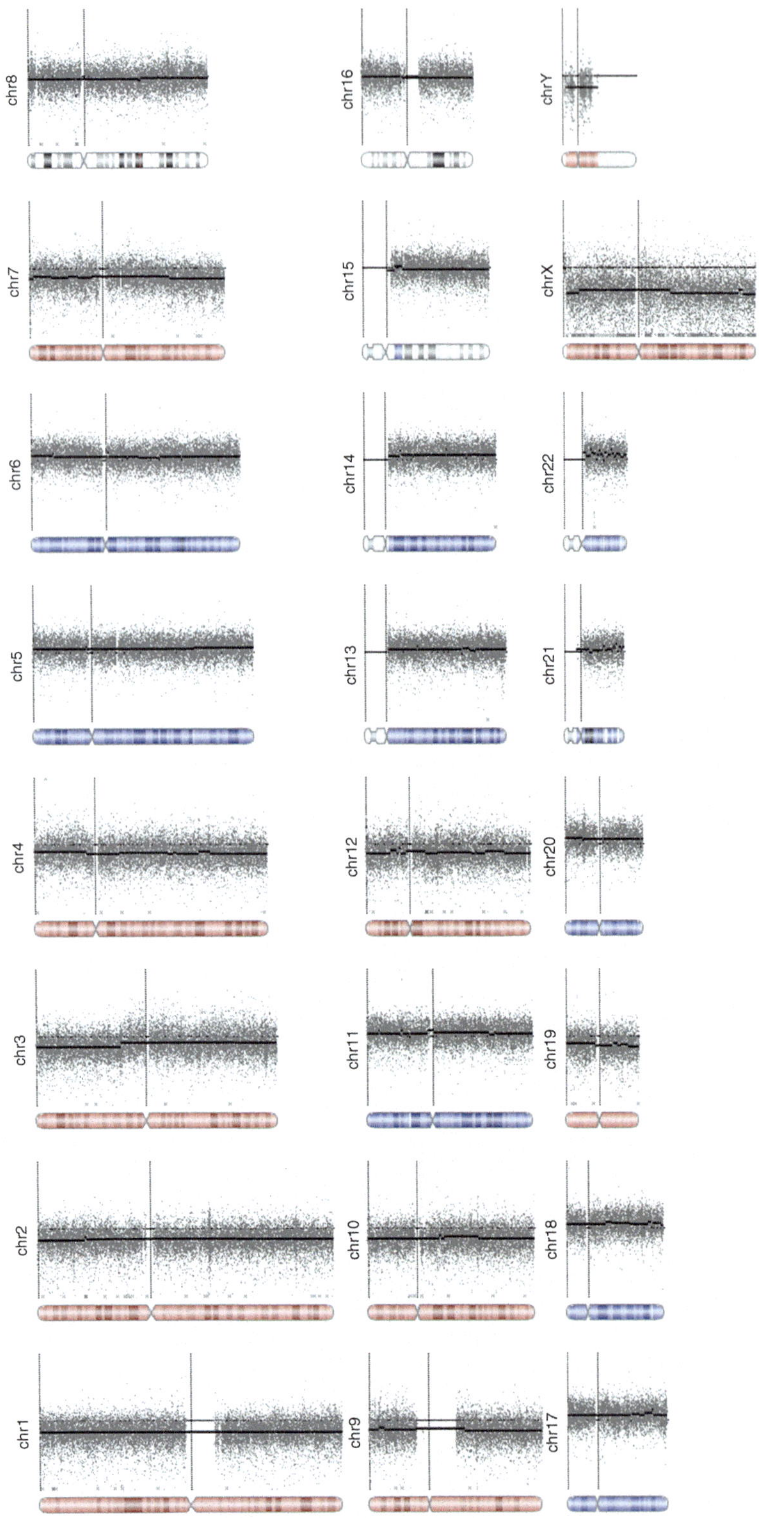

Fig. 4 Chromosomal copy number profile of an olfactory neuroblastoma exclusively carrying gains (in blue) and losses (in red) of whole chromosomes

Contrary to these results, three previous works had claimed ONB to be tumors with a high rate of chromosomal instability involving deletions of 1p, 3p/q, 9p, and 10p/q, and amplifications of 17q, 17p13, 20p, and 22q were frequent [85–88]. It is difficult to find a common denominator in these data, except perhaps for the frequent finding of whole chromosome events and the gains at chromosome arm 20q, which appeared in most studies. On the one hand, the heterogeneous map of copy number alterations may be explained by the difficulty to diagnose ONB correctly, especially the high-grade tumors. On the other hand, it is possible that the series of ONBs in the above publications differed with respect to Hyams grade.

In addition to fairly simple karyotypes, ONB also appear to carry few mutations. Two sets of sequencing data, both on 20 ONB by a 400/560 cancer-related gene panels, revealed only two cases with TP53 and two cases with DNMT3A mutation in one study and no recurrent mutations in the other [52, 84]. Gay et al. studied 41 refractory or recurrent ONB samples, many of which treated previously by radio/chemotherapy. Their results showed TP53 mutation in 17% of cases, while mutations in PIK3CA, NF1, and IDH2 were noted in two cases each [89]. Three studies have reported mutations in single cases of ONB. Weiss and collaborators found mutations in TP53, MAP 4K2, and TAOK2 in a primary ONB, whereas the corresponding metastasis acquired four more mutations in KDR, MYC, SIN3B, and NLRC4, suggesting a role for these mutations in metastatic development [90]. Another metastatic ONB recognized 8 candidate cancer genes: BRINP1, CARD11, CDKN2C, MEIS1, MINK1, PPP6C, TGFBR2, and TP53 [91]. A case of recurrent ONB was found to carry mutations in EGFR, KDR, FGFR2, and RET [92].

Genome-wide methylation patterns in a series of 66 ONB were studied by Capper et al. [52]. Cluster analysis revealed four groups of tumors with distinct methylation profiles, only one of which (42 cases) identified as "true" ONB, another as IDH2-mutated SNUC and the two remaining as miscellaneous sinonasal tumors. This 42 ONB group showed the lowest level of overall CpG methylation and tended to display a low-grade histology with not a single case fulfilling the criteria for a Hyams grade IV.

Ewing Sarcoma/Primitive Neuroectodermal Tumor

Similar to most sarcomas, also Ewing sarcomas and primitive neuroectodermal tumors are characterized by the presence of chromosomal rearrangements (Fig. 5) between the EWSR1 gene at 22q12 and several members of the ETS family of

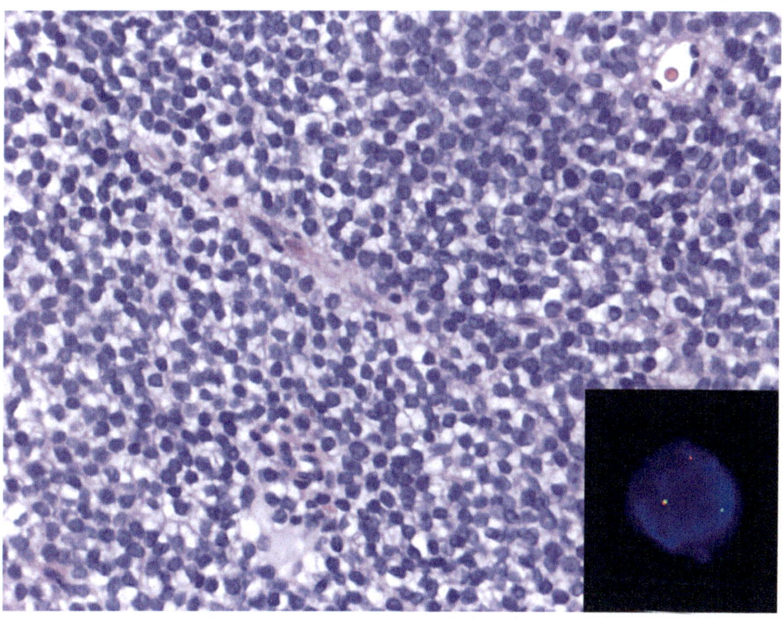

Fig. 5 Photomicrograph of an H&E stained Ewing sarcoma presenting undifferentiated round cells. The insert shows chromosomal rearrangement of the EWS gene detected with a break apart FISH probe

genes, the most common (approx. 90% of cases) being t(11;22)(q24;q12) resulting in EWSR1-FLI1 fusion [93].

Malignant Mucosal Melanoma (MMM)

Cutaneous, acral, uveal, and mucosal melanomas are cytogenetically different, showing more frequent aneuploidy, CNAs and chromosomal rearrangements in acral and mucosal melanoma genomes than in cutaneous melanoma [94]. Microarray CGH analysis of 14 sinonasal MMM indicated highly frequent gains of whole chromosome arms 1q, 6p, and 8q (100%, 93%, and 57%, respectively). Recurrent losses of whole arms 9p and 6q (both 50%) and whole chromosome 10 (43%) were observed. A third of cases appeared diploid or near-diploid and carried very few gains and losses [95]. In oral MMM, Zhou et al. reported frequent gains at 1p12, 4q12, 5p15, 11q13, and 12q13–15 and losses on 9p21 and 17p13. Notably, they found regions 5p15 and 12q13–15, with candidate genes hTERT and CDK4, respectively, also showing concurrent high-level amplification and translocation, although no formal translocation between these two genes was postulated [96]. Amplification of these two regions and particularly these two genes was also detected by Curtin et al. [97] and Lyu et al. [98]. It is not known whether these copy number alterations also occur in sinonasal MMM.

A relatively large number of mutation studies focusing on genes known to play a role in cutaneous mucosal melanoma have been dedicated to sinonasal MMM [99–104], sometimes as part of a series of head and neck MMM [105, 106]. The following frequencies of mutations were found: 7–30% NRAS, 0–25% KIT, 8–11% TERT, 3–10% BRAF (in one study 36%), and 7% SF3B1. These frequencies are very similar from those seen in head and neck mucosal melanoma [96, 106–109], suggesting a common tumorigenesis. However, there are apparent differences with cutaneous and acral mucosal melanomas; most frequent mutations in cutaneous melanoma are BRAF, CDKN2A, NRAS, in acral melanoma BRAF and NF1, and in mucosal melanoma KIT and SF3B1. Mutations affecting the TERT promoter are frequent in all melanomas [94]. Recently, several translocations involving BRAF have been described in mucosal melanoma (including head and neck) that activate the MAPK signalling pathway and may define a new molecular subset. Fusion partners of BRAF were ZNF767, NFIC, TMEM178B, and DGKI [110].

Mesenchymal Tumors

NF1 inactivating mutations have been reported in up to 40% of malignant peripheral nerve sheath tumors [111–113], and a second hit may be heterozygous deletions of CDKN2A [114]. Microarray comparative genomic hybridization-based studies have shown highly complex copy number alterations, with four regions of copy number gain including candidate genes SOX5 (12p12.1), NOL1 and MLF2 (12p13.31), FOXM1 and FKBP1 (12p13.33), and CDK4 and TSPAN31 (12q14.1). CDK4 gain/amplification appears an independent predictor for poor survival in malignant peripheral nerve sheath tumor patients [115]. NF1 mutations also occur in pediatric rhabdomyosarcoma [116]. In about 10% of sinonasal neurofibromas, NF1 is altered in the germline as part of the neurofibromatosis type 1 tumor predisposition syndrome [117, 118].

CTNNB1 mutations are found in a majority of sporadic desmoid tumors [119, 120], while 10–15% of cases are associated with germline mutations of APC as in familial adenomatous polyposis and Gardner syndrome. It is now established that alterations in the Wnt pathway underlie all desmoid tumors; gene alterations other than APC and CTNNB1 include chromosome 6 loss and BMI1 mutation [121]. In a similar fashion, similar CTNNB1 mutation is a characterizing genetic event in glomangiopericytoma, found in virtually all tumors studied [122, 123]. Immunohistochemical staining of β-catenin can be used as indicator of CTNNB1 mutation, and nuclear positivity has been observed in most cases [124]. Nuclear and cytoplasmatic β-catenin in up to 90% of cases has also been reported in biphenotypic sinonasal sarcoma [125, 126] and in synovial sarcoma [124, 127], but to date no CTNNB1 mutations have been reported in these tumors.

Chromosomal translocations are common in mesenchymal tumors and indeed are used in classification of specific types of cancer. Moreover, the fusion sequence may be used for monitoring disease by liquid biopsy testing of cell-free circulating DNA in blood [128].

Solitary fibrous tumor typically harbors the NAB2-STAT6 gene fusion, leading to EGR1 activation, and is a driving event in initiation of these tumors. In addition, chromosomal deletion on arms 13q and 17p and TP53 mutations in combination with TERT promoter mutations seem to play a role in the high-grade transformation [129–133].

Synovial sarcoma is consistently associated with translocation t(X;18)(p11;q11) fusing SYT-SXX genes [134–136]. Using in vitro experiments, Kadoch and Crabtree observed that expression of the fusion oncogene induced depletion of the SMARCB1 subunit from the SWI-SNF complex, in addition to SMARCB1 loss in synovial sarcoma cell lines [137]. APC-inactivating and β-catenin-stabilizing mutations have been described in approximately 20% of cases [138, 139], while nuclear accumulation of β-catenin was detected in 30–60% of synovial sarcomas [140]. Two different studies showed that nuclear β-catenin accumulation can be induced by SYT-SSX which may explain why nuclear β-catenin accumulation is more frequent than APC/CTNNB1 mutation [141, 142].

Biphenotypic sinonasal sarcoma carries rearrangements involving PAX3 and several partner genes. The most common genetic event is PAX3-MAML3 fusion (60% or more), followed by PAX3-FOXO1, PAX3-NCOA1 (4–8%), PAX3-WWTR1, and PAX3-NCOA2 [143, 144]. PAX3 is a transcription factor that controls differentiation of cells of melanocytic, neural, and myogenic lineage which may explain the divergent differentiation pattern of these tumors [144]. A role for the related PAX7 gene has not been claimed in biphenotypic sinonasal sarcoma. Nuclear and cytoplasmatic β-catenin has been reported in biphenotypic sinonasal sarcoma; however, its role in tumorigenesis is not yet understood [125, 126].

Rhabdomyosarcoma has been associated with PAX3 translocations as well. Particularly, PAX3-FOXO1 is found in approximately 70–80% of alveolar rhabdomyosarcoma, and also PAX7-FOXO1 fusions have been described [145]. Rearrangements NCOA2-SRF and NCOA2-TEAD1 were described in spindle cell rhabdomyosarcoma [146]. To date, embryonal and pleomorphic have not been associated with chromosomal translocations. Alveolar rhabdomyosarcoma with PAX7-FOXO1 fusion has been shown to carry amplification of the 13q31 chromosomal region, and gene copy number gain and overexpression of ALK in a majority of cases [147, 148]. In general, embryonal rhabdomyosarcomas carry more complex genetic events including mutations in GLI1, NF1, RAS, FGFR4, PIK3CA, and CTNNB1 [116].

References

1. El-Naggar AK, et al. WHO classification of tumors pathology and genetics of head and neck tumors. 4th ed. Lyon: IARC Press; 2017.
2. Hanahan D, Weinberg RA. The hallmarks of cancer. Cell. 2000;100(1):57–70.
3. Hanahan D, Weinberg RA. Hallmarks of cancer: the next generation. Cell. 2011;144(5):646–74.
4. Llorente JL, López F, Suárez C, Hermsen M. Sinonasal carcinoma: clinical, pathological and genetic advances for new therapeutic opportunities. Nat Rev Clin Oncol. 2014;11(8):460–72.
5. López F, Llorente JL, García-Inclán C, Alonso-Guervós M, Cuesta-Albalad MP, Fresno MF, Alvarez-Marcos C, Suárez C, Hermsen MA. Genomic profiling of sinonasal squamous cell carcinoma. Head Neck. 2011;33(2):145–53.
6. García-Inclán C, López-Hernández A, Alonso-Guervós M, Allonca E, Potes S, López F, Llorente JL, Hermsen M. Establishment and genetic characterization of six unique tumor cell lines as preclinical models for sinonasal squamous cell carcinoma. Sci Rep. 2014;4:4925.
7. López F, Llorente JL, Martín Oviedo C, Vivanco B, Álvarez Marcos C, García-Inclán C, Scola B, Hermsen MA. Gene amplification and protein overexpression of EGFR and ERBB2 in sinonasal squamous cell carcinoma. Cancer. 2012;118(7):1818–26.

8. Schröck A, Göke F, Wagner P, et al. Fibroblast growth factor receptor-1 as a potential therapeutic target in sinonasal cancer. Head Neck. 2014;36(9):1253–7.
9. Schröck A, Göke F, Wagner P, Bode M, Franzen A, Braun M, Huss S, Agaimy A, Ihrler S, Menon R, Kirsten R, Kristiansen G, Bootz F, Lengerke C, Perner S. Sex determining region Y-Box 2 (*SOX2*) amplification is an independent indicator of disease recurrence in sinonasal cancer. PLoS One. 2013;8(3):e59201.
10. Holmila R, Bornholdt J, Heikkilä P, Suitiala T, Févotte J, Cyr D, Hansen J, Snellman SM, Dictor M, Steiniche T, Schlünssen V, Schneider T, Pukkala E, Savolainen K, Wolff H, Wallin H, Luce D, Husgafvel-Pursiainen K. Mutations in TP53 tumor suppressor gene in wood dust-related sinonasal cancer. Int J Cancer. 2010;127(3):578–88.
11. López F, García Inclán C, Pérez-Escuredo J, Alvarez Marcos C, Scola B, Suárez C, Llorente JL, Hermsen MA. KRAS and BRAF mutations in sinonasal cancer. Oral Oncol. 2012;48(8):692–7.
12. Bornholdt J, Hansen J, Steiniche T, Dictor M, Antonsen A, Wolff H, Schlünssen V, Holmila R, Luce D, Vogel U, Husgafvel-Pursiainen K, Wallin H. K-ras mutations in sinonasal cancers in relation to wood dust exposure. BMC Cancer. 2008;8:53.
13. Udager AM, McHugh JB, Betz BL, Montone KT, Livolsi VA, Seethala RR, Yakirevich E, Iwenofu OH, Perez-Ordonez B, DuRoss KE, Weigelin HC, Lim MS, Elenitoba-Johnson KS, Brown NA. Activating KRAS mutations are characteristic of oncocytic sinonasal papilloma and associated sinonasal squamous cell carcinoma. J Pathol. 2016;239(4):394–8.
14. Udager AM, Rolland DCM, McHugh JB, Betz BL, Murga-Zamalloa C, Carey TE, Marentette LJ, Hermsen MA, DuRoss KE, Lim MS, Elenitoba-Johnson KSJ, Brown NA. High frequency targetable EGFR mutations in inverted sinonasal papilloma and associated sinonasal squamous cell carcinoma. Cancer Res. 2015;75(13):2600–6.
15. Udager AM, McHugh JB, Goudsmit CM, Weigelin HC, Lim MS, Elenitoba-Johnson KSJ, Betz BL, Carey TE, Brown NA. Human papillomavirus (HPV) and somatic EGFR mutations are essential, mutually exclusive oncogenic mechanisms for inverted sinonasal papillomas and associated sinonasal squamous cell carcinomas. Ann Oncol. 2018;29(2):466–71.
16. Sahnane N, Ottini G, Turri-Zanoni M, Furlan D, Battaglia P, Karligkiotis A, Albeni C, Cerutti R, Mura E, Chiaravalli AM, Castelnuovo P, Sessa F, Facco C. Comprehensive analysis of HPV infection, EGFR exon 20 mutations and LINE1 hypomethylation as risk factors for malignant transformation of sinonasal-inverted papilloma to squamous cell carcinoma. Int J Cancer. 2019;144(6):1313–20.
17. Sasaki E, Nishikawa D, Hanai N, Hasegawa Y, Yatabe Y. Sinonasal squamous cell carcinoma and EGFR mutations: a molecular footprint of a benign lesion. Histopathology. 2018;73(6):953–62.
18. Stransky N, Egloff AM, Tward AD, Kostic AD, Cibulskis K, Sivachenko A, Kryukov GV, Lawrence MS, Sougnez C, McKenna A, Shefler E, Ramos AH, Stojanov P, Carter SL, Voet D, Cortés ML, Auclair D, Berger MF, Saksena G, Guiducci C, Onofrio RC, Parkin M, Romkes M, Weissfeld JL, Seethala RR, Wang L, Rangel-Escareño C, Fernandez-Lopez JC, Hidalgo-Miranda A, Melendez-Zajgla J, Winckler W, Ardlie K, Gabriel SB, Meyerson M, Lander ES, Getz G, Golub TR, Garraway LA, Grandis JR. The mutational landscape of head and neck squamous cell carcinoma. Science. 2011;333(6046):1157–60.
19. Martínez JG, Pérez-Escuredo J, López F, Suárez C, Alvarez-Marcos C, Llorente JL, Hermsen MA. Microsatellite instability analysis of sinonasal carcinomas. Otolaryngol Head Neck Surg. 2009;140(1):55–60.
20. Uryu H, Oda Y, Shiratsuchi H, et al. Microsatellite instability and proliferating activity in sinonasal carcinoma: molecular genetic and immunohistochemical comparison with oral squamous cell carcinoma. Oncol Rep. 2005;14:1133–42.
21. Costales M, López-Hernández A, García-Inclán C, Vivanco B, López F, Llorente JL, Hermsen MA. Gene methylation profiling in sinonasal adenocarcinoma and squamous cell carcinoma. Otolaryngol Head Neck Surg. 2016;155(5):808–15.
22. Syrjänen K, Syrjänen S. Detection of human papillomavirus in sinonasal papillomas: systematic review and meta-analysis. Laryngoscope. 2013;123(1):181–92.
23. Bishop JA, Guo TW, Smith DF, Wang H, Ogawa T, Pai SI, Westra WH. Human papillomavirus-related carcinomas of the sinonasal tract. Am J Surg Pathol. 2013;37(2):185–92.
24. Gray ST. Treatment outcomes and prognostic factors, including human papillomavirus, for sinonasal undifferentiated carcinoma: a retrospective review. Head Neck. 2015;37:366–74.
25. El-Mofty SK, Lu DW. Prevalence of high-risk human papillomavirus DNA in nonkeratinizing (cylindrical cell) carcinoma of the sinonasal tract: a distinct clinicopathologic and molecular disease entity. Am J Surg Pathol. 2005;29:1367–72.
26. Alos L, Moyano S, Nadal A, Alobid I, Blanch JL, Ayala E, Lloveras B, Quint W, Cardesa A, Ordi J. Human papillomaviruses are identified in a subgroup of sinonasal squamous cell carcinomas with favorable outcome. Cancer. 2009;115:2701–9.
27. Larque AB, Hakim S, Ordi J, Nadal A, Diaz A, del Pino M, Marimon L, Alobid I, Cardesa A, Alos L. High-risk human papillomavirus is transcriptionally active in a subset of sinonasal squamous cell carcinomas. Mod Pathol. 2014;27(3):343–51.
28. Laco J, Sieglová K, Vošmiková H, Dundr P, Němejcová K, Michálek J, Čelakovský P, Chrobok V, Mottl R, Mottlová A, Tuček L, Slezák R, Chmelařová M, Sirák I, Vošmik M, Ryška A. The presence of high-risk human papillomavirus (HPV) E6/E7 mRNA transcripts in a subset of sinonasal

carcinomas is evidence of involvement of HPV in its etiopathogenesis. Virchows Arch. 2015;467:405–15.
29. Ariza M, Llorente JL, Alvarez-Marcas C, Baragaño L, Salas A, Rodriguez Prado N, Hermsen M, Suárez C, Sampedro A. Comparative genomic hybridization of primary sinonasal adenocarcinomas. Cancer. 2004;100(2):335–41.
30. Korinth D, Pacyna-Gengelbach M, Deutschmann N, Hattenberger S, Bockmühl U, Dietel M, Schroeder HG, Donhuijsen K, Petersen I. Chromosomal imbalances in wood dust-related adenocarcinomas of the inner nose and their associations with pathological parameters. J Pathol. 2005;207(2):207–15.
31. Hermsen MA, Llorente JL, Pérez-Escuredo J, López F, Ylstra B, Alvarez-Marcos C, Suárez C. Genome-wide analysis of genetic changes in intestinal-type sinonasal adenocarcinoma. Head Neck. 2009;31(3):290–7.
32. Pérez-Escuredo J, López-Hernández A, Costales M, López F, Potes Ares S, Vivanco B, Llorente JL, Hermsen MA. Recurrent DNA copy number alterations in intestinal-type sinonasal adenocarcinoma. Rhinology. 2016;54(3):278–86.
33. López-Hernández A, Pérez-Escuredo J, Vivanco B, García-Inclán C, Potes-Ares S, Cabal VN, Riobello C, Costales M, López F, Llorente JL, Hermsen MA. Genomic profiling of intestinal-type sinonasal adenocarcinoma reveals subgroups of patients with distinct clinical outcomes. Head Neck. 2018;40(2):259–73.
34. Franchi A, Fondi C, Paglierani M, Pepi M, Gallo O, Santucci M. Epidermal growth factor receptor expression and gene copy number in sinonasal intestinal type adenocarcinoma. Oral Oncol. 2009;45:835–8.
35. Franchi A, Innocenti DR, Palomba A, et al. Low prevalence of K-RAS, EGFR and BRAF mutations in sinonasal adenocarcinomas. Implications for anti-EGFR treatments. Pathol Oncol Res. 2014;20:571–9.
36. Projetti F, Mesturoux L, Coulibaly B, et al. Study of MET protein levels and MET gene copy number in 72 sinonasal intestinal-type adenocarcinomas. Head Neck. 2015;37(11):1563–8.
37. Pacheco E, Llorente JL, López-Hernández A, et al. Absence of chromosomal translocations and protein expression of ALK in sinonasal adenocarcinomas. Acta Otorrinolaringol Esp. 2017;68(1):9–14.
38. Franchi A, Palomba A, Fondi C, et al. Immunohistochemical investigation of tumorigenic pathways in sinonasal intestinal-type adenocarcinoma. A tissue microarray analysis of 62 cases. Histopathology. 2011;59:98–105.
39. Perrone F, Oggionni M, Birindelli S, et al. TP53, p14ARF, p16INK4a and H-ras gene molecular analysis in intestinal-type adenocarcinoma of the nasal cavity and paranasal sinuses. Int J Cancer. 2003;105:196–203.
40. Yom SS, Rashid A, Rosenthal DI, et al. Genetic analysis of sinonasal adenocarcinoma phenotypes: distinct alterations of histogenetic significance. Mod Pathol. 2005;18(3):315–9.
41. Pérez-Escuredo J, Martínez JG, Vivanco B, et al. Wood dust-related mutational profile of TP53 in intestinal-type sinonasal adenocarcinoma. Hum Pathol. 2012;43:1894–901.
42. Bossi P, Perrone F, Miceli R, et al. TP53 status as guide for the management of ethmoid sinus intestinal-type adenocarcinoma. Oral Oncol. 2013;49:413–9.
43. Pérez-Escuredo J, García Martínez J, García-Inclán C, Vivanco B, Costales M, Álvarez Marcos C, Llorente JL, Hermsen MA. Establishment and genetic characterization of an immortal tumor cell line derived from intestinal-type sinonasal adenocarcinoma. Cell Oncol (Dordr). 2011;34(1):23–31.
44. Perez-Ordonez B, Huynh NN, Berean KW, Jordan RC. Expression of mismatch repair proteins, β-catenin, and cadherin in intestinal-type sinonasal adenocarcinoma. J Clin Pathol. 2004;57(10):1080–3.
45. Díaz-Molina JP, Llorente JL, Vivanco B, Martínez-Camblor P, Fresno MF, Pérez-Escuredo J, Álvarez-Marcos C, Hermsen MA. Wnt-pathway activation in intestinal-type sinonasal adenocarcinoma. Rhinology. 2011;49(5):593–9.
46. Frattini M, Perrone F, Suardi S, Balestra D, Caramuta S, Colombo F, Licitra L, Cantù G, Pierotti MA, Pilotti S. Phenotype-genotype correlation: challenge of intestinal-type adenocarcinoma of the nasal cavity and paranasal sinuses. Head Neck. 2006;28(10):909–15.
47. García-Inclán C, López F, Pérez-Escuredo J, Cuesta-Albalad MP, Vivanco B, Centeno I, Balbín M, Suárez C, Llorente JL, Hermsen MA. EGFR status and KRAS/BRAF mutations in intestinal-type sinonasal adenocarcinomas. Cell Oncol (Dordr). 2012;35(6):443–50.
48. Projetti F, Durand K, Chaunavel A, et al. Epidermal growth factor receptor expression and KRAS and BRAF mutations: study of 39 sinonasal intestinal-type adenocarcinomas. Hum Pathol. 2013;44:2116–25.
49. López-Hernández A, Vivanco B, Franchi A, Bloemena E, Cabal VN, Potes-Ares S, Riobello C, García-Inclán C, López F, Llorente JL, Hermsen M. Genetic profiling of poorly differentiated sinonasal tumors. Sci Rep. 2018;8(1):3998.
50. Jo VY, Chau NG, Hornick JL, Krane JF, Sholl LM. Recurrent IDH2 R172X mutations in sinonasal undifferentiated carcinoma. Mod Pathol. 2017;30(5):650–9.
51. Dogan S, Chute DJ, Xu B, Ptashkin RN, Chandramohan R, Casanova-Murphy J, Nafa K, Bishop JA, Chiosea SI, Stelow EB, Ganly I, Pfister DG, Katabi N, Ghossein RA, Berger MF. Frequent IDH2 R172 mutations in undifferentiated and poorly-differentiated sinonasal carcinomas. J Pathol. 2017;242(4):400–8.
52. Capper D, Engel NW, Stichel D, Lechner M, Glöss S, Schmid S, Koelsche C, Schrimpf D, Niesen J,

Wefers AK, Jones DTW, Sill M, Weigert O, Ligon KL, Olar A, Koch A, Forster M, Moran S, Tirado OM, Sáinz-Jaspeado M, Mora J, Esteller M, Alonso J, Del Muro XG, Paulus W, Felsberg J, Reifenberger G, Glatzel M, Frank S, Monoranu CM, Lund VJ, von Deimling A, Pfister S, Buslei R, Ribbat-Idel J, Perner S, Gudziol V, Meinhardt M, Schüller U. DNA methylation-based reclassification of olfactory neuroblastoma. Acta Neuropathol. 2018;136(2):255–71.

53. Takahashi Y, Kupferman ME, Bell D, Jiffar T, Lee JG, Xie TX, Li NW, Zhao M, Frederick MJ, Gelbard A, Myers JN, Hanna EY. Establishment and characterization of novel cell lines from sinonasal undifferentiated carcinoma. Clin Cancer Res. 2012;18(22):6178–87.
54. Gelbard A, Hale KS, Takahashi Y, Davies M, Kupferman ME, El-Naggar AK, Myers JN, Hanna EY. Molecular profiling of sinonasal undifferentiated carcinoma. Head Neck. 2014;36(1):15–21.
55. Mito JK, Bishop JA, Sadow PM, Stelow EB, Faquin WC, Mills SE, Krane JF, French CA, Fletcher CDM, Hornick JL, Sholl LM, Jo VY. Immunohistochemical detection and molecular characterization of IDH-mutant sinonasal undifferentiated carcinomas. Am J Surg Pathol. 2018;42(8):1067–75.
56. Lu C, Ward PS, Kapoor GS, Rohle D, Turcan S, Abdel-Wahab O, Edwards CR, Khanin R, Figueroa ME, Melnick A, Wellen KE, O'Rourke DM, Berger SL, Chan TA, Levine RL, Mellinghoff IK, Thompson CB. IDH mutation impairs histone demethylation and results in a block to cell differentiation. Nature. 2012;483(7390):474–8.
57. Jackson EM, Sievert AJ, Gai X, Hakonarson H, Judkins AR, Tooke L, Perin JC, Xie H, Shaikh TH, Biegel JA. Genomic analysis using high-density single nucleotide polymorphism-based oligonucleotide arrays and multiplex ligation-dependent probe amplification provides a comprehensive analysis of INI1/SMARCB1 in malignant rhabdoid tumors. Clin Cancer Res. 2009;15(6):1923–30.
58. Agaimy A, Hartmann A, Antonescu CR, Chiosea SI, El-Mofty SK, Geddert H, Iro H, Lewis JS Jr, Märkl B, Mills SE, Riener MO, Robertson T, Sandison A, Semrau S, Simpson RH, Stelow E, Westra WH, Bishop JA. SMARCB1 (INI-1)-deficient sinonasal carcinoma: a series of 39 cases expanding the morphologic and clinicopathologic spectrum of a recently described entity. Am J Surg Pathol. 2017;41(4):458–71.
59. Kohashi K, Oda Y, Yamamoto H, et al. Reduced expression of SMARCB1/INI1 protein in synovial sarcoma. Mod Pathol. 2010;23:981–90.
60. French CA, Miyoshi I, Kubonishi I, Grier HE, Perez-Atayde AR, Fletcher JA. BRD4-NUT fusion oncogene: a novel mechanism in aggressive carcinoma. Cancer Res. 2003;63(2):304–7.
61. French CA, Ramirez CL, Kolmakova J, Hickman TT, Cameron MJ, Thyne ME, Kutok JL, Toretsky JA, Tadavarthy AK, Kees UR, Fletcher JA, Aster JC. BRD-NUT oncoproteins: a family of closely related nuclear proteins that block epithelial differentiation and maintain the growth of carcinoma cells. Oncogene. 2008;27(15):2237–42.
62. French C. NUT midline carcinoma. Nat Rev Cancer. 2014;14:149–50.
63. Alekseyenko AA, Walsh EM, Zee BM, Pakozdi T, Hsi P, Lemieux ME, Dal Cin P, Ince TA, Kharchenko PV, Kuroda MI, French CA. Ectopic protein interactions within BRD4-chromatin complexes drive oncogenic megadomain formation in NUT midline carcinoma. Proc Natl Acad Sci U S A. 2017;114(21):E4184–92.
64. Shiota H, Elya JE, Alekseyenko AA, Chou PM, Gorman SA, Barbash O, Becht K, Danga K, Kuroda MI, Nardi V, French CA. 'Z4' complex member fusions in NUT carcinoma: Implications for a novel oncogenic mechanism. Mol Cancer Res. 2018;16(12):1826–33.
65. Schaefer IM, Dal Cin P, Landry LM, Fletcher CDM, Hanna GJ, French CA. CIC-NUTM1 fusion: a case which expands the spectrum of NUT-rearranged epithelioid malignancies. Genes Chromosomes Cancer. 2018;57(9):446–51.
66. French CA. NUT Carcinoma: clinicopathologic features, pathogenesis, and treatment. Pathol Int. 2018;68(11):583–95.
67. Lee JK, Louzada S, An Y, et al. Complex chromosomal rearrangements by single catastrophic pathogenesis in NUT midline carcinoma. Ann Oncol. 2017;28:890–7.
68. Shah AA, Lamarre ED, Bishop JA. Human papillomavirus-related multiphenotypic sinonasal carcinoma: a case report documenting the potential for very late tumor recurrence. Head Neck Pathol. 2018;12:623–8.
69. Adamane SA, Mittal N, Teni T, Pawar S, Waghole R, Bal M. Human papillomavirus-related multiphenotypic sinonasal carcinoma with unique HPV type 52 association: a case report with review of literature. Head Neck Pathol. 2019;13(3):331–8.
70. Bishop JA, Ogawa T, Stelow EB, Moskaluk CA, Koch WM, Pai SI, et al. Human papillomavirus-related carcinoma with adenoid cystic-like features: a peculiar variant of head and neck cancer restricted to the sinonasal tract. Am J Surg Pathol. 2013;37:836–44.
71. Bishop JA, Andreasen S, Hang JF, Bullock MJ, Chen TY, Franchi A, et al. HPV-related multiphenotypic sinonasal carcinoma: an expanded series of 49 cases of the tumor formerly known as HPV-related carcinoma with adenoid cystic carcinoma-like features. Am J Surg Pathol. 2017;41:1690–701.
72. Hang JF, Hsieh MS, Li WY, Chen JY, Lin SY, Liu SH, et al. Human papillomavirus-related carcinoma with adenoid cysticlike features: a series of five cases expanding the pathological spectrum. Histopathology. 2017;71(6):887–96.
73. Andreasen S, Skalova A, Agaimy A, Bishop JA, Laco J, Leivo I, et al. ETV6 gene rearrangements characterize a morphologically distinct subset of sinonasal low-grade non–intestinal-type adenocarcinoma: a novel translocation-associated carcinoma restricted to the sinonasal tract. Am J Surg Pathol. 2017;41:1552–60.
74. Andreasen S, Kiss K, Melchior LC, Laco J. The ETV6-RET gene fusion is found in ETV6-

rearranged low-grade sinonasal adenocarcinoma without NTRK3 involvement. Am J Surg Pathol. 2018;42:985–8.

75. Skalova A, Vanecek T, Martinek P, Weinreb I, Stevens TM, Simpson RHW, et al. Molecular profiling of mammary analog secretory carcinoma revealed a subset of tumors harboring a novel ETV6-RET translocation: report of 10 cases. Am J Surg Pathol. 2018;42:234–46.
76. Baneckova M, Agaimy A, Andreasen S, Vanecek T, Steiner P, Slouka D, et al. Mammary analog secretory carcinoma of the nasal cavity. Am J Surg Pathol. 2018;42:735–43.
77. Soon GST, Chang KTE, Kuick CH, Petersson F. A case of nasal low-grade non-intestinal-type adenocarcinoma with aberrant CDX2 expression and a novel SYN2-PPARG gene fusion in a 13-year-old girl. Virchows Arch. 2019;474(5):619–23.
78. Villatoro TM, Mardekian SK. Two cases of sinonasal nonintestinal-type adenocarcinoma with squamoid morules expressing nuclear β-catenin and CDX2: a curious morphologic finding supported by molecular analysis. Case Rep Pathol. 2018;2018:8741017.
79. Vranic S, Caughron SK, Djuricic S, Bilalovic N, Zaman S, Suljevic I, Lydiatt WM, Emanuel J, Gatalica Z. Hamartomas, teratomas and teratocarcinosarcomas of the head and neck: Report of 3 new cases with clinico-pathologic correlation, cytogenetic analysis, and review of the literature. BMC Ear Nose Throat Disord. 2008;8:8.
80. Thomas J, Adegboyega P, Iloabachie K, Mooring JW, Lian T. Sinonasal teratocarcinosarcoma with yolk sac elements: a neoplasm of somatic or germ cell origin? Ann Diagn Pathol. 2011;15(2):135–9.
81. Birkeland AC, Burgin SJ, Yanik M, Scott MV, Bradford CR, McHugh JB, McLean SA, Sullivan SE, Nor JE, McKean EL, Brenner JC. Pathogenetic analysis of sinonasal teratocarcinosarcomas reveal actionable β-catenin overexpression and a β-catenin mutation. J Neurol Surg B Skull Base. 2017;78(4):346–52.
82. Franchi A, Rocchetta D, Palomba A, Innocenti DRD, Castiglione F, Spinelli G. Primary combined neuroendocrine and squamous cell carcinoma of the maxillary sinus: report of a case with immunohistochemical and molecular characterization. Head Neck Pathol. 2015;9(1):107–13.
83. Bockmuhl U, You X, Pacyna-Gengelbach M, et al. CGH pattern of esthesioneuroblastoma and their metastases. Brain Pathol. 2004;14:158–63.
84. Lazo de la Vega L, McHugh JB, Cani AK, Kunder K, Walocko FM, Liu CJ, Hovelson DH, Robinson D, Chinnaiyan AM, Tomlins SA, Harms PW. Comprehensive molecular profiling of olfactory neuroblastoma identifies potentially targetable FGFR3 amplifications. Mol Cancer Res. 2017;15(11):1551–7.
85. Holland H, Koschny R, Krupp W, et al. Comprehensive cytogenetic characterization of an esthesioneuroblastoma. Cancer Genet Cytogenet. 2007;173:89–96.
86. Riazimand SH, Brieger J, Jacob R, et al. Analysis of cytogenetic aberrations in esthesioneuroblastomas by comparative genomic hybridization. Cancer Genet Cytogenet. 2002;136:53–7.
87. Guled M, Myllykangas S, Frierson HFJ, et al. Array comparative genomic hybridization analysis of olfactory neuroblastoma. Mod Pathol. 2008;21:770–8.
88. Valli R, De Bernardi F, Frattini A, Volpi L, Bignami M, Facchetti F, Pasquali F, Castelnuovo P, Maserati E. Comparative genomic hybridization on microarray (a-CGH) in olfactory neuroblastoma: analysis of ten cases and review of the literature. Genes Chromosomes Cancer. 2015;54(12):771–5.
89. Gay LM, Kim S, Fedorchak K, et al. Comprehensive genomic profiling of esthesioneuroblastoma reveals additional treatment options. Oncologist. 2017;22(7):834–42.
90. Weiss GJ, Liang WS, Izatt T, et al. Paired tumor and normal whole genome sequencing of metastatic olfactory neuroblastoma. PLoS One. 2012;7:e37029.
91. Cha S, Lee J, Shin J-Y, Kim J-Y, Sim SH, Keam B, Kim TM, Kim D-W, Heo DS, Lee S-H, Kim J-I. Clinical application of genomic profiling to find druggable targets for adolescent and young adult (AYA) cancer patients with metastasis. BMC Cancer. 2016;16:170.
92. Wang L, Ding Y, Wei L, Zhao D, Wang R, Zhang Y, Gu X, Wang Z. Recurrent olfactory neuroblastoma treated with cetuximab and sunitinib: a case report. Medicine (Baltimore). 2016;95:e3536.
93. Weiss SW, Goldblum JR. Enzinger and Weiss's soft tissue tumors. 5th ed. Philadelphia: Mosby Elsevier; 2008.
94. Hayward NK, Wilmott JS, Waddell N, Johansson PA, Field MA, Nones K, Patch AM, Kakavand H, Alexandrov LB, Burke H, Jakrot V, Kazakoff S, Holmes O, Leonard C, Sabarinathan R, Mularoni L, Wood S, Xu Q, Waddell N, Tembe V, Pupo GM, De Paoli-Iseppi R, Vilain RE, Shang P, LMS L, Dagg RA, Schramm SJ, Pritchard A, Dutton-Regester K, Newell F, Fitzgerald A, Shang CA, Grimmond SM, Pickett HA, Yang JY, Stretch JR, Behren A, Kefford RF, Hersey P, Long GV, Cebon J, Shackleton M, Spillane AJ, RPM S, López-Bigas N, Pearson JV, Thompson JF, Scolyer RA, Mann GJ. Whole-genome landscapes of major melanoma subtypes. Nature. 2017;545(7653):175–80.
95. Van Dijk M, Sprenger S, Rombout P, Marres H, Kaanders J, Jeuken J, Ruiter D. Distinct chromosomal aberrations in sinonasal mucosal melanoma as detected by comparative genomic hybridization. Genes Chromosomes Cancer. 2003;36(2):151–8.
96. Zhou R, Shi C, Tao W, Li J, Wu J, Han Y, Yang G, Gu Z, Xu S, Wang Y, Wang L, Wang Y, Zhou G, Zhang C, Zhang Z, Sun S. Analysis of mucosal melanoma whole-genome landscapes reveals clinically relevant genomic aberrations. Clin Cancer Res. 2019;25(12):3548–60.
97. Curtin JA, Fridlyand J, Kageshita T, Patel HN, Busam KJ, Kutzner H, Cho KH, Aiba S, Bröcker EB, LeBoit PE, Pinkel D, Bastian BC. Distinct sets of genetic alterations in melanoma. N Engl J Med. 2005;353(20):2135–47.

98. Lyu J, Song Z, Chen J, Shepard MJ, Song H, Ren G, et al. Whole-exome sequencing of oral mucosal melanoma reveals mutational profile and therapeutic targets. J Pathol. 2018;244:358–66.
99. Zebary A, Jangard M, Omholt K, et al. KIT, NRAS and BRAF mutations in sinonasal mucosal melanoma: a study of 56 cases. Br J Cancer. 2013;109:559–64.
100. Amit M, Tam S, Abdelmeguid AS, Roberts DB, Takahashi Y, Raza SM, Su SY, Kupferman ME, DeMonte F, Hanna EY. Mutation status among patients with sinonasal mucosal melanoma and its impact on survival. Br J Cancer. 2017;116(12):1564–71.
101. Colombino M, Lissia A, Franco R, Botti G, Ascierto PA, Manca A, Sini MC, Pisano M, Paliogiannis P, Tanda F, Palmieri G, Cossu A. Unexpected distribution of cKIT and BRAF mutations among southern Italian patients with sinonasal melanoma. Dermatology. 2013;226(3):279–84.
102. Jangard M, Zebary A, Ragnarsson-Olding B, Hansson J. TERT promoter mutations in sinonasal malignant melanoma: a study of 49 cases. Melanoma Res. 2014;25:185–8.
103. Turri-Zanoni M, Medicina D, Lombardi D, et al. Sinonasal mucosal melanoma: molecular profile and therapeutic implications from a series of 32 cases. Head Neck. 2013;35:1066–77.
104. Öztürk Sari Ş, Yilmaz İ, Taşkin OÇ, Narli G, Şen F, Çomoğlu Ş, Firat P, Bİlgİç B, Yilmazbayhan D, Özlük Y, Büyükbabanİ N. BRAF, NRAS, KIT, TERT, GNAQ/GNA11 mutation profile analysis of head and neck mucosal melanomas: a study of 42 cases. Pathology. 2017;49(1):55–61.
105. Wroblewska JP, Mull J, Wu CL, Fujimoto M, Ogawa T, Marszalek A, Hoang MP. SF3B1, NRAS, KIT, and BRAF Mutation; CD117 and cMYC Expression; and Tumoral pigmentation in sinonasal melanomas: an analysis with newly found molecular alterations and some population-based molecular differences. Am J Surg Pathol. 2019;43(2):168–77.
106. Maldonado-Mendoza J, Ramírez-Amador V, Anaya-Saavedra G, Ruíz-García E, Maldonado-Martínez H, Fernández Figueroa E, Meneses-García A. CD117 immunoexpression in oral and sinonasal mucosal melanoma does not correlate with somatic driver mutations in the MAPK pathway. J Oral Pathol Med. 2019;48(5):382–8.
107. Hintzsche JD, Gorden NT, Amato CM, Kim J, Wuensch KE, Robinson SE, et al. Whole-exome sequencing identifies recurrent SF3B1 R625 mutation and comutation of NF1 and KIT in mucosal melanoma. Melanoma Res. 2017;27:189–99.
108. Cosgarea I, Ugurel S, Sucker A, Livingstone E, Zimmer L, Ziemer M, Utikal J, Mohr P, Pfeiffer C, Pföhler C, Hillen U, Horn S, Schadendorf D, Griewank KG, Roesch A. Targeted next generation sequencing of mucosal melanomas identifies frequent NF1 and RAS mutations. Oncotarget. 2017;8(25):40683–92.
109. Lyu J, Wu Y, Li C, Wang R, Song H, Ren G, et al. Mutation scanning of BRAF, NRAS, KIT, and GNAQ/GNA11 in oral mucosal melanoma: a study of 57 cases. J Oral Pathol Med. 2016;45:295–301.
110. Kim HS, Jung M, Kang HN, Kim H, Park CW, Kim SM, Shin SJ, Kim SH, Kim SG, Kim EK, Yun MR, Zheng Z, Chung KY, Greenbowe J, Ali SM, Kim TM, Cho BC. Oncogenic BRAF fusions in mucosal melanomas activate the MAPK pathway and are sensitive to MEK/PI3K inhibition or MEK/CDK4/6 inhibition. Oncogene. 2017;36(23):3334–45.
111. D'Orazio JA. Inherited cancer syndromes in children and young adults. J Pediatr Hematol Oncol. 2010;32(3):195–228.
112. Sohier P, Luscan A, Lloyd A, Ashelford K, Laurendeau I, Briand-Suleau A, Vidaud D, Ortonne N, Pasmant E, Upadhyaya M. Confirmation of mutation landscape of NF1-associated malignant peripheral nerve sheath tumors. Genes Chromosomes Cancer. 2017;56(5):421–6.
113. Lee W, Teckie S, Wiesner T, et al. PRC2 is recurrently inactivated through EED or SUZ12 loss in malignant peripheral nerve sheath tumors. Nat Genet. 2014;46:1227–32.
114. Thway K, Fisher C. Malignant peripheral nerve sheath tumor: pathology and genetics. Ann Diagn Pathol. 2014;18(2):109–16.
115. Yu J, Deshmukh H, Payton JE, et al. Array-based comparative genomic hybridization identifies CDK4 and FOXM1 alterations as independent predictors of survival in malignant peripheral nerve sheath tumor. Clin Cancer Res. 2011;17:1924–34.
116. Hawkins DS, Gupta AA, Rudzinski ER. What is new in the biology and treatment of pediatric rhabdomyosarcoma? Curr Opin Pediatr. 2014;26(1):50–6.
117. Philpott C, Tovell H, Frayling IM, Cooper DN, Upadhyaya M. The NF1 somatic mutational landscape in sporadic human cancers. Hum Genomics. 2017;11(1):13.
118. Abramowicz A, Gos M. Neurofibromin in neurofibromatosis type 1—mutations in NF1gene as a cause of disease. Dev Period Med. 2014;18(3):297–306.
119. Le Guellec S, Soubeyran I, Rochaix P, Filleron T, Neuville A, Hostein I, Coindre JM. CTNNB1 mutation analysis is a useful tool for the diagnosis of desmoid tumors: a study of 260 desmoid tumors and 191 potential morphologic mimics. Mod Pathol. 2012;25(12):1551–8.
120. Penel N, Chibon F, Salas S. Adult desmoid tumors: biology, management and ongoing trials. Curr Opin Oncol. 2017;29(4):268–74.
121. Crago AM, Chmielecki J, Rosenberg M, et al. Near universal detection of alterations in CTNNB1 and wnt pathway regulators in desmoid-type fibromatosis by whole-exome sequencing and genomic analysis. Genes Chromosomes Cancer. 2015;54:606–15.
122. Lasota J, Felisiak-Golabek A, Aly FZ, Wang ZF, Thompson LD. MiettinenM. Nuclear expression and gain-of-function betacatenin mutation in glomangiopericytoma (sinonasal-type hemangiopericytoma): insight into pathogenesis and a diagnostic marker. Mod Pathol. 2015;28(5):715–20.
123. Haller F, Bieg M, Moskalev EA, et al. Recurrent mutations within the amino-terminal region of beta-

catenin are probable key molecular driver events in sinonasal hemangiopericytoma. Am J Pathol. 2015;185:563–71.
124. Jo VY, Fletcher CDM. Nuclear β-catenin expression is frequent in sinonasal hemangiopericytoma and its mimics. Head Neck Pathol. 2017;11(2):119–23.
125. Rooper LM, Huang SC, Antonescu CR, et al. Biphenotypic sinonasal sarcoma: an expanded immunoprofile including consistent nuclear beta-catenin positivity and absence of SOX10 expression. Hum Pathol. 2016;55:44–50.
126. Kakkar A, Rajeshwari M, Sakthivel P, Sharma MC, Sharma SC. Biphenotypic sinonasal sarcoma: a series of six cases with evaluation of role of β-catenin immunohistochemistry in differential diagnosis. Ann Diagn Pathol. 2018;33:6–10.
127. Briski LM, Thomas DG, Patel RM, Lawlor ER, Chugh R, McHugh JB, Lucas DR. Canonical Wnt/β-catenin signaling activation in soft-tissue sarcomas: a comparative study of synovial sarcoma and leiomyosarcoma. Rare Tumors. 2018;10:2036361318813431.
128. Eguchi-Ishimae M, Tezuka M, Kokeguchi T, Nagai K, Moritani K, Yonezawa S, Tauchi H, Tokuda K, Ishida Y, Ishii E, Eguchi M. Early detection of the PAX3-FOXO1 fusion gene in circulating tumor-derived DNA in a case of alveolar rhabdomyosarcoma. Genes Chromosomes Cancer. 2019;58(8):521–9.
129. Thway K, Ng W, Noujaim J, Jones RL, Fisher C. The current status of solitary fibrous tumor: diagnostic features, variants, and genetics. Int J Surg Pathol. 2016;24(4):281–92.
130. Thompson LDR, Fanburg-Smith JC. Update on select benign mesenchymal and meningothelial sinonasal tract lesions. Head Neck Pathol. 2016;10(1):95–108.
131. Akaike K, Kurisaki-Arakawa A, Hara K, et al. Distinct clinicopathological features of NAB2-STAT6 fusion gene variants in solitary fibrous tumor with emphasis on the acquisition of highly malignant potential. Hum Pathol. 2015;46:347–56.
132. Dagrada GP, Spagnuolo RD, Mauro V, et al. Solitary fibrous tumors: loss of chimeric protein expression and genomic instability mark dedifferentiation. Mod Pathol. 2015;28:1074–83.
133. Mohajeri A, Tayebwa J, Collin A, et al. Comprehensive genetic analysis identifies a pathognomonic NAB2/STAT6 fusion gene, nonrandom secondary genomic imbalances, and a characteristic gene expression profile in solitary fibrous tumor. Genes Chromosomes Cancer. 2013;52:873–86.
134. El Beaino M, Araujo DM, Lazar AJ, Lin PP. Synovial sarcoma: advances in diagnosis and treatment identification of new biologic targets to improve multimodal therapy. Ann Surg Oncol. 2017;24(8):2145–54.
135. Clark J, Rocques PJ, Crew AJ, Gill S, Shipley J, Chan AM, Gusterson BA, Cooper CS. Identification of novel genes, SYT and SSX, involved in the t(X;18)(p11.2;q11.2) translocation found in human synovial sarcoma. Nat Genet. 1994;7(4):502–8.
136. Nielsen TO, Poulin NM, Ladanyi M. Synovial sarcoma: recent discoveries as a roadmap to new avenues for therapy. Cancer Discov. 2015;5(2):124–34.
137. Kadoch C, Crabtree GR. Reversible disruption of mSWI/SNF (BAF) complexes by the SS18-SSX oncogenic fusion in synovial sarcoma. Cell. 2013;153:71–85.
138. Saito T, Oda Y, Sakamoto A, Kawaguchi K, Tanaka K, Matsuda S, Tamiya S, Iwamoto Y, Tsuneyoshi M. APC mutations in synovial sarcoma. J Pathol. 2002;196(4):445–9.
139. Subramaniam MM, Calabuig-Fariñas S, Pellin A, Llombart-Bosch A. Mutational analysis of E-cadherin, β-catenin and APC genes in synovial sarcomas. Histopathology. 2010;57(3):482–6.
140. Ng TL, Gown AM, Barry TS, Cheang MC, Chan AK, Turbin DA, et al. Nuclear beta-catenin in mesenchymal tumors. Mod Pathol. 2005;18:68–74.
141. Barham W, Frump AL, Sherrill TP, Garcia CB, Saito-Diaz K, VanSaun MN, et al. Targeting the Wnt pathway in synovial sarcoma models. Cancer Discov. 2013;3:1286–301.
142. Trautmann M, Sievers E, Aretz S, Kindler D, Michels S, Friedrichs N, et al. SS18-SSX fusion protein-induced Wnt/beta-catenin signaling is a therapeutic target in synovial sarcoma. Oncogene. 2013;33:5006–16.
143. Le Loarer F, Laffont S, Lesluyes T, Tirode F, Antonescu C, Baglin AC, Delespaul L, Soubeyran I, Hostein I, Pérot G, Chibon F, Baud J, Le Guellec S, Karanian M, Costes-Martineau V, Castain C, Eimer S, Le Bail B, Wassef M, Coindre JM. Clinicopathologic and molecular features of a series of 41 biphenotypic sinonasal sarcomas expanding their molecular spectrum. Am J Surg Pathol. 2019;43(6):747–54.
144. Andreasen S, Bishop JA, Hellquist H, Hunt J, Kiss K, Rinaldo A, et al. Biphenotypic sinonasal sarcoma: demographics, clinicopathological characteristics, molecular features, and prognosis of a recently described entity. Virchows Arch. 2018;473(5):615–26.
145. Yasuda T, Perry KD, Nelson M, et al. Alveolar rhabdomyosarcoma of the head and neck region in older adults: genetic characterization and a review of the literature. Hum Pathol. 2009;40:341–8.
146. Mosquera JM, Sboner A, Zhang L, Kitabayashi N, Chen CL, Sung YS, Wexler LH, LaQuaglia MP, Edelman M, Sreekantaiah C, Rubin MA, Antonescu CR. Recurrent NCOA2 gene rearrangements in congenital/infantile spindle cell rhabdomyosarcoma. Genes Chromosomes Cancer. 2013;52:538–50.
147. Reichek JL, Duan F, Smith LM, et al. Genomic and clinical analysis of amplification of the 13q31 chromosomal region in alveolar rhabdomyosarcoma: a report from the Children's Oncology Group. Clin Cancer Res. 2011;17:1463–73.
148. Van Gaal JC, Flucke UE, Roeffen MH, et al. Anaplastic lymphoma kinase aberrations in rhabdomyosarcoma: clinical and prognostic implications. J Clin Oncol. 2012;30:308–15.

Clinical Aspects and Surgical Treatment

Giandomenico Maggiore, Maria Silvia Lazio, and Oreste Gallo

Clinical Aspects

Benign Tumors

Many benign masses are slow-growing tumors with non-specific symptoms probably due to an adaptation on the part of patients. Unilateral nasal obstruction is the most common symptom in patients with either benign or malignant tumors of the sinonasal tract associated with nasal discharge, epistaxis, facial pain, and headache [1, 2]. Although epistaxis is generally associated with malignant disease, it may also be a presenting symptom of a benign tumor due to the crusting and small areas of mucositis and mucosal excoriation. It is the most common presenting symptom in vascular benign tumors such as the juvenile nasopharyngeal angiofibroma (Fig. 1) and lobular capillary hemangioma [3]. The pain experienced is rarely severe and may be the result of ostial obstruction. A deep retro orbital pain and occipital, frontal, and bitemporal headache can be observed in the schwannomas with extension into the sphenoid sinus [4]. The endoscopic examination of the nasal cavity is necessary to evaluate the borders, the features, and the extent of the lesion. In many cases, the tumors appear macroscopically like specific masses such as inverted papilloma that at the endoscopic examination is represented like a polypoid lesion with a papillary appearance that protrudes from the middle meatus; the schwannomas like a gelatinous or cystic, well-encapsulated masses [4]; or osteomas that appear as hard, white, and multilobulated masses. The preoperative diagnostic workup includes imaging studies. If a diagnosis cannot be established by imaging studies, then the endoscopic biopsy is indicated.

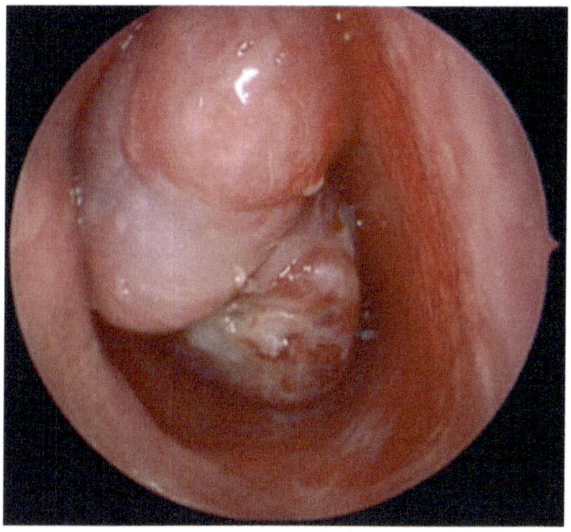

Fig. 1 Juvenile nasopharyngeal angiofibroma

G. Maggiore (✉) · M. S. Lazio · O. Gallo
Clinic of Otolaryngology, Head and Neck Surgery, Department of Surgery and Translational Medicine, Careggi University Hospital, Florence, Italy
e-mail: oreste.gallo@unifi.it

A. Franchi (ed.), *Pathology of Sinonasal Tumors and Tumor-Like Lesions*,
https://doi.org/10.1007/978-3-030-29848-7_3

Malignant Tumors

Sinonasal malignancies are a diverse group of uncommon tumors that represent challenging entities to treat. Diagnostic evaluation and workup should be performed by a multidisciplinary team with involvement of an otolaryngologist—head and neck surgeon, neurosurgeon, medical and radiation oncologists, neuroradiologist, and pathologist. These tumors are rare diseases that arise from a variety of tissues of origin, defined as epithelial or non-epithelial. The most frequent tumors have epithelial origin and poor prognosis, such as squamous cell carcinoma, intestinal-type adenocarcinoma (ITAC) (Fig. 2), undifferentiated carcinoma, and neuroendocrine carcinoma. It is not uncommon that these tumors are asymptomatic or presenting with nonspecific symptoms in their early stages such as nasal discharge and epistaxis. Pain, paraesthesia or anesthesia, swelling of the palate or face, and loosening of the teeth may be the presenting symptoms. The latter complaints may be present when an adenoid cystic carcinoma, the most frequent malignant salivary gland-type tumor of the sinonasal tract, subsisted and are due to the typical high propensity for perineural spread (e.g., trigeminal branches) and bony invasion. This feature can lead to skull base involvement and intracranial extension, including cavernous sinus and anterior and middle cranial fossa. The impairment or the loss of smell may be a clinical symptom of the esthesioneuroblastoma (Fig. 3), although it is not common as might be expected, in part because olfaction is preserved on the contralateral side in some tumors and in part because some patients do not report the gradual loss [5]. Endoscopic examination is necessary and generally reveals a mass within the nasal cavity. High-resolution preoperative imaging is used to determine the extent of disease, the possibility to resect the lesion, and the surgical approach [6]. A combination of computed tomography (CT) and magnetic resonance imaging (MRI) is now established as the optimum assessment; they can be used for computer-aided surgery and preoperative planning. When clinical and radiological information have been obtained, the endoscopic-assisted biopsy of the sinonasal lesion is mandatory in order to clearly identify the specific histotype of cancer that associated with the molecular pattern of the tumor can guide the type of treatment to be administered. If the risk of massive bleeding subsists, then the biopsy should be carried out under general anesthesia.

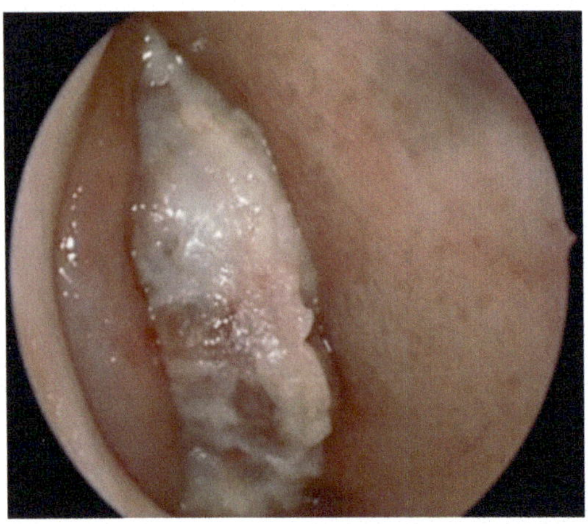

Fig. 2 Intestinal-type adenocarcinoma (ITAC)

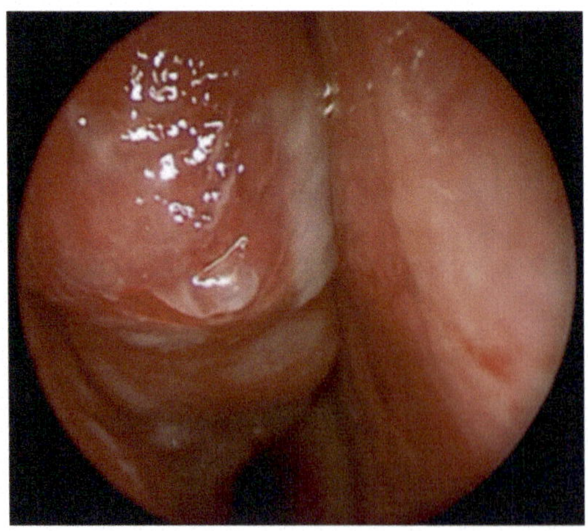

Fig. 3 Esthesioneuroblastoma

Surgical Treatment

Definitive treatment of paranasal sinus tumors is complex, and it typically requires multidisciplinary expertise with involvement of an otolaryngologist-head and neck surgeon, neurosurgeon, medical and radiation oncologists, neuroradiologist, and pathologist, and the selected surgical approach should be planned and executed to accomplish a specific goal. With small tumors, the goal should be identifying the attachment site and obtaining negative margins around this area. Larger tumors tend to have an element of expansive remodeling rather than frank erosion. The advances in endoscopy have changed the management of sinonasal and skull base lesions. Many masses that traditionally required open approaches are now amenable to purely endoscopic endonasal resection, providing less invasive surgery with lower morbidity but with comparable oncologic outcomes in terms of survival rates [7].

Indications for an endoscopic endonasal approach (EEA) have been extended from 2003 to the last years. In fact, if at the beginning the infiltration of the external bony boundaries of the ethmoid, such as lamina papyracea, cribriform plate, and ethmoid roof, represented contraindications for this treatment, today also selected intradural lesions have been treated. An EEA is contraindicated when the lateral extension over the orbit roof or extensive involvement of the brain is present. The approach consists of different steps: the operation is usually started by debulking of the tumor to more clearly defining the site of origin of the lesion (Fig. 4); subperiosteal dissection of the nasoethmoidal–sphenoidal complex is performed and the surgical specimen is removed either transnasally or transorally. During this time, multiple biopsy specimens from surgical margins are routinely examined by frozen sections in order to map the negative surgical field; the lamina papyracea, the posterior two-thirds of the nasal septum, and the ethmoid roof including the cribriform plate need to be removed when the lesion involves their mucosal covering; and the resection of the dura, olfactory bulb, or periorbita is performed when these structures are radiological or intraoperative suspected or with an olfactory neuroblastoma diagnosis because of its high propensity to spread along olfactory phyla (Fig. 5). A massive infiltration of the dura, its involvement in close proximity to the lamina papyracea (which requires an extensive dural resection far lateral over the orbital roof(s)), or an extensive brain contact/involvement represents the indications

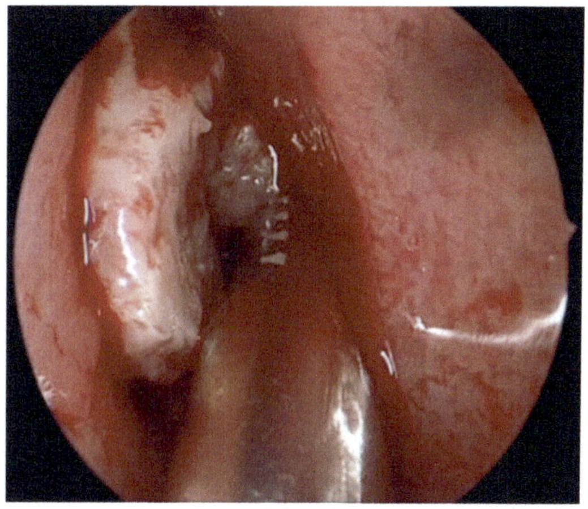

Fig. 4 Sinonasal lesion debulking

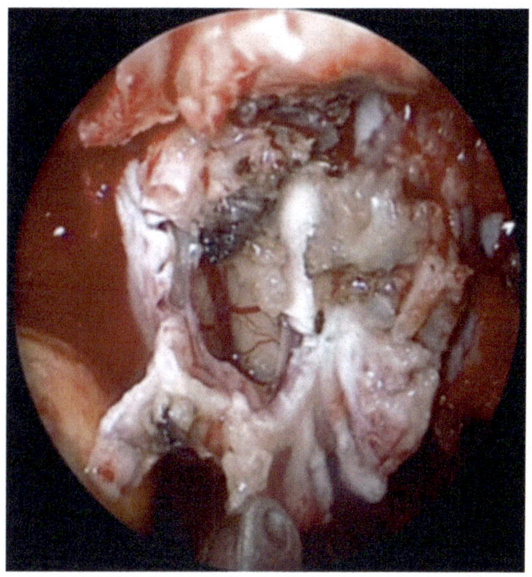

Fig. 5 Resection of the dura and olfactory bulb

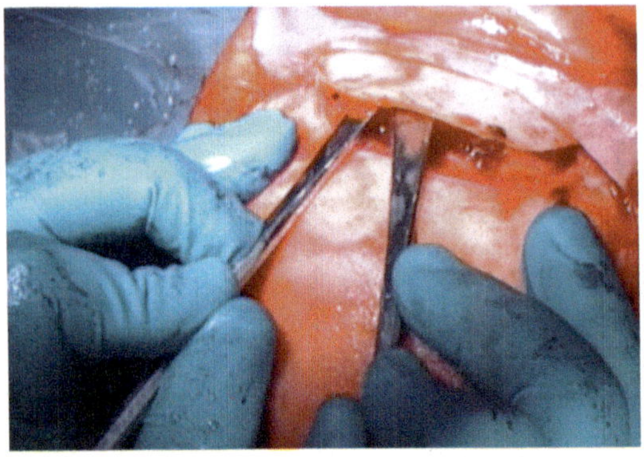

Fig. 6 Transcranial surgical phase

for a combined cranioendoscopic approach (CEA). In this case, a double surgical team (neurosurgical and ear, nose, and throat (ENT)) is required, and surgery consists of an endoscopic phase and a transcranial one (Fig. 6). It begins with the endoscopic debulking of the intranasal portion of the lesion, the osteotomies of the nasal septum, and the dissection of the lamina papyracea from the periorbita on both sides. The floor, the anterior wall, and the intersinusal septum of the sphenoid sinus are then resected; osteotomy is performed along the superior margin of the frontal sinus; a bony volet including the anterior wall of the frontal sinus and the superomedial contour of the orbits is removed after preplating, and the posterior wall of the frontal sinus is drilled out; the exposed dura is incised and the orbital roof to check the intradural extension of the lesion, the superior part of the frontoethmoidal sphenoidal bony complex is isolated; at this stage, the neurosurgical and otolaryngological teams work in parallel in order to control all the margins of the ethmoidal box during its resection. The skull base reconstruction is generally managed with an intradural graft of pericranium or temporal fascia and an extradural pedicle pericranial flap with an endoscopic guide and control. Contraindications for CEA are represented by an invasion of the following structures: palatal, lacrimal sac, bony walls of the maxillary sinus (except of the medial wall), posterior wall of the sphenoid sinus, nasal pyramid, or an extension into the pterygopalatine or infratemporal fossa [8–10] (Tables 1 and 2).

Considering benign sinonasal masses, surgical removal should be contemplated when they are causing symptoms or pending complications or when the suspicion of malignancy exists. Even though most benign tumors of the sinonasal tract can now be managed through an endoscopic approach, certain situations still require an external or a combined procedure. Osteomas for examples are slow-growing lesions, and a general consensus in the literature advocates for a "wait and see" policy for any lesion that is asymptomatic, does not encroach upon critical structures such as the optic nerve, and does not extensively invade the anterior skull base or the orbit. If a surgical treatment is required, then cavitation is a surgical trick that helps resect even large osteomas through the nose with an endoscopic approach [9, 10]. Although inverted papilloma is a benign tumor (Fig. 7), it presents a local aggression which makes necessary the operation with the aim to dissect the involved mucosa along the subperiosteal plane and to drill the underlying bone. The extension of the operation is tailored to defined characteristics of the lesions such as the site and the area of mucosa involved [11]. Surgery is also considered the mainstay in the management of juvenile angiofibroma (Fig. 8), following the preoperative embolization which is commonly performed 48 h before surgery [12]. Despite the surgery techniques have changed over time in order to give a curative solution and reduce surgical morbidity and mortality, the prognosis for patients with this kind of tumors remains poor.

Table 1 Surgery indications and contraindications

Endoscopic endonasal approach	Cranioendoscopic approach	Multiportal approaches	Open approach
Indications:	**Indications:**	**Indications:**	**Indications:**
• Advanced lesions in contact with or minimally infiltrating in dura	• Sinonasal lesions with endonasal and endocranial extension requiring a dural resection extending over the orbital roof(s)	• Tumors with anterior extension:	• Soft tissue or skin involvement of the face or forehead
• Selected intradural lesions without brain infiltration		– Nasal spine (sublabial corridor)	• Frontal sinus bone involvement
		– Nasal bone and anterior portion of medial orbital wall and/or lacrimal sac (transorbital corridor)	• Palate involvement • Dural involvement lateral to the orbit
Contraindications:	**Contraindications:**		
• Lateral extension over the orbital roof	• Lacrimal sac involvement		• Internal carotid artery encasement
• Extensive involvement of the brain	• Involvement of the orbital content		• Involvement of the mandible
• Extensive lacrimal pathway infiltration	• Involvement of the bony walls of the maxillary sinus with the exception of the medial one		• Significant orbital involvement or invasion into extraocular muscles and/or optic nerve
• Involvement of the anterior wall and lateral portion of the frontal sinus	• Extension into the pterygopalatine or infratemporal fossa		
• Infiltrating of the bony walls of the maxillary sinus with the exception of the medial one	• Involvement of the posterior wall of the sphenoid sinus		• Invasion into the cavernous sinus
	• Extension to the hard palate		
• Infiltration of the hard palate	• Nasal pyramid involvement		
• Erosion of the nasal bone			

Table 2 Type of treatment according to cancer extension

T1	T2	T3	T4
Surgery	Surgery +/− Radiotherapy	Surgery + (Chemo)radiotherapy	(Chemo)radiotherapy +/− Surgery + (Chemo)radiotherapy

Surgery:

- Endonasal endoscopic resection (EER)
- Endoscopic resection with transnasal craniectomy (ERTC)
- Cranio-endoscopic resection (CER)
- Multiportal approaches (transorbital, sublabial)

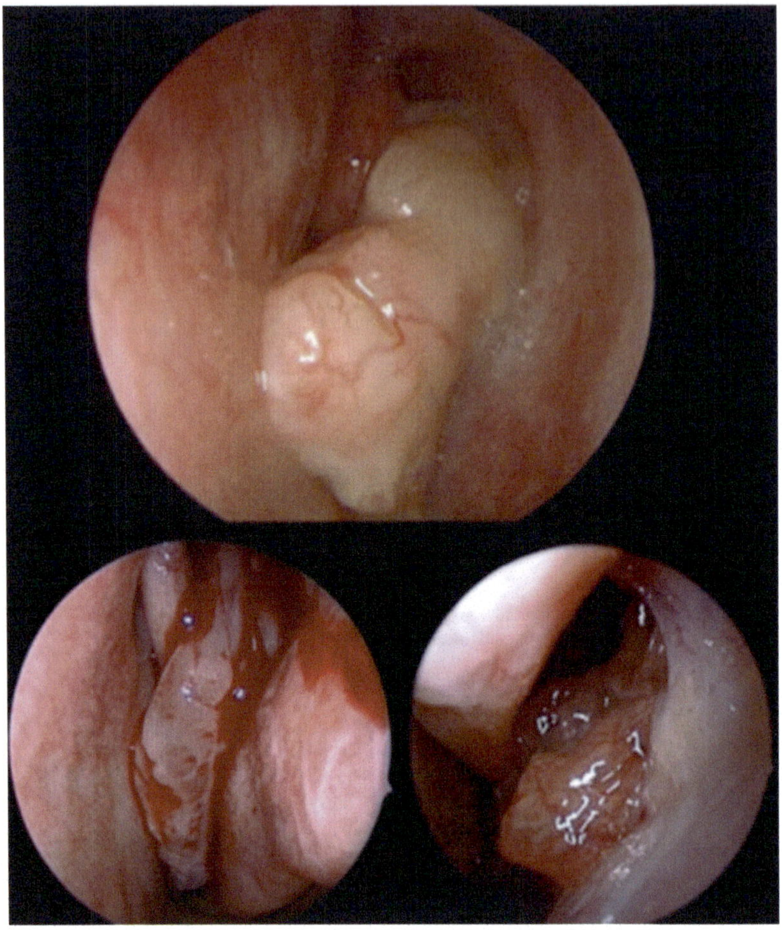

Fig. 7 Inverted papilloma

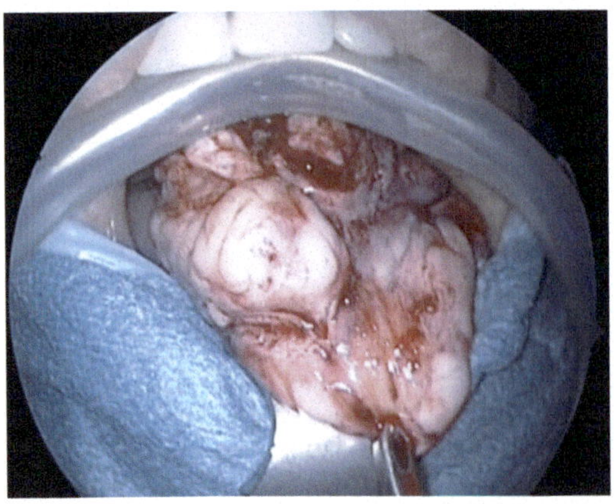

Fig. 8 Transoral exeresis of juvenile nasopharyngeal angiofibroma

Skull Base Reconstruction

After the surgical approach to remove masses that involve the anterior cranial fossa, there are different techniques and materials available for reconstruction of the skull base. The duraplasty with a "three-layer" technique is largely used, and it is generally performed using autologous material: fascia lata for the intracranial intradural and extradural layers (underlay) and nasal mucoperiosteum obtained from the contralateral fossa for the extracranial layer (overlay) stabilized with fibrin glue (Fig. 9). This technique proposed by Nicolai et al. in 2008 [13, 14] is a safe, effective, and always available reconstructive

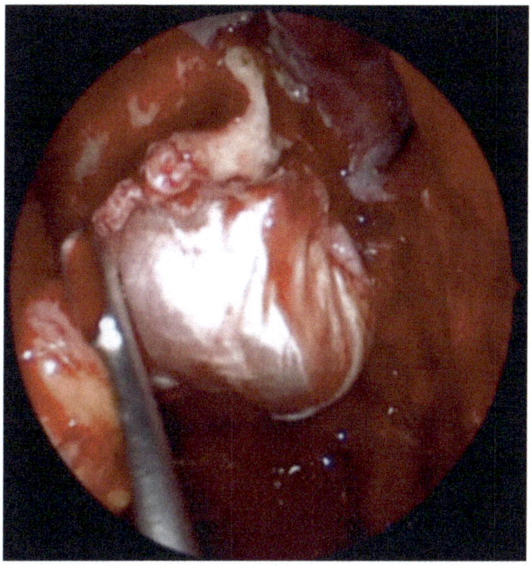

Fig. 9 Duraplasty with a "three-layer" technique

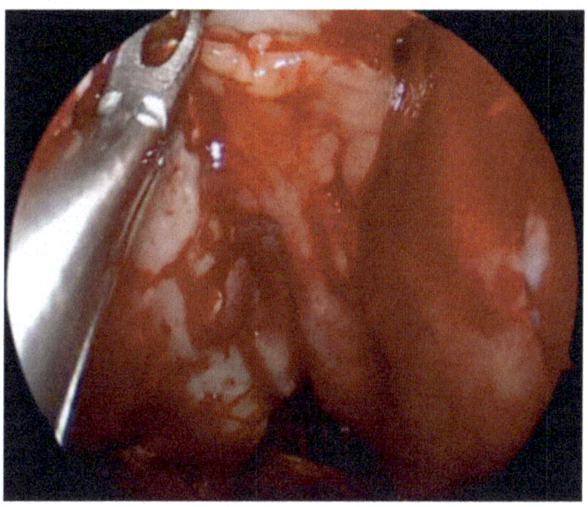

Fig. 10 Nasoseptal flap

option for large defects of the anterior skull base with acceptable complication rate and donor site morbidity [15]. Vascularized local pedicled flaps, such as the nasoseptal flap, could be used if the tumor involvement does not interest these structures (Fig. 10).

Surgical Management of the Neck and Orbit

Elective treatment of the neck lymph nodes is not routinely performed in sinonasal malignances because the risk of regional metastases is low for

Table 3 Type of treatment according to Kadish staging system

Kadish A	Kadish B	Kadish C–D
Surgery	Surgery + (Chemo) radiotherapy	(Chemo) radiotherapy + Surgery + (Chemo) radiotherapy

Lund V, Stammberger H, Nicolai P, et al. *European position paper on endoscopic management of tumours of the nose and paranasal sinuses and skull base. Rhinology 2010; Suppl 22:30–31*

the early stage tumors or in histological type such as adenocarcinoma. However, for a locally advanced lesion (T3–T4) squamous cell carcinoma or in esthesioneuroblastoma with intracranial disease at presentation (Kadish C), concomitant neck dissection and/or postoperative radiotherapy should be considered because of the increment frequency of cervical lymph node metastases [16] (Table 3). Management of orbital disease is still discussed, and orbital invasion has been shown to be an independent prognostic factor. It is determinant in order to carry out an entirely endoscopic endonasal approach [13, 17]. To identify the involvement of this structure, a preoperative accurate imaging studies with CT and MRI is required associated with the frozen section during the surgical procedures to prove if the orbit is free from disease. However, eye-sparing protocols have been developed, and radiation or chemotherapy may be employed when the tumor does not violate the periorbita [18].

Complications

Any surgical procedure to approach the skull base malignancies has the potential to cause complications. These could be identified with the following impairments: systemic, central nervous system, orbital, vascular, and skull base defects after duraplasty. In particular, central nervous system complications such as brain edema, intracranial abscess, and hematoma result in neurological symptoms, and they should be managed in cooperation with the neurosurgeon. Cerebrospinal fluid leak is one of the most common complications

(<5%) [12, 16], and it can be resolved with an endoscopic revision of the duraplasty or with a lumbar drainage placement. After surgical procedures with craniotomy, a CT scan is generally required in order to evaluate the presence of pneumocephalus and its degree when it subsists to exclude brain compression. Nowadays, expanded endonasal endoscopic approaches are associated with lower morbidity rather than traditional open craniofacial ones (9–11% vs. 30%) [13, 17, 19].

Importance of Frozen Section Analysis in Surgical Resection of Sinonasal Malignancies

The histology of the primary tumor associated with its intracranial extent and the status of surgical margins represent the independent predictors of recurrence-free survival, overall survival, and disease-specific survival. The incidence of positive tumor margins is reported to be similar in patients with advanced anterior skull base disease undergoing either endoscopic resection or traditional craniofacial resection [20]. Although the margins to visible tumor distance has not been defined for most anterior skull base malignancies, these should be taken with sufficient distance from the tumor preserving as much structure as possible. To ensure the optimum oncological results, the primary tumor must be completely removed and margins checked by frozen section to obtain mucosa free from disease [21].

Outcomes

Despite the rarity of the sinonasal malignancies, the knowledge about these pathologies was expanded during the last years. The 5-year overall survival varies as a function of stage, histological type, and treatment options. Among the malignant lesions, histological types such as squamous cell carcinoma, adenocarcinoma, olfactory neuroblastoma, and adenoid cystic carcinoma registered better outcomes if well treated and when at a lower stage at the presentation. For the abovementioned lesions, when the use of the endoscopic techniques finds indications, it demonstrated an improvement of the 5-year disease-specific survival of 91% compared with 59% of the cranioendoscopic approach [13]. On the one hand, this kind of treatment requires experienced hands and selected patients for the best oncological outcomes in relation to specific histologies and should be associated with adjuvant therapy when it is indicated. On the other hand, poor prognostic lesions such as mucosal melanoma or undifferentiated sinonasal carcinoma need biological studies to evaluate the possibility to use immunological therapy or protocol of neoadjuvant treatment with chemotherapy in association or not with the radiation therapy. The multimodality treatment is required to reduce the pathological mass and when it is feasible to give an adequate radical surgery resection in a second step.

Conclusions

Sinonasal tumors and tumorlike lesions are rare entities with a wide variety of histopathologic diagnoses. The histological, immunohistochemical, and molecular studies are needed in order to achieve the best protocol treatment. Surgery has an important role for the management of both benign and malignant lesions. The different approach is determined by many factors such as stage, localization, histology, and morbidity of the patient. Postoperative radiation therapy is indicated in the majority of malignant lesions, and systemic chemotherapy could be used as neoadjuvant therapy in certain protocols in order to reduce the mass of the tumor before surgery or associated with RT in the postoperative setting. Although the optimal strategy is yet to be determined, individualized treatment that evaluates the stage of tumor, patient comorbidities, and histologic characteristics can achieve better survival.

References

1. Melroy CT, Senior BA. Benign sinonasal neoplasms: a focus on inverting papilloma. Otolaryngol Clin N Am. 2006;39(3):601–17.
2. Tufano RP, Thaler ER, Lanza DC, et al. Endoscopic management of sinonasal inverted papilloma. Am J Rhinol. 1999;13(6):423–6.

3. Gullane PJ, Davidson J, O'Dwyer T, et al. Juvenile angiofibroma: a review of the literature and a case series report. Laryngoscope. 1992;102:928–33.
4. Fanburg-Smith JC, Thompson LDR. Benign soft tissue tumors. In: Barnes L, Eveson JW, Reichart P, et al., editors. Pathology and genetics of head and neck tumours. Lyon: IARC Press; 2005.
5. Maggiore G, Lazio MS, Gallo O. Treatment of pediatric esthesioneuroblastoma with smell preservation. Auris Nasus Larynx. 2018;45(5):1107–12.
6. Blitz AM, Choudhri AF, Chonka ZD, et al. Anatomic considerations, nomenclature, and advanced cross-sectional imaging techniques for visualization of the cranial nerve segments by MR imaging. Neuroimaging Clin N Am. 2014;24:1–15.
7. Castelnuovo P, Lepera D, Turri-Zanoni M, et al. Quality of life following endoscopic endonasal resection of anterior skull base cancers. J Neurosurg. 2013;119(6):1401–9.
8. Nicolai P, Castelnuovo P, Lombardi D, et al. Role of endoscopic surgery in the management of selected malignant epithelial neoplasms of the naso-ethmoidal complex. Head Neck. 2007;29:1075–82.
9. Castelnuovo P, Battaglia P, Locatelli D, et al. Endonasal micro-endoscopic treatment of the malignant tumors of paranasal sinuses and anterior skull base. Oper Tech Otolayngol Head Neck Surg. 2006;17:152–67.
10. Bignami M, Dallan I, Terranova P, et al. Frontal sinus osteomas: the window of endonasal endoscopic approach. Rhinology. 2007;45:315–20.
11. Lombardi D, Tomenzoli D, Buttà L, et al. Limitations and complications of endoscopic surgery for treatment for sinonasal inverted papilloma: a reassessment after 212 cases. Head Neck. 2011;33:1154–61.
12. Robertson GH, Biller H, Sessions DG, et al. Presurgical internal maxillary artery embolization in juvenile angiofibroma. Laryngoscope. 1972;82:1524–32.
13. Nicolai P, Battaglia P, Bignami M, et al. Endoscopic surgery for malignant tumors of the sinonasal tract and adjacent skull base: a 10-year experience. Am J Rhinol. 2008;22(3):308–16.
14. Villaret AB, Yakirevitch A, Bizzoni A, et al. Endoscopic transnasal craniectomy in the management of selected sinonasal malignancies. Am J Rhinol Allergy. 2010;24(1):60–5.
15. Mattavelli D, Schreiber A, Bolzoni Villaret A, et al. Complications and donor site morbidity of 3-layer reconstruction with iliotibial tract of the anterior skull base: retrospective analysis of 186 patients. Head Neck. 2017;40:63–9.
16. Lund VJ, Stammberger H, Nicolai P, et al. European position paper on endoscopic management of tumours of the nose, paranasal sinuses and skull base. Rhinology Suppl. 2010;22:1–143.
17. Hanna E, DeMonte F, Ibrahim S, et al. Endoscopic resection of sinonasal cancers with and without craniotomy: oncologic results. Arch Otolaryngol Head Neck Surg. 2009;135:1219–24.
18. Perry C, Levine PA, Williamson BR, et al. Preservation of the eye in paranasal sinus cancer surgery. Arch Otolaryngol Head Neck Surg. 1988;114:632–4.
19. Ganly I, Patel SG, Singh B, et al. Craniofacial resection for malignant paranasal sinus tumors: report of an international collaborative study. Head Neck. 2005;27:575–84.
20. Roxbury CR, Ishii M, Richmon JD, et al. Endonasal endoscopic surgery in the management of sinonasal and anterior skull base malignancies. Head Neck Pathol. 2016;10(1):13–22.
21. Lund VJ, Clarke PM, Swift AC, et al. Nose and paranasal sinus tumours. UK National Multidisciplinary Guidelines. J Laryngol Otol. 2016;130(Suppl. S2):S111–8.

Radiotherapy and Medical Treatment

Ester Orlandi, Domenico Romanello, Donata Galbiati, and Lisa Licitra

Introduction

Sinonasal cancers (SNC) are rare diseases (<1 case/100,000 annually) [1] comprising a highly heterogeneity of histologies. Due to the rarity and variety of histological types, there is paucity of data regarding their optimal management. Furthermore, the anatomy of the sinonasal region, close to important structures, adds complexity to the treatment planning.

A multidisciplinary approach in SNC is essential and is generally based in complete surgical resection with postoperative radiotherapy (RT) [2]. However, despite the use of sophisticated surgical approaches and new radiation techniques [3–5], the prognosis of patients with locally advanced SNC remains generally dismal [6]. In some selected histotypes, chemotherapy is considered within multimodal treatment with curative purposes. While for advanced cancers not amenable to local treatment or in metastatic patients, systemic treatment has a palliative intent.

The following chapter goes through the evidences available in the literature on the role of systemic treatment (chemotherapy and targeted therapy) and RT in the management of SNCs.

Radiotherapy

As for the other head and neck cancers, RT is a cornerstone in the treatment of this pathology, either in a definitive setting or in a postoperative one, with a role in recurrent disease as well.

For T1–T2 N0, after radical surgery, RT is recommended when risk factors are present, such as positive or close margins, perineural invasion (PNI), vascular emboli, or in case of unfavorable histologies [7], such as adenoid cystic carcinoma (ACC) [8].

For resectable T3–T4 N0 and N+, surgery followed by RT is the gold standard [9–12]. Elective ipsilateral neck RT is recommended for T3–T4 squamocellular carcinomas (SCC): Le et al. reported a 12% lymph node relapse at 5 years in a cohort of 97 patients with maxillary sinus tumors, 56 of whom had surgery first and 41 had

Domenico Romanello and Donata Galbiati contributed equally to this work.

E. Orlandi (✉) · D. Romanello
Radiotherapy 2 Unit, Fondazione IRCCS Istituto Nazionale dei Tumori, Milan, Italy
e-mail: ester.orlandi@istitutotumori.mi.it; domenico.romanello@istitutotumori.mi.it

D. Galbiati
Head and Neck Medical Oncology Unit, Fondazione IRCCS IstitutoTumori, Milan, Italy

L. Licitra
Head and Neck Medical Oncology Unit, Fondazione IRCCS IstitutoTumori, Milan, Italy

University of Milan, Milan, Italy
e-mail: Lisa.Licitra@istitutotumori.mi.it

A. Franchi (ed.), *Pathology of Sinonasal Tumors and Tumor-Like Lesions*,
https://doi.org/10.1007/978-3-030-29848-7_4

pre-op or definitive RT; none of the patient receiving RT had nodal recurrence [13]. Preoperative RT, however, could have a negative impact on recurrence-free survival (RFS), probably because it is more difficult to clearly define the extent of the resection margin in irradiated patients [14].

In unresectable or inoperable diseases, RT or chemoradiotherapy (CRT) is the treatment of choice [15, 16]. A radiation dose of more than 65 Gy appears to be the only significant prognostic factor predicting local control (LC) and overall survival (OS) [16]. New techniques of intensity-modulated RT (IMRT), such as volumetric-modulated arc therapy (VMAT), could overcome the augment of toxicity related to the dose escalation, especially when large, complex volumes—even with nodal involvement—have to be irradiated [17].

RT Techniques, Volumes, and Doses

Three-Dimensional Conformal RT (3D CRT)

Due to the proximity of critical structures (brain, optical chiasm, optical nerves, etc.) RT for the treatment of SNCs has always been characterized by significant complications. With conventional techniques, it has been reported 30% unilateral and 10% bilateral blindness [8, 9, 18]. 3D CRT gave the important contribution to reduce the dose to the organs at risk (OARs) without jeopardizing the result of the treatment [19–21]. With 3D CRT, dose conformality is guaranteed by a "forward planned" system, in which beam angles and modulators are manually optimized. This technique includes unmodulated arc therapy as well.

IMRT

During the last years, IMRT has become state of the art. By delivering nonuniform photon fluency from any given position to the treatment beam, IMRT permits a very precise isodose shaping. This measure, with the aid of image-guided radiation therapy (IGRT) which uses a precise targeting system before each RT fraction, allows the generation of steep gradients between high- and low-dose regions. The result is the concentration of the dose at the target, sparing the various close sensitive anatomic structures. Using multi-leaf collimators, beam intensity is modulated over the radiation field, and an "inverse planned" system is used to define the beam angles and the fluency map, given the dose to the target and the constraints to the OARs. A variant of IMRT, VMAT, uses modulated arcs to improve the speed of treatment delivery.

Chen et al. reported, among 127 patients, important reduction of severe toxicities (≥ Grade 3) among the 1960s, 1970s, 1980s, 1990s, and 2000s, with no significant difference in 5-year OS rates [22].

Hadron Therapy

Protons and carbon ions are heavily charged particles that penetrate specific distances, which are dependent on their energy. They share the advantage of lacking in exit doses, concentrating most of their energy at the end of their range in a physic phenomenon known as the Bragg Peak. The energy of these particles can be modified by using a variety of filters, so that the Bragg Peak can be eventually widened: this allows a more precise conformation of dose than it is possible with photons, and thus it permits to dose-escalate. Mock et al. performed a dosimetric comparison involving five patients, whose proton plans were compared with conventional RT, 3D CRT, and IMRT; on the one hand, proton therapy reduced the dose to OARs up to 65% and to 62% compared with 3D CRT and IMRT, respectively; on the other hand, photon plans resulted in greater volumes of irradiated nontarget tissues at the 10–70% dose level compared with corresponding proton plans [23].

Furthermore, having a high linear energy transfer (LET), protons and carbon ions can give an increased biologically effective dose compared to photons, characterized by a low LET

[24]: this suggests an interesting role in the treatment of unresectable/inoperable diseases. Truong et al. retrospectively analyzed 20 patients treated with proton therapy between 1991 and 2005; with a median prescription dose of 76 Gy (RBE) and a median follow-up of 27 months, the 2-year local, regional, and freedom from distant metastases rates were 86%, 86%, and 50%, respectively [25]. In a meta-analysis by Patel et al., patients undergoing hadron therapy, either in definitive or adjuvant setting, showed a higher 5-year disease-free survival (DFS) than those who underwent IMRT (relative risk 1.44, 95% CI 1.01–2.05, $p = 0.045$); LC as well appeared to be higher ($p = 0.0011$). In spite of these encouraging data, hadron therapy seems to be affected by a higher neurological toxicity rate ($p = 0.0002$) than IMRT, although this could be as well a selection bias (most difficult cases were redirected to hadron therapy centers) [22]. Miyawaki reported a 17% and a 64% incidence of MRI-detected radiation-induced brain changes in patients treated with protons and carbon ions, respectively. Though the median follow-up—33 months—is limited, the incidence of radiation-induced brain changes appears to be increasing with time and to be worsening in patients treated with carbon ions compared with those treated with protons [26].

In definitive cases, the gross tumor volume (GTV) is represented by the macroscopic disease on TC/MRI images; the clinical target volume (CTV) comprehends the GTV and the areas at risk of subclinical microscopic disease. The high-risk CTV (HDCTV) is GTV plus a margin of 0.5–1.0 cm; it does not include intact bone or uninvolved cranial nerves, but in case of macroscopic involvement of bony structures that do not offer a resistance to the spread of the disease (e.g., orbit, base of skull, masticator, or parapharyngeal spaces), the entire compartment is to be added to HDCTV [27]. Involved nodes should be part of HDCTV as well. An intermediate risk CTV (IDCTV) is to be contoured when PNI is described, it is larger than HDCTV, and it includes the base of skull and foramina. Low-risk CTV (LDCTV) comprehends elective nodes (levels IB, II, III) and the lateral retropharyngeal nodes [13, 28, 29]. HDCTV should receive 66–70 Gy/2 Gy per fraction, IDCTV 60 Gy/2 Gy per fraction, and LDCTV 50–54 Gy/2 Gy per fraction. Planning treatment volume (PTV) is a volume that takes into account any eventual setup error: it is obtained by adding a 3–5 mm to CTV, depending on image guidance (portal images, cone beam CT, etc.).

In postoperative cases, HDCTV is made of the edges of resection plus variable margins edited on bases of the compartmental criteria described above, including every ECE+ nodes. If PNI and/or ECE-positive nodes are described, IDCTV should include these nodes and the base of the skull with the foramina. LDCTV comprehends elective nodes. HDCTV should receive 66 Gy/2 Gy per fraction, IDCTV 60 Gy/2 Gy per fraction, and LDCTV 50–54 Gy/2 Gy per fraction [27].

RT for Recurrent Disease

Most of recurrences are in the previous treatment field [30, 31]. On the one hand, no universal consensus is established on the proper treatment of recurrent SNCs, and only 20% of these patients are candidate to surgery: that is, due to the proximity of critical structures, either involved by the disease or responsible for iatrogenic dysfunctions. Chemotherapy, on the other hand, is limited by short-lasting effects and is reserved for palliative purposes. As for re-irradiation, Lagendijk et al. reported 3-year OS rate of 10–20% and LCR of 20–30% [32]; Spencer et al. reported better OS and LC by adding chemotherapy to re-irradiation, even though this is related to higher severe toxicity rate [33, 34]. Recurrences seem to be more radio-resistant than the primitive cancer, because of the effects the radiation has on the micro-environment, especially on blood vessels. Stereotactic RT (SRT) appears to be an interesting technique to perform re-irradiation: it is characterized by one or a few—less than five—fractions with a higher dose per fraction than conventional fractionation; it can be delivered either with a linear accelerator (LINAC) or a specific machine, such as the Cyberknife. Ozyigit et al. retrospectively analyzed 27 SNC patients including recurrent patients treated with Cyberknife, most of whom (44%) had squamocellular carcinoma (SCC) [35]. With a median dose to the target of 31 Gy (range, 15–37.5 Gy) and a median of 5 fractions (range, 3–5 fractions), after a median follow-up of 21.4 months (range, 3–59 months), 76% of the patients did not show signs of local relapse. Survival rates of 1 and 2 years for the entire group were 95.2% and 77.1%, respectively. Brain necrosis, visual disorders, and bone necrosis were observed in two patients each. Iwata et al. reported a series of 51 recurrent nasal or paranasal carcinomas, especially SCC, treated with Cyberknife in 3–5 fractions [36]. With a median previous dose of 60 Gy in conventional fractionation and a median follow-up of 21 months (range, 12–52) the 1-year OS was 67%, and the 1-year LC was 62%. No statistically significant difference in outcome was observed, concerning histology (SCC vs. non-SCC), tumor volume (≥ vs. <20 mL), and the time from previous RT (≥ vs. <1 year). Severe toxicity (≥ Grade 3) was reported in 23%.

Toxicity

In retrospective studies analyzing postoperative conventional or 3D CRT, acute toxicity was related to proximity of important structures, especially the eyes and the brain, and these side effects appear not to occur with IMRT [3, 19, 37–39]. This is because IMRT allows to better observe dose constraints without jeopardizing the target coverage.

RT complications may be either acute or late; the former includes mucositis, skin erythema, nasal dryness, and xerostomia; the latter comprehends xerostomia, chronic keratitis and iritis, cataracts, blindness, osteoradionecrosis, brain necrosis, and radiation-induced hypopituitarism.

As regards acute toxicity, the damage to the lachrymal gland and the cornea is dose-dependent: Wiegner reported a 78% of risk of acute toxicity with a mean dose of 30 Gy to the cornea and an 86% incidence of toxicity with a median dose of 25.6 Gy to the lachrymal gland [39]. On the one hand, ocular toxicity is more severe with conventional RT, with several older studies reporting blindness, retinopathy, and optic neuropathy up to 47% of patients [40–42]. On the other hand, the development of IMRT allowed a better spare of the OAR without jeopardizing the coverage of the targets: similar to other studies, Chen et al. reported no Grade 3 toxicities compared with conventional (20%) and conformal (9%) techniques. IMRT spares moreover retinas, optic nerves, and chiasm, with a lower incidence of optic neuropathy, a condition that usually starts within 4 years after treatment [30].

Concerning late toxicity, RT can cause xerophthalmia, lacrimal canal stenosis, corneal ulceration, brain, and osteoradionecrosis. As for acute toxicity, IMRT appears to prevent dry-eye syndrome, a condition that usually develops within the first year after RT. Brain necrosis and osteoradionecrosis are much less frequent with IMRT: Hawkings et al. reported an 11% incidence of these toxicities with non-IMRT techniques [43], while Daly et al. only 3% with IMRT [44].

Chemotherapy

Neoadjuvant chemotherapy combined with surgery and/or CRT showed promising results in patients with advanced SNCs. However, this data are based on single institution studies with limited number of patients. The choice of the type of chemotherapy according to histologic tumor type has not been specifically addressed, but the most used drugs were platinum-based chemotherapy in combination with either 5-fluorouracil, taxane, ifosfamide, or vincristine.

One of the earliest reported experience in this setting is a small American study where 16 untreated patient with advanced SNC (predominantly squamous cell type) received platinum base-chemotherapy followed by surgery and/or RT obtaining an overall response rate of 82% (complete response = 44%) [45].

In 1992, induction chemotherapy was used for the first time in an organ preservation strategy. Twelve patients with advanced epithelial non-adenocarcinoma of the paranasal sinus and nasal fossa were treated with cisplatin and 5-fluoruracil (PF) followed by external RT (48 Gy) and limited surgery. LC was obtained in 92% of patients avoiding surgical mutilation and functional or cosmetic loss. After a median follow-up of 27 months, ten patients were alive and disease free [46].

Lee et al. reported data on 16 patients with stage III or IV SNC who received induction chemotherapy with three cycles of PF followed by surgical resection or debulking. Fifteen out of 16 patients thereafter received concomitant chemoradiotherapy with hydroxyurea and 5-fluorouracil. Induction chemotherapy achieved a clinical response in 87% with a complete histological response of 31%. The 10-year OS, DFS, and LC rates (LCR) were 56%, 73%, and 79%, respectively [47].

In an Italian series of 49 patients with resectable paranasal cancers, treatment with PF plus leucovorin (PFL) was active as an induction to anterior craniofacial resection with or without RT. Patients who attained a pathological complete remission had a favorable prognosis, and 3-year OS was 69% [48].

A retrospective study of MD Anderson Cancer Center reported data of 46 patients with SCC of the paranasal sinus treated with induction chemotherapy followed by either surgery and RT (or CRT) or with definitive RT (or CRT), with salvage surgery for residual disease. The majority of patients (80%) had a stage IV disease at presentation, with orbital invasion (67%) and nodal metastasis (26%). Thirty-seven patients (80%) received a combination of platinum and taxane, the remaining 9 patients (20%) had taxane and 5-floururacil. Despite the advanced disease extension, LC was high, and conservative surgery with orbital preservation was achieved in 87% of patients. Furthermore, response to induction chemotherapy was associated with better survival and a reasonable chance of organ preservation [49].

Chemotherapy administered concurrently with RT (CCRT) has been less studied in this disease, and SNC has not been included in the trials evaluating the impact of chemotherapy as radio sensitizer. Therefore, experience in this setting derives from retrospective studies.

Thirty-nine patients with unresectable stage IVB SNCs (46% SCC) were treated at the Memorial Sloan-Kettering Cancer Center from January 1990 to December 2006, 35 with CCRT (82% with cisplatin), and 4 with radiation alone. At a median follow-up of 90 months, 5-year local PFS, regional PFS, distant metastasis-free survival, DFS, and OS were 21%, 61%, 51%, 14%, and 15%, respectively [31]. Despite aggressive treatment with CRT, both disease control and OS were poor. Furthermore, the primary cause of death was local recurrence, occurring in 64% of patients, and was typically located within the irradiated field. The only factor associated with improved local PFS and OS was a biologically equivalent dose of radiation of ≥65 Gy.

Recently, Chopra et al. reported a case series of 23 locally advanced SNCs with mixed histotypes nonsurgically treated concluding that curative IMRT associated with platinum-base regimens may have a potential curative role [50].

Intra-arterial chemotherapy concurred with or followed by locoregional treatment showed conflicting results in terms of outcome and toxicities [51–53]. Therefore, in absence of a multi-institution trial providing the safety and efficacy of this approach, it cannot be recommended for clinical practice.

Chemotherapy in patients with local-regional recurrence not amenable to surgical salvage or re-irradiation has a palliative intent. In this setting, there are no trials comparing chemotherapy with best supportive care. Generally, the decision of giving chemotherapy or not depends on performance status, age, previous treatment received, time to disease recurrence, and amount of benefit expected from systemic treatment. The chemotherapy regime should be selected according to the chemosensitivity of each single histological type.

In the following paragraphs, the role of chemotherapy is considered on individual histological types with the main focus on malignant epithelial tumors.

Sinonasal Undifferentiated Carcinoma (SNUC)

SNUC is an aggressive disease with frequent locoregional failures and a tendency to metastatize to regional nodes and distant sites. It is a chemo-sensitive histotype; therefore, systemic therapy may have a role in improving locoregional control and reducing distant metastatization.

A meta-analysis of 30 published trials including 167 patients with SNUC showed a survival benefit from the addiction of chemotherapy to surgery, especially in patients with locoregional advanced disease [54]. No indication of the best chemotherapy protocol (pre- or postoperative adjuvant therapy) or regimen was stated, though CAV (cyclophosphamide, doxorubicin and vincristine) was the most frequent scheme used.

A suitable approach in locally advanced tumors is induction chemotherapy (platinum-based) followed by surgery and postoperative radiation, as reported by some single institution series showing the feasibility and the activity of this multimodal treatment. Agents most commonly combined with cisplatin were doxorubicin and vincristine or docetaxel and 5-fluorouracil [55–57].

Sinonasal Neuroendocrine Carcinoma (SNEC)

Among neuroendocrine cancers, small-cell carcinomas are the disease with the worst prognosis, with high rates of local recurrences and distant metastases. Multimodality approach, including chemotherapy, should be the cornerstone of treatment [58, 59].

In a prospective study with mixed series (olfactory neuroblastomas, SNEC and mixed tumors with some neuroendocrine features), a favorable survival (74% at 5 years) and a control rate of 88% were achieved with an induction chemotherapy with cisplatin and etoposide followed by proton/photon RT or surgery (in the case of unresponsiveness) and adjuvant chemotherapy [60].

In a large series of malignancies with neuroendocrine differentiation, 18 patients with NEC were treated in a similar way to SNUC (8/18 received induction chemotherapy followed by surgery or radiation) and showed almost identical outcomes with 64% 5-year OS, 73% 5-year LCR, and 14% distant metastasis rate [59].

Intestinal-Type Adenocarcinoma (ITAC)

Patients with advanced ITAC can be selected to receive induction chemotherapy with cisplatin, 5-fluorouracil, and leucovorin (PFL) according to tumor p53 status. In tumors with functional p53 protein (i.e., tumor with wild-type TP53 or with a partially/fully functional TP53 mutation), the PFL regimen achieved a higher response rate and better prognosis in comparison with p53 mutated tumors [61, 62].

Olfactory Neuroblastoma (ONB) or Esthesioneuroblastoma

Multiple studies reported the value of multimodal treatment in ONB. Although, the optimal role and sequencing of systemic therapy and drugs to be used is not clearly identified in the literature. Response to chemotherapy of this histotype is related to tumor dedifferentiation, with higher-grade tumors more responsive to systemic therapy [63].

Neoadjuvant chemotherapy was investigated by Loy et al. on a cohort of 50 patients with ONB. Patients with Kadish C stage (64%) were treated with induction chemotherapy and radiation followed by surgery [64]. Overall, they reported favorable long-term results, with a 5-year and 15-year DFS of 87% and 83%, respectively. The local–regional recurrence was 24%, and distant recurrence was 10%.

A small retrospective trial suggested the use of adjuvant chemotherapy after locoregional treatment in higher-grade and advanced stage tumors [65].

In regard to the chemotherapy regimen, different institutions reported the use of platinum-based chemotherapy [66, 67], while others considered the use of cyclophosphamide, vincristine, and doxorubicin [64].

NUT Midline Carcinoma

NUT midline carcinoma (NMC) is an aggressive subtype of poorly differentiated squamous cell carcinoma driven by the BRD4–NUT fusion oncoprotein. Most patients present with locally advanced or metastatic disease at diagnosis. Despite aggressive chemotherapy and RT, the mean survival is 6.7 months. Stathis et al. reported impressive and rapid antitumor activity targeting

BRD4–NUT. OTX015/MK-862 (a synthetic small molecule inhibitor of BRD2, BRD3, and BRD4) was administered to four patients with advanced NMC after failure of previous therapies. Two patients responded rapidly with tumor regression and symptomatic relief, and a third had a disease stabilization. These findings provide a rationale supporting the development of this novel targeted approach in NMC, alone or in combination with other therapeutic agents [68].

Carcinomas of Salivary Type

Salivary gland type are chemo-resistant tumors; therefore, systemic chemotherapy is reserved only for advanced cases not amenable to surgery and RT and with a palliative intent. The most used drug combinations are platinum-based, anthracycline, and cyclophosphamide, but modest activities of taxanes and vinorelbine have been reported [69]. Androgen-blockage strategy could be adopted in adenocarcinoma or ductal carcinoma expressing androgen receptors [70, 71].

Targeted Therapy

SNCs were not included in most studies with targeted agents. Thus, it is not possible to extrapolate the results with anti-EGFR agents obtained at other HNSCC sites, both in curative and palliative settings, to SNC.

The most frequent alterations in targetable molecular pathways include EGFR and HER2 overexpression, KRAS mutation (mainly in ITAC), overexpression of VEGFr- and NFkB-encoding genes, FGFR1 amplification, and COX2 overexpression [72]. HPV has been detected in about 30% SNC, and a trend toward a better prognosis was observed in these patients [73]. However, it is not clear yet whether this finding has any bearing on treatment decision for this disease.

As abovementioned, promising encouraging results come from targeting BRD4–NUT with a bromodomain and extra-terminal (BET) inhibitor [68].

Conclusion

A multidisciplinary approach to diagnosis and treatment is essential for SNC management. Despite the absence of randomized trials, data from multiple studies suggest that systemic therapy may play an important role in prolonging survival with a possible role in organ/structure preservation. Further studies are needed to define the role and appropriate sequencing of systemic therapy in SNC. Promising results are coming by the use of particle therapy. Finally, advances in molecular profiling of these diseases may help predict the prognosis and tailor the treatment to individual patients.

References

1. Turner JH, Reh DD. Incidence and survival in patients with sinonasal cancer: a historical analysis of population-based data. Head Neck. 2012;34:877. https://doi.org/10.1002/hed.21830.
2. Llorente JL, López F, Suárez C, Hermsen MA. Sinonasal carcinoma: clinical, pathological, genetic and therapeutic advances. Nat Rev Clin Oncol. 2014;11(8):460–72. https://doi.org/10.1038/nrclinonc.2014.97.
3. Duprez F, Madani I, Morbée L, et al. IMRT for sinonasal tumors minimizes severe late ocular toxicity and preserves disease control and survival. Int J Radiat Oncol Biol Phys. 2012;83(1):252–9. https://doi.org/10.1016/j.ijrobp.2011.06.1977.
4. Marta GN, Silva V, De Andrade CH, et al. Intensity-modulated radiation therapy for head and neck cancer: systematic review and meta-analysis. Radiother Oncol. 2014;110(1):9–15. https://doi.org/10.1016/j.radonc.2013.11.010.
5. Alonso-Basanta M, Lustig RA, Kennedy DW. Proton beam therapy in skull base pathology. Otolaryngol Clin N Am. 2011;44(5):1173–83. https://doi.org/10.1016/j.otc.2011.08.012.
6. Ansa B, Goodman M, Ward K, et al. Paranasal sinus squamous cell carcinoma incidence and survival based on surveillance, epidemiology, and end results data, 1973 to 2009. Cancer. 2013;119(14):2602–10. https://doi.org/10.1002/cncr.28108.
7. Nicolai P, Castelnuovo P, Lombardi D, et al. Role of endoscopic surgery in the management of selected malignant epithelial neoplasms of the naso-ethmoidal complex. Head Neck. 2007;29(12):1075–82. https://doi.org/10.1002/hed.20636.
8. Seong SY, Hyun DW, Kim YS, et al. Treatment outcomes of sinonasal adenoid cystic carcinoma: 30 cases from a single institution. J Craniomaxillofac Surg. 2014;42(5):e171–5. https://doi.org/10.1016/j.jcms.2013.08.002.

9. Hu YH, Tu GY, Qi YQ, et al. Comparison of pre- and postoperative radiation in the combined treatment of carcinoma of maxillary sinus. Int J Radiat Oncol Biol Phys. 1982;8(6):1045–9.
10. Sisson GAS, Toriumi DM, Atiyah RA. Paranasal sinus malignancy: a comprehensive update. Laryngoscope. 1989;99(2):143–50. https://doi.org/10.1288/00005537-198902000-00005.
11. Waldron J, Witterick I. Paranasal sinus cancer: caveats and controversies. World J Surg. 2003;27(7):849–55. https://doi.org/10.1007/s00268-003-7111-8.
12. Bristol IJ, Ahamad A, Garden AS, et al. Postoperative radiotherapy for maxillary sinus cancer: long-term outcomes and toxicities of treatment. Int J Radiat Oncol Biol Phys. 2007;68(3):719–30. https://doi.org/10.1016/j.ijrobp.2007.01.032.
13. Guan X, Wang X, Liu Y, Hu C, Zhu G. Lymph node metastasis in sinonasal squamous cell carcinoma treated with IMRT/3D-CRT. Oral Oncol. 2013;49(1):60–5. https://doi.org/10.1016/j.oraloncology.2012.07.009.
14. Ganly I, Patel S, Bilsky M, Shah J, Kraus D. Complications of craniofacial resection for malignant tumors of the skull base: report of an international collaborative study. Otolaryngol Head Neck Surg. 2009;140:218–23.
15. Duthoy W, Boterberg T, Claus F, et al. Postoperative intensity-modulated radiotherapy in sinonasal carcinoma: clinical results in 39 patients. Cancer. 2005;104:71. https://doi.org/10.1002/cncr.21100.
16. Hoppe BS, Stegman LD, Zelefsky MJ, et al. Treatment of nasal cavity and paranasal sinus cancer with modern radiotherapy techniques in the postoperative setting-the MSKCC experience. Int J Radiat Oncol Biol Phys. 2007;67(3):691–702. https://doi.org/10.1016/j.ijrobp.2006.09.023.
17. Orlandi E, Giandini T, Iannacone E, et al. Radiotherapy for unresectable sinonasal cancers: dosimetric comparison of intensity modulated radiation therapy with coplanar and non-coplanar volumetric modulated arc therapy. Radiother Oncol. 2014;113(2):260–6. https://doi.org/10.1016/j.radonc.2014.11.024.
18. Lindeman P, Eklund U, Petruson B. Survival after surgical treatment in maxillary neoplasms of epithelial origin. J Laryngol Otol. 1987;101(6):564–8.
19. Roa WH, Hazuka MB, Sandler HM, et al. Results of primary and adjuvant CT-based 3-dimensional radiotherapy for malignant tumors of the paranasal sinuses. Int J Radiat Oncol Biol Phys. 1994;28(4):857–65.
20. Pommier P, Ginestet C, Sunyach M, et al. Conformal radiotherapy for paranasal sinus and nasal cavity tumors: three-dimensional treatment planning and preliminary results in 40 patients. Int J Radiat Oncol Biol Phys. 2000;48(2):485–93.
21. Gabriele AM, Airoldi M, Garzaro M, et al. Stage III-IV sinonasal and nasal cavity carcinoma treated with three-dimensional conformal radiotherapy. Tumori. 2008;94(3):320–6. https://doi.org/10.1177/030089160809400306.
22. Patel SH, Wang Z, Wong WW, et al. Charged particle therapy versus photon therapy for paranasal sinus and nasal cavity malignant diseases: a systematic review and meta-analysis. Lancet Oncol. 2014;15(9):1027–38. https://doi.org/10.1016/S1470-2045(14)70268-2.
23. Mock U, Georg D, Bogner J, Auberger T, Pötter R. Treatment planning comparison of conventional, 3D conformal, and intensity-modulated photon (IMRT) and proton therapy for paranasal sinus carcinoma. Int J Radiat Oncol Biol Phys. 2004;58:147–54. https://doi.org/10.1016/S0360-3016(03)01452-4.
24. Zenda S, Kohno R, Kawashima M, et al. Proton beam therapy for unresectable malignancies of the nasal cavity and paranasal sinuses. Int J Radiat Oncol Biol Phys. 2011;81(5):1473–8. https://doi.org/10.1016/j.ijrobp.2010.08.009.
25. Truong MT, Kamat UR, Liebsch NJ, et al. Proton radiation therapy for primary sphenoid sinus malignancies: treatment outcome and prognostic factors. Head Neck. 2009;31:1297. https://doi.org/10.1002/hed.21092.
26. Miyawaki D, Murakami M, Demizu Y, et al. Brain injury after proton therapy or carbon ion therapy for head-and-neck cancer and skull base tumors. Int J Radiat Oncol Biol Phys. 2009;75:378. https://doi.org/10.1016/j.ijrobp.2008.12.092.
27. Claus F, De Gersem W, De Wagter C, et al. An implementation strategy for IMRT of ethmoid sinus cancer with bilateral sparing of the optic pathways. Int J Radiat Oncol Biol Phys. 2001;51(2):318–31. https://doi.org/10.1016/S0360-3016(01)01627-3.
28. Cantù G, Bimbi G, Miceli R, et al. Lymph node metastases in malignant tumors of the paranasal sinuses: prognostic value and treatment. Arch Otolaryngol Head Neck Surg. 2008;134(2):170–7. https://doi.org/10.1001/archoto.2007.30.
29. Kraus DH, Maghami E. Cancer of the nasal cavity and paranasal sinuses. Expert Rev Anticancer Ther. 2004;4(3):411–24. https://doi.org/10.1586/14737140.4.3.411.
30. Chen AM, Daly ME, Bucci MK, et al. Carcinomas of the paranasal sinuses and nasal cavity treated with radiotherapy at a single institution over five decades: are we making improvement? Int J Radiat Oncol Biol Phys. 2007;69(1):141–7. https://doi.org/10.1016/j.ijrobp.2007.02.031.
31. Hoppe BS, Nelson CJ, Gomez DR, et al. Unresectable carcinoma of the paranasal sinuses: outcomes and toxicities. Int J Radiat Oncol Biol Phys. 2008;72(3):763–9. https://doi.org/10.1016/j.ijrobp.2008.01.038.
32. Langendijk JA, Kasperts N, Leemans CR, Doornaert P, Slotman BJ. A phase II study of primary reirradiation in squamous cell carcinoma of head and neck. Radiother Oncol. 2006;78(3):306–12. https://doi.org/10.1016/j.radonc.2006.02.003.
33. Spencer SA, Harris J, Wheeler RH, et al. Final report of RTOG 9610, a multi-institutional trial of reirradiation and chemotherapy for unresectable recurrent squamous cell carcinoma of the head and neck. Head

Neck. 2008;30(3):281–8. https://doi.org/10.1002/hed.20697.

34. Langer CJ, Harris J, Horwitz EM, et al. Phase II study of low-dose paclitaxel and cisplatin in combination with split-course concomitant twice-daily reirradiation in recurrent squamous cell carcinoma of the head and neck: results of Radiation Therapy Oncology Group Protocol 9911. J Clin Oncol. 2007;25(30):4800–5. https://doi.org/10.1200/JCO.2006.07.9194.
35. Ozyigit G, Cengiz M, Hurmuz P, et al. Robotic stereotactic radiosurgery in patients with nasal cavity and paranasal sinus tumors. Technol Cancer Res Treat. 2014;13(5):409–13. https://doi.org/10.7785/tcrtexpress.2013.600264.
36. Iwata H, Tatewaki K, Inoue M, Yokota N, Sato K, Shibamoto Y. Salvage stereotactic reirradiation using the CyberKnife for the local recurrence of nasal or paranasal carcinoma. Radiother Oncol. 2012;104(3):355–60. https://doi.org/10.1016/j.radonc.2012.01.017.
37. Jiang GL, Ang KK, Peters LJ, Wendt CD, Oswald MJ, Goepfert H. Maxillary sinus carcinomas: natural history and results of postoperative radiotherapy. Radiother Oncol. 1991;21:193. https://doi.org/10.1016/0167-8140(91)90037-H.
38. Karim AB, Kralendonk JH, Njo KH, Tabak JM, Elsenaar WH, van Balen AT. Ethmoid and upper nasal cavity carcinoma: treatment, results and complications. Radiother Oncol. 1990;19(2):109–20.
39. Wiegner EA, Daly ME, Murphy JD, et al. Intensity-modulated radiotherapy for tumors of the nasal cavity and paranasal sinuses: clinical outcomes and patterns of failure. Int J Radiat Oncol Biol Phys. 2012;83:243–51. https://doi.org/10.1016/j.ijrobp.2011.05.044.
40. Katz TS, Mendenhall WM, Morris CG, Amdur RJ, Hinerman RW, Villaret DB. Malignant tumors of the nasal cavity and paranasal sinuses. Head Neck. 2002;24(9):821–9. https://doi.org/10.1002/hed.10143.
41. Parsons JT, Bova FJ, Fitzgerald CR, Mendenhall WM, Million RR. Severe dry-eye syndrome following external beam irradiation. Int J Radiat Oncol Biol Phys. 1994;30(4):775–80. https://doi.org/10.1016/0360-3016(94)90348-4.
42. Takeda A, Shigematsu N, Suzuki S, et al. Late retinal complications of radiation therapy for nasal and paranasal malignancies: relationship between irradiated-dose area and severity. Int J Radiat Oncol Biol Phys. 1999;44(3):599–605. https://doi.org/10.1016/S0360-3016(99)00057-7.
43. Hawkins RB, Wynstra JH, Pilepich MV, Fields JN. Carcinoma of the nasal cavity—results of primary and adjuvant radiotherapy. Int J Radiat Oncol Biol Phys. 1988;15(5):1129–33. https://doi.org/10.1016/0360-3016(88)90194-0.
44. Daly ME, Chen AM, Bucci MK, et al. Intensity-modulated radiation therapy for malignancies of the nasal cavity and paranasal sinuses. Int J Radiat Oncol Biol Phys. 2007;67(1):151–7. https://doi.org/10.1016/j.ijrobp.2006.07.1389.
45. Lorusso P, Tapazoglou E, Kish JA, et al. Chemotherapy for paranasal sinus carcinoma. A 10-year experience at Wayne State University. Cancer. 1988;62(1):1–5. https://doi.org/10.1002/1097-0142(19880701)62:1<1::AID-CNCR2820620102>3.0.CO;2-F.
46. Björk-Eriksson T, Mercke C, Petruson B, Ekholm S. Potential impact on tumor control and organ preservation with cisplatin and 5-fluorouracil for patients with advanced tumors of the paranasal sinuses and nasal fossa. A prospective pilot study. Cancer. 1992;70:2615. https://doi.org/10.1002/1097-0142(19921201)70:11<2615::AID-CNCR2820701108>3.0.CO;2-G.
47. Lee MM, Vokes EE, Rosen A, Witt ME, Weichselbaum RR, Haraf DJ. Multimodality therapy in advanced paranasal sinus carcinoma: superior long-term results. Cancer J Sci Am. 1999;42:327. https://doi.org/10.1016/S0360-3016(98)80506-3.
48. Licitra L, Locati LD, Cavina R, et al. Primary chemotherapy followed by anterior craniofacial resection and radiotherapy for paranasal cancer. Ann Oncol. 2003;14:367–72. https://doi.org/10.1093/annonc/mdg113.
49. Hanna EY, Cardenas AD, DeMonte F, et al. Induction chemotherapy for advanced squamous cell carcinoma of the paranasal sinuses. Arch Otolaryngol Head Neck Surg. 2011;137:78–81. https://doi.org/10.1001/archoto.2010.231.
50. Chopra S, Kamdar DP, Cohen DS, et al. Outcomes of nonsurgical management of locally advanced carcinomas of the sinonasal cavity. Laryngoscope. 2017;127(4):855–61. https://doi.org/10.1002/lary.26228.
51. Papadimitrakopoulou VA, Ginsberg LE, Garden AS, et al. Intraarterial cisplatin with intravenous paclitaxel and ifosfamide as an organ-preservation approach in patients with paranasal sinus carcinoma. Cancer. 2003;98(10):2214–23. https://doi.org/10.1002/cncr.11771.
52. Samant S, Robbins KT, Vang M, Wan J, Robertson J. Intra-arterial cisplatin and concomitant radiation therapy followed by surgery for advanced paranasal sinus cancer. Arch Otolaryngol Head Neck Surg. 2004;130(8):948–55. https://doi.org/10.1001/archotol.130.8.948.
53. Homma A, Sakashita T, Yoshida D, et al. Superselective intra-arterial cisplatin infusion and concomitant radiotherapy for maxillary sinus cancer. Br J Cancer. 2013;109(12):2980–6. https://doi.org/10.1038/bjc.2013.663.
54. Reiersen DA, Pahilan ME, Devaiah AK. Meta-analysis of treatment outcomes for sinonasal undifferentiated carcinoma. Otolaryngol Head Neck Surg. 2012;147(1):7–14. https://doi.org/10.1177/0194599812440932.
55. Musy PY, Reibel JF, Levine PA. Sinonasal undifferentiated carcinoma: the search for a better outcome. Laryngoscope. 2002;112:1450. https://doi.org/10.1097/00005537-200208000-00023.

56. Mourad WF, Hauerstock D, Shourbaji RA, et al. Trimodality management of sinonasal undifferentiated carcinoma and review of the literature. Am J Clin Oncol. 2013;36:584–8. https://doi.org/10.1097/COC.0b013e31825eb3a5.
57. Rischin D, Porceddu S, Peters L, Martin J, Corry J, Weih LA. Promising results with chemoradiation in patients with sinonasal undifferentiated carcinoma. Head Neck. 2004;26(5):435–41. https://doi.org/10.1002/hed.10396.
58. Likhacheva A, Rosenthal D, Hanna E, Kupferman M, Demonte F, El-Naggar A. Sinonasal neuroendocrine carcinoma: Impact of differentiation status on response and outcome. Head Neck Oncol. 2011;3(1):32. https://doi.org/10.1186/1758-3284-3-32.
59. Rosenthal DI, Barker JL, El-Naggar AK, et al. Sinonasal malignancies with neuroendocrine differentiation: patterns of failure according to histologic phenotype. Cancer. 2004;101(11):2567–73. https://doi.org/10.1002/cncr.20693.
60. Fitzek MM, Thornton AF, Varvares M, et al. Neuroendocrine tumors of the sinonasal tract: results of a prospective study incorporating chemotherapy, surgery, and combined proton-photon radiotherapy. Cancer. 2002;94(10):2623–34. https://doi.org/10.1002/cncr.10537.
61. Licitra L, Suardi S, Bossi P, et al. Prediction of TP53 status for primary cisplatin, fluorouracil, and leucovorin chemotherapy in ethmoid sinus intestinal-type adenocarcinoma. J Clin Oncol. 2004;22(24):4901–6. https://doi.org/10.1200/JCO.2004.05.071.
62. Bossi P, Perrone F, Miceli R, et al. Tp53 status as guide for the management of ethmoid sinus intestinal-type adenocarcinoma. Oral Oncol. 2013;49(5):413–9. https://doi.org/10.1016/j.oraloncology.2012.12.011.
63. McElroy EA, Buckner JC, Lewis JE. Chemotherapy for advanced esthesioneuroblastoma: the Mayo Clinic experience. Neurosurgery. 1998;42(5):1023–7. ; discussion 1027–1028. https://doi.org/10.1097/00006123-199805000-00040.
64. Loy AH, Reibel JF, Read PW, et al. Esthesioneuroblastoma: continued follow-up of a single institution's experience. Arch Otolaryngol Head Neck Surg. 2006;132(2):134–8. https://doi.org/10.1001/archotol.132.2.134.
65. Porter AB, Bernold DM, Giannini C, et al. Retrospective review of adjuvant chemotherapy for esthesioneuroblastoma. J Neuro-Oncol. 2008;90(2):201–4. https://doi.org/10.1007/s11060-008-9645-y.
66. Bell D, Saade R, Roberts D, et al. Prognostic utility of Hyams histological grading and Kadish-Morita staging systems for esthesioneuroblastoma outcomes. Head Neck Pathol. 2015;9(1):51–9. https://doi.org/10.1007/s12105-014-0547-3.
67. Resto VA, Eisele DW, Forastiere A, Zahurak M, Lee DJ, Westra WH. Esthesioneuroblastoma: the Johns Hopkins experience. Head Neck. 2000;22(6):550–8. https://doi.org/10.1002/1097-0347(200009)22:6<550::AID-HED2>3.0.CO;2-0.
68. Stathis A, Zucca E, Bekradda M, et al. Clinical response of carcinomas harboring the BRD4–NUT oncoprotein to the targeted bromodomain inhibitor OTX015/MK-8628. Cancer Discov. 2016;6(5):492–500. https://doi.org/10.1158/2159-8290.CD-15-1335.
69. Laurie SA, Licitra L. Systemic therapy in the palliative management of advanced salivary gland cancers. J Clin Oncol. 2006;24(17):2673–8. https://doi.org/10.1200/JCO.2005.05.3025.
70. Jaspers HCJ, Verbist BM, Schoffelen R, et al. Androgen receptor-positive salivary duct carcinoma: a disease entity with promising new treatment options. J Clin Oncol. 2011;29(16):e473–6. https://doi.org/10.1200/JCO.2010.32.8351.
71. Locati LD, Perrone F, Cortelazzi B, et al. Clinical activity of androgen deprivation therapy in patients with metastatic/relapsed androgen receptor-positive salivary gland cancers. Head Neck. 2016;38(5):724–31. https://doi.org/10.1002/hed.23940.
72. Bossi P, Saba NF, Vermorken JB, et al. The role of systemic therapy in the management of sinonasal cancer: a critical review. Cancer Treat Rev. 2015;41(10):836–43. https://doi.org/10.1016/j.ctrv.2015.07.004.
73. Thavaraj S. Human papillomavirus-associated neoplasms of the sinonasal tract and nasopharynx. Semin Diagn Pathol. 2016;33(2):104–11. https://doi.org/10.1053/j.semdp.2015.09.011.

Part II

Sinonasal Tumor-Like Lesions

Sinonasal Tumor-Like Lesions

Alessandro Franchi

Sinonasal Polyps

Inflammatory Polyp

Definition

An inflammatory polyp (IP) is a non-neoplastic growth of the sinonasal mucosa due to the presence of marked edema and inflammation.

Clinical Features

IPs occur at all ages, being most common over 20 years of age. They are single and unilateral or multiple and bilateral and most commonly arise from the middle meatus and ethmoid sinuses. Presenting symptoms include nasal obstruction, headaches, rhinorrhea, and epistaxis. They are associated with several conditions including allergy, vasomotor rhinitis, infections, cystic fibrosis, Kartagener's syndrome, diabetes mellitus, aspirin intolerance, and nickel exposure. Presence of nasal IPs with eosinophils, aspirin intolerance, and asthma is known as Samter's triad or aspirin exacerbated respiratory disease (AERD) and affects up to 9% of asthmatics patients [1].

Pathologic Features

IPs appear as polypoid translucent and soft, myxoid lesions, measuring from few millimeters to several centimeters. They are covered by respiratory type epithelium, often with goblet cell hyperplasia, but areas of squamous metaplasia may be present. The basement membrane is thickened and hyaline (Fig. 1). The core of the polyp consists of myxoid edematous stroma with pseudocysts containing eosinophilic proteinaceous fluid and a variably cellular infiltrate of inflammatory cells, usually rich in eosinophils, accompanied by variable number of lymphocytes, plasma cells, and some mast cells [2] (Figs. 2, 3, and 4). Seromucous glands are usually absent. Some differences in the histologic appearance of IP have been reported according to the etiopathogenesis of the lesion. For example, polyps arising in asthmatic patients present a marked chronic inflammatory reaction, as well as more prominent membrane thickening and goblet cell hyperplasia (Fig. 5), compared to those arising in non-asthmatic patients [3].

A number of secondary changes may occur in sinonasal IP, and some of these may cause concern for malignancy at histologic examination. The most commonly observed is the presence of

A. Franchi (✉)
Department of Translational Research and of New Technologies in Medicine and Surgery, University of Pisa, Pisa, Italy
e-mail: alessandro.franchi@unipi.it

A. Franchi (ed.), *Pathology of Sinonasal Tumors and Tumor-Like Lesions*,
https://doi.org/10.1007/978-3-030-29848-7_5

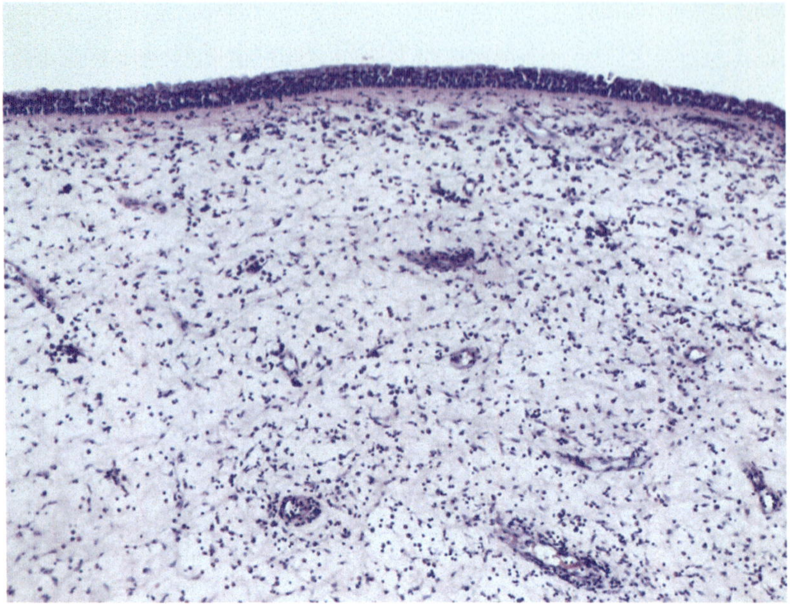

Fig. 1 The surface of this inflammatory polyp is covered by respiratory-type epithelium. The basement membrane is thick and hyaline

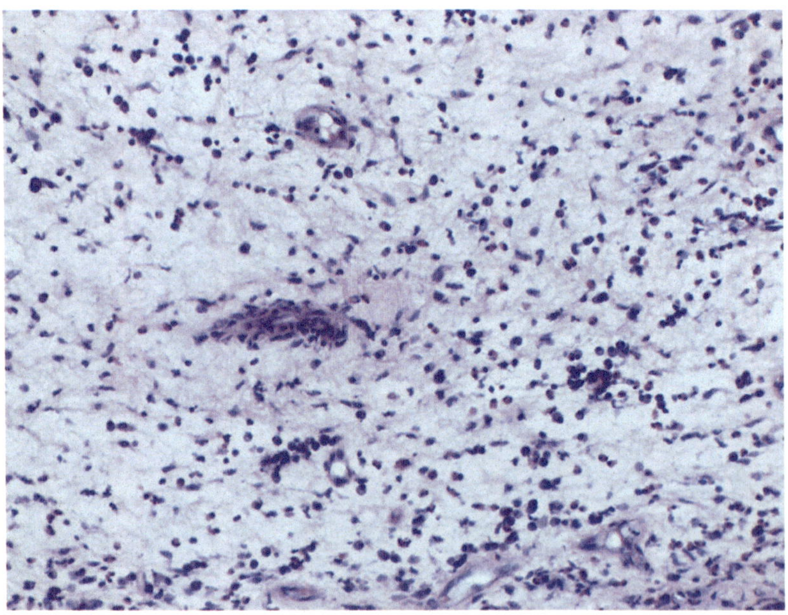

Fig. 2 The core of the polyp consists of myxoid edematous stroma with an inflammatory infiltrate rich in eosinophils, accompanied by lymphocytes and plasma cells

atypical stromal cells (Figs. 6 and 7). These are large bizarre spindle or stellate cells, with hyperchromatic nuclei and prominent nucleoli. They tend to concentrate in areas showing reactive changes including necrosis, hemorrhage vascular thrombosis, fibrosis, or ulceration. Based on immunohistochemical and ultrastructural findings, they have been interpreted as reactive fibroblasts/myofibroblasts [4–7]. The so-called angiomatoid change consists of a conspicuous proliferation capillary within the myxoid background of the polyp stalk, often with vessel thrombosis, fibrin deposition, foci of necrosis, hemorrhage, and presence of atypical stromal

Fig. 3 Collections of macrophages are rarely seen

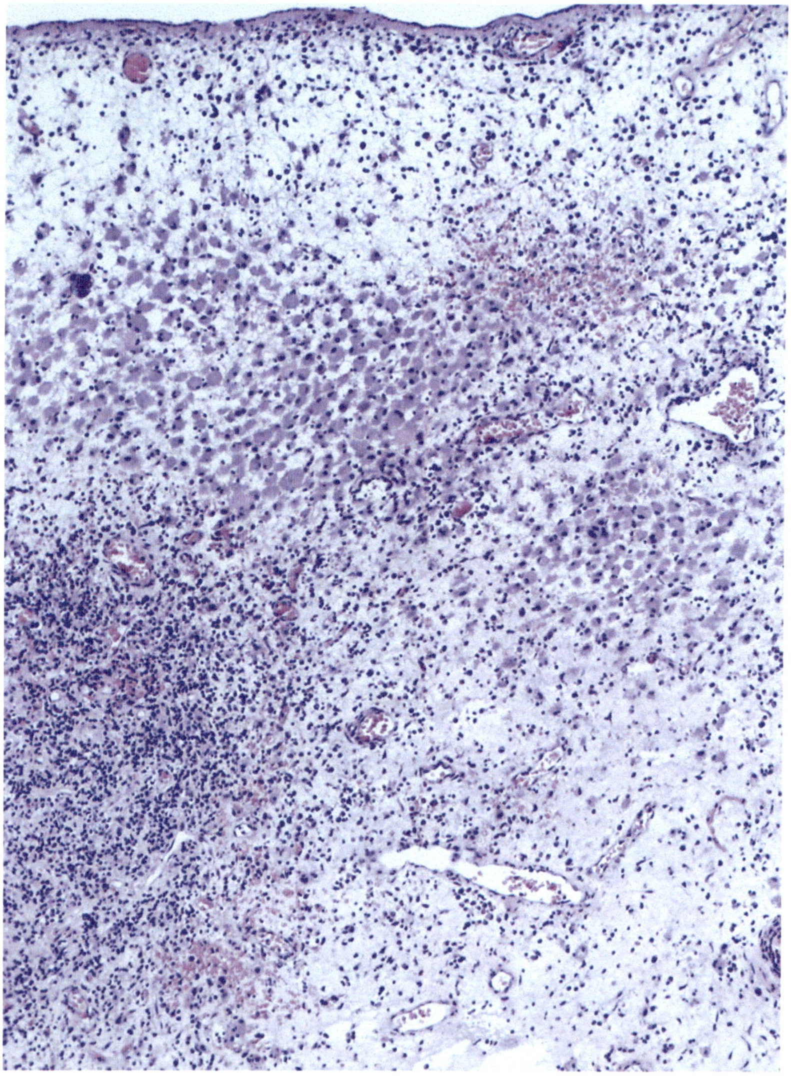

Fig. 4 Glands are usually absent in inflammatory polyps, but they may be present and markedly dilated

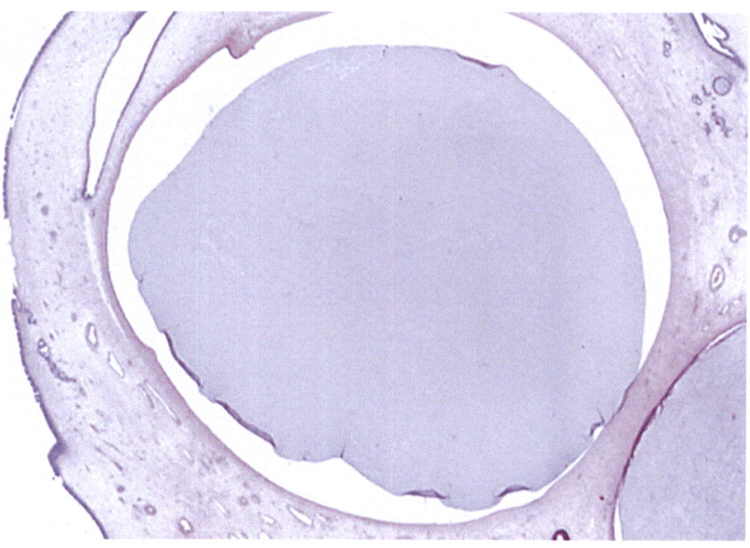

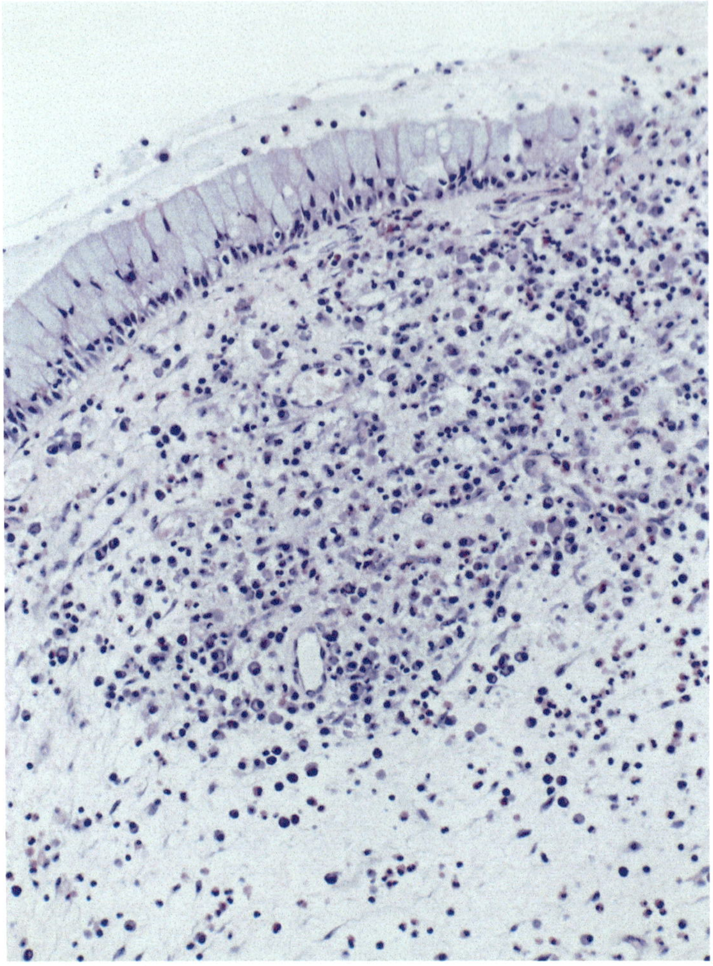

Fig. 5 Goblet cell hyperplasia of the surface epithelium

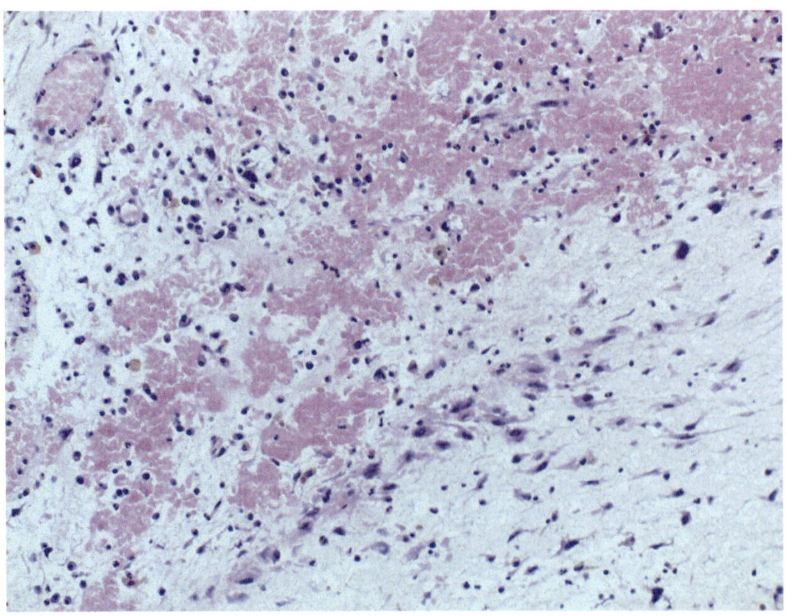

Fig. 6 Atypical spindle cells with hyper chromatic nuclei are seen in association with hemorrhage

Fig. 7 Multinucleated atypical cells in the stroma of an inflammatory polyp

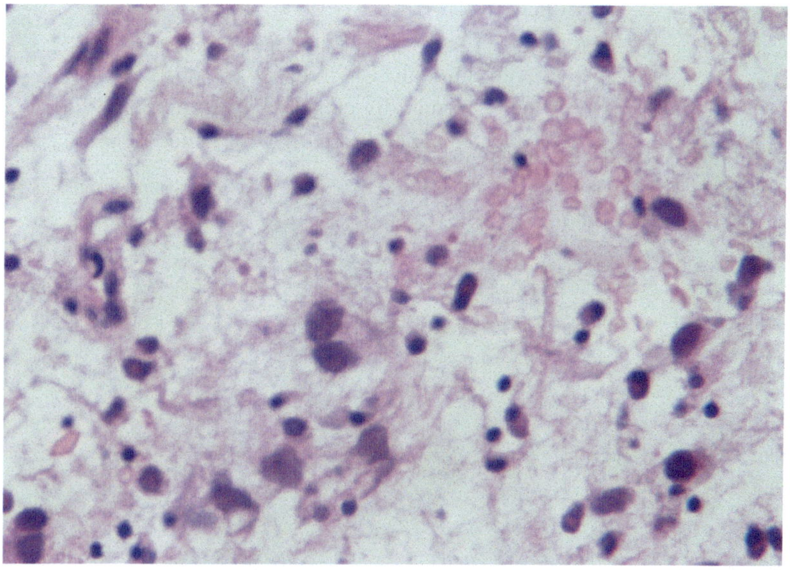

cells that simulate the appearance of an angiosarcoma [8–11]. Other secondary changes include fibrosis, ulceration of the surface epithelium, stromal deposition of amyloid-like material, osseous, or cartilaginous metaplasia. Granulomas may be seen in polyps treated with intranasal injection, application of steroids, or other oily medications, as well as for rupture of mucous cysts.

Immunohistochemical Findings

Stromal cells, including atypical bizarre elements, are positive for vimentin and frequently for actins [5, 6]. Cytokeratin immunoreactivity has also been reported [6].

Differential Diagnosis

The presence of atypical stromal cells may lead to consider a diagnosis of sarcoma, including rhabdomyosarcoma and angiosarcoma. However, in IP these atypical cells are localized in limited areas of the lesion and do not present mitotic figures. Since stromal elements may seldom be positive for cytokeratins, spindle cell squamous cell carcinoma may also be considered in the differential diagnosis.

Sinonasal papilloma frequently shows an inflammatory background with edema and may be confused with IP. However, sinonasal papillomas are unilateral lesions, lack the mucoid gross appearance of IP, and present a thick epithelium with transmigrating neutrophils, mucous cysts, and microabscesses that are not seen in IP.

Treatment and Prognosis

Treatment consists of endoscopic surgery [12], associated with various medical therapies [13–16]. Some forms of IP, in particular those associated with conditions like allergy, asthma, and aspirin sensitivity, show a greater degree of local aggressiveness, a weak response to drugs, and high recurrence rates after surgical treatment [17].

Antrochoanal Polyp

Definition

Anthrocoanal polyp (AP) is an IP variant which takes origin from the maxillary sinus and extends through the middle meatus into the nasal cavity, with posterior extension into the choana.

Clinical Features

AP occurs at a younger age as compared to IP, involves more frequently male subjects, and more frequently presents with unilateral nasal obstruction and nasal discharge [18, 19]. AP is frequently associated with chronic rhinosinusitis and allergy [18].

Pathologic Features

AP presents a smooth surface and a long and thin stalk that originates from the mucosa of the maxillary antrum. Microscopically, it is similar to a conventional IP, but the inflammatory infiltrate usually lacks a marked eosinophilic infiltrate, and the background is more fibrous and collagenized (Figs. 8 and 9). Atypical stromal cells are present as well, often with other reactive changes. These include hemorrhage and necrosis due to torsion of the long stalk.

Differential Diagnosis

Similar to IP, the most important differential diagnosis is with sarcomas. Sinonasal-inverted papilloma has also to be considered.

Treatment and Prognosis

Surgical removal with endoscopic surgery is the generally accepted treatment of choice for APs. The rate of recurrence is low, ranging between 5 and 10% [18, 20, 21].

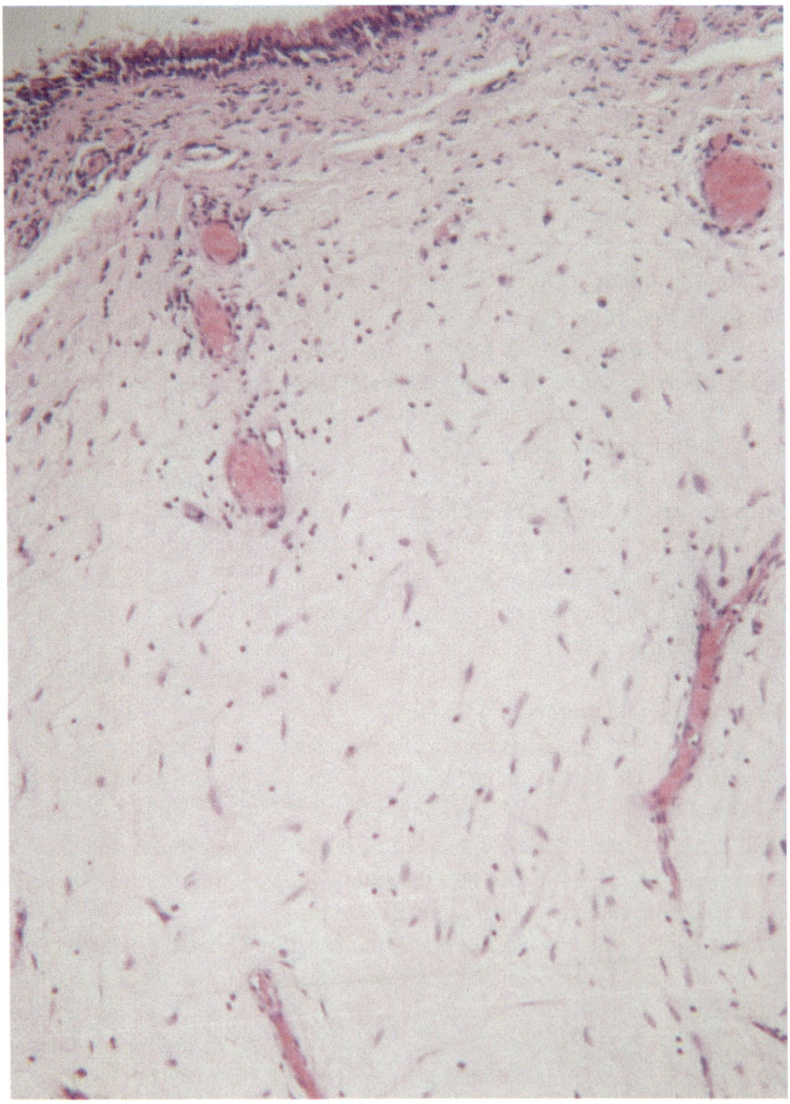

Fig. 8 Antrochoanal polyp. The stromal background of the antrochoanal polyp is often more collagenized than other inflammatory polyps

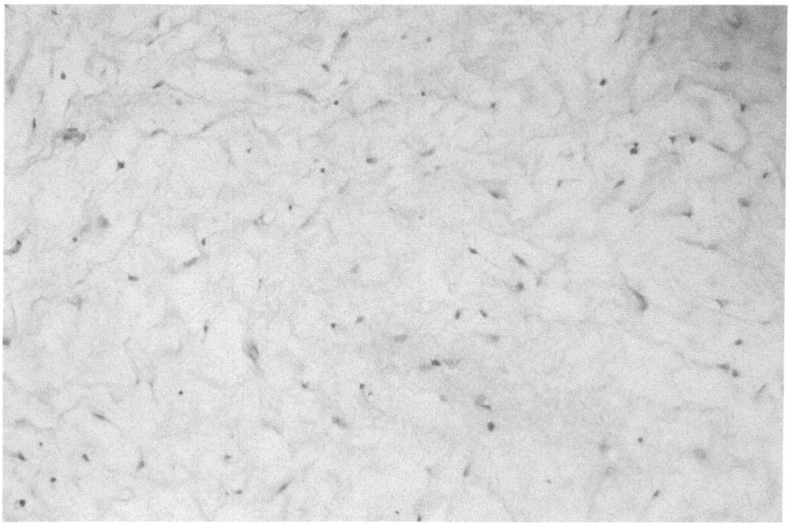

Fig. 9 A population of fibroblasts with no significant atypia is present in the stroma of this antrochoanal polyp

Sinonasal Heterotopias and Hamartomas

Nasal Glial Heterotopia and Encephalocele

Definition

Nasal glial heterotopia (NGH) (synonym: heterotypic neuroglial tissue) is a developmental displacement of neuroglial tissue. The term NGH appears to be more appropriate than nasal glioma, which implies a neoplastic proliferation. The term encephalocele is used to indicate a protrusion of brain tissue through a skull base defect that is connected to the rest of the brain by a pedicle.

Multiple mechanisms have been proposed to explain the pathogenesis of NGH, including the displacement of totipotent neuroectodermal cells that mature in the brain tissue, an aberrant fusion of the chondrocranium that results in separation of neural elements from the developing brain, an encephalocele that loses the connection to the brain, or entrapment or migration of neuroglial cells from the olfactory bulb [22].

Clinical Features

NGH may involve the external nose (approximately 60%), the nasal cavities (30%), or both sites (10%). Intracranial extension may also be present. Most frequently, intranasal GH presents in the newborn period with airway obstruction, but in rare instances it may also present later in life [23]. Patients may have other craniofacial anomalies, such as cleft palate, micrognathia, and choanal atresia [24].

Encephalocele has similar clinical presentation, with symptoms of nasal obstruction and respiratory distress, and intracranial extension is usually detected by imaging [25].

Pathologic Features

Histologically, NGH consists of fibrous tissue with a nested proliferation of glial cells in a fibrillary background [23] (Fig. 10). Gemistocytic astrocytes can be present. True neuronal cells are variably present, but sometimes cannot be identified. The presence of choroid plexus elements, ependymal cells, pigmented retinal cells, and calcifications has also been reported [23] (Figs. 11 and 12). Encephaloceles are histologically identical to normal brain with meningeal coverings, but usually present dysplastic changes and degenerative aspects, including hemorrhage, inflammation, and fibrosis.

Immunohistochemical Findings

The glial components show immunoreactivity for glial fibrillary acidic protein (GFAP) and S100, while the neuronal elements are positive for neurofilaments and neuron-specific enolase [23].

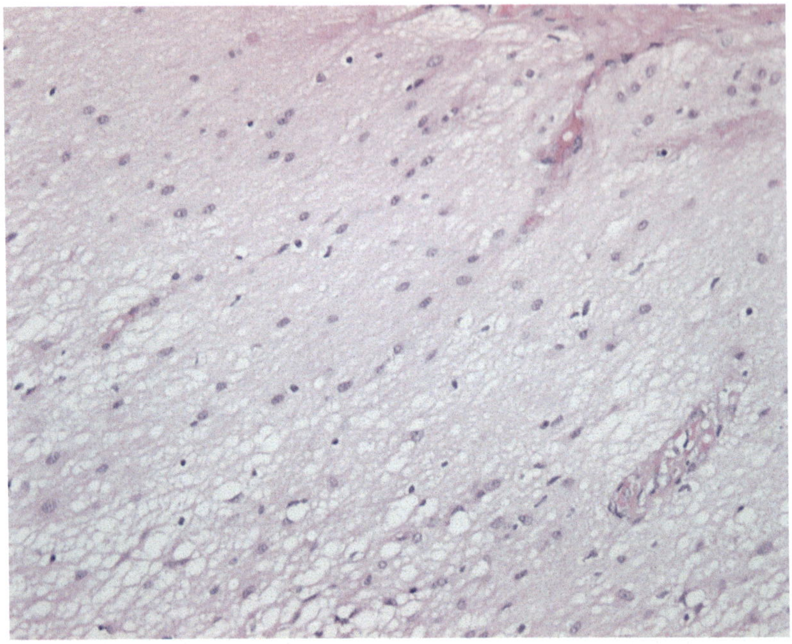

Fig. 10 Nasal glial heterotopia presents as a proliferation of glial cells in a fibrillary background

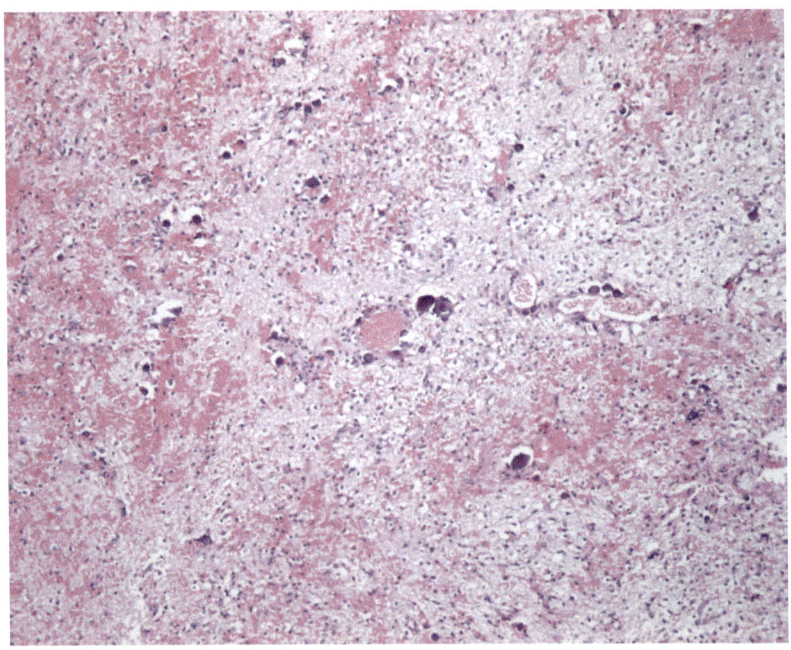

Fig. 11 Hemorrhage and calcification are frequently seen in glial heterotopia

Differential Diagnosis

The diagnosis of NGH is relatively easy in a young child, because the clinical suspicion for NGH is usually high and immunohistochemistry supports the correct diagnosis. Presence of choroid plexus and ependymal and pigmented retinal elements may complicate the picture.

The diagnosis of NGH may be more challenging in the setting of an older patient because this entity may not be considered in the differential diagnoses due to the clinical presentation and because neural tissue may be very difficult to identify because of marked replacement by fibrous tissue [26]. However, immunohistochem-

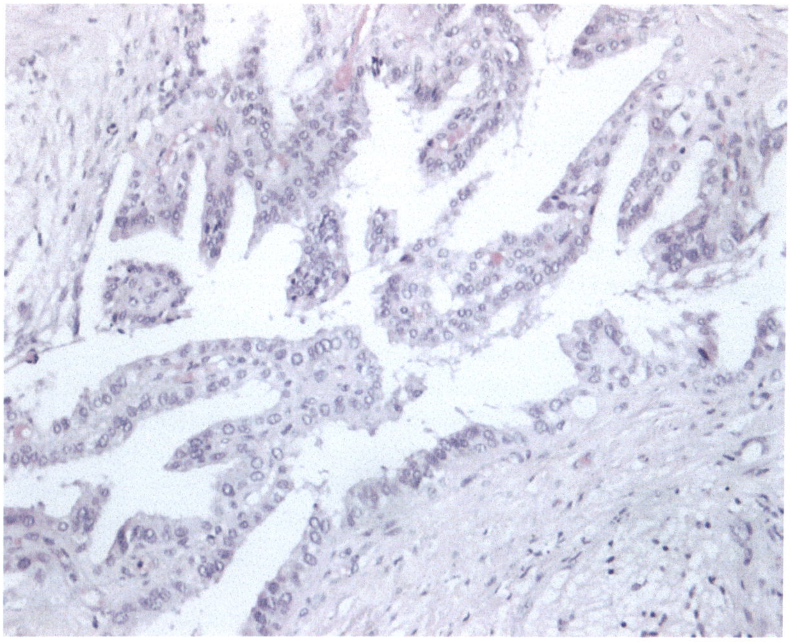

Fig. 12 Choroid plexus elements in glial heterotopia

istry brings to light the different constitutive elements of NGH, helping to recognize the entity.

The distinction between NGH and encephalocele is mainly based on clinicoradiographic correlations.

Treatment and Prognosis

The treatment of choice of NGH is complete surgical excision through an endonasal endoscopic approach [25]. Local recurrences are rarely reported. Similarly, encephaloceles are treated with a transnasal endoscopic approach and/or transcranial endoscopic approach [25]. Reconstruction of the cranial base defect is necessary in patients with intracranial extension [25].

One example of sinonasal undifferentiated carcinoma arising in the background of extensive, multifocal NGH has been reported [27]. Bona fide gliomas may also develop from NGH [28].

Hamartomas

Respiratory Epithelial Lesions

The fourth edition of the WHO classification has grouped two rare benign acquired lesions of the sinonasal tract, *respiratory epithelial adenomatoid hamartoma* (REAH) and *seromucinous hamartoma* (SH) under the heading "respiratory epithelial lesions" [29, 30]. Indeed, these lesions present some histologic similarities and hybrid cases presenting features of both REAH and SH have been reported, suggesting that they may represent a spectrum of the same lesion rather than different entities. Recently, another subtype of sinonasal epithelial hamartoma has been described, that has been designated *olfactory epithelial hamartoma*. It is characterized by features of seromucinous hamartoma, with the additional presence of areas of olfactory epithelium in the surface lining and gland-like ductal invaginations [31].

Respiratory Epithelial Adenomatoid Hamartoma

Definition

Respiratory epithelial adenomatoid hamartoma (REAH; synonym: glandular hamartoma) is a benign-acquired glandular overgrowth of the sinonasal tract arising from the surface epithelium [32]. Although initially considered a non-neoplastic hamartomatous epithelial proliferation, loss of heterozygosity studies rather supports the hypothesis that REAH may indeed be a benign neoplasm [33].

Clinical Features

REAH typically occurs in adult patients with a preference for male subjects and a mean age of 58 years [34]. Headache, nasal obstruction, rhinorrhea, and hyposmia are the most common presenting symptoms [35]. Concurrent inflammatory pathology is detected in approximately 2/3 of the patients [35]. REAH may indeed present either as solitary lesion or in association with nasal polyps [36, 37]. Both types are more frequently bilateral. Solitary REAH typically arises from the posterior septum and the olfactory cleft, whereas lesions associated with nasal polyps may also involve the ethmoid labyrinth [37].

Pathologic Features

Macroscopically, REAH presents as a firm, polypoid, yellow to gray white mass, with a relatively uneven surface, measuring up to 4 cm [37]. Histologically, it consists of medium to large gland-like structures arising in continuity with the surface epithelium, lined by multilayered ciliated respiratory epithelium, often with admixed mucous-producing cells (Figs. 13 and 14). Larger, cystically dilated tubules may be present as well. These glands are characteristically surrounded by a thick eosinophilic basement membrane. In rare instances, the lining epithelium may show florid mucinous metaplasia (Fig. 15). An inflammatory background, with edema and fibrosis, is frequently observed. Osseous or cartilaginous elements can be present in the stromal component, and the term chondro-osseous respiratory epithelial hamartoma (COREAH) has been used to report such cases [38, 39].

REAH may be found in association with other sinonasal lesions, mainly nasal polyps and seromucinous hamartoma. However, sporadic cases have been described in association with sinonasal inverted papilloma, sinonasal adenocarcinoma, and solitary fibrous tumor [32, 40].

Immunohistochemical Findings

The gland-like structures of REAH are positive for cytokeratin 7, with p63- and p40-positive basal cells [37, 41]. Cytokeratin 20, CDX2, smooth muscle actin, calponin, and S100 are negative [42]. Ki-67 labeling index is low, with staining only localized to the basal layer [41]. The distinctive hyalinized basement membrane that surrounds the ciliated epithelium is positive for collagen IV [41].

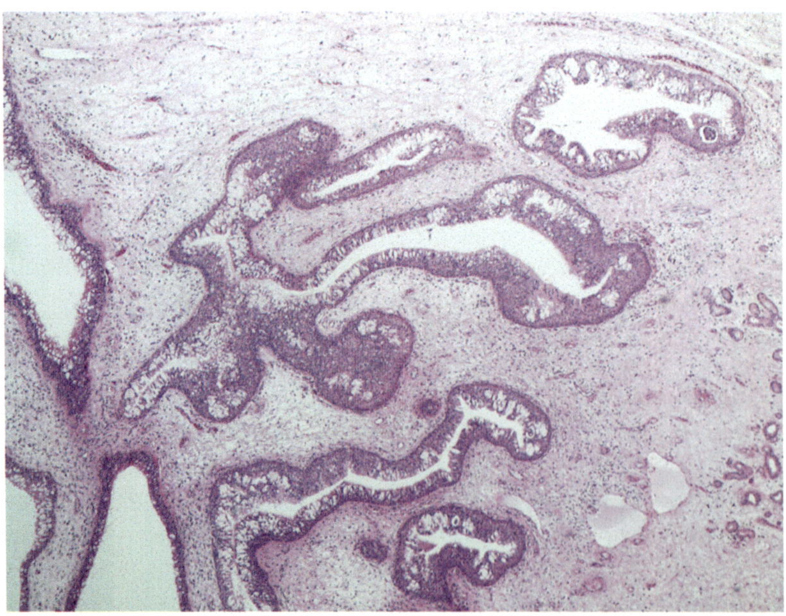

Fig. 13 The glandular proliferation of REAH is connected with surface epithelium

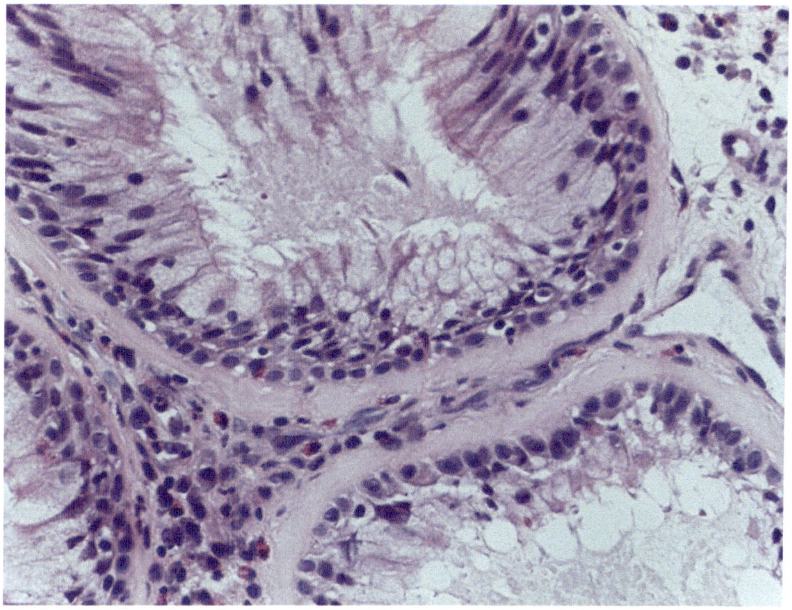

Fig. 14 Glands are surrounded by a thickened hyaline basement membrane

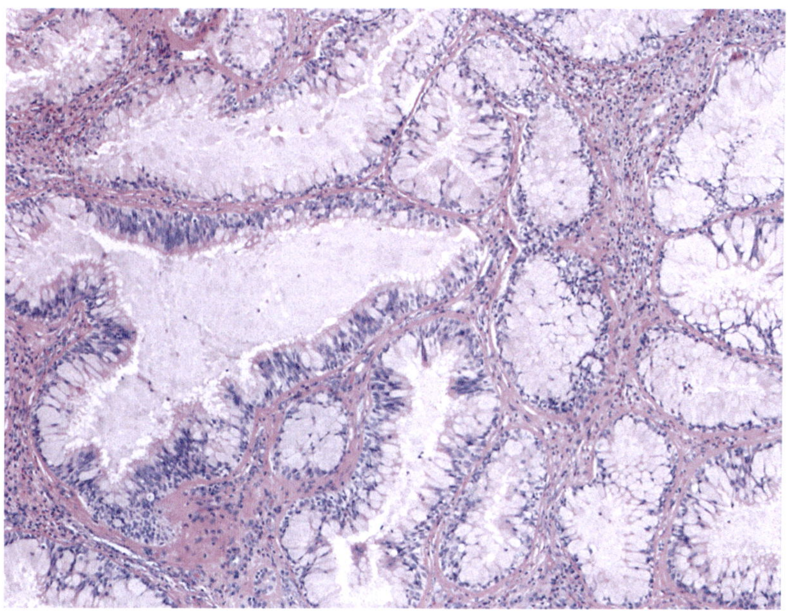

Fig. 15 The gland epithelium in this REAH shows mucinous features

Molecular Features

Loss of heterozygosity studies have demonstrated a fractional allelic loss of 31% in REAH [33]. This rate has been considered high for a non-neoplastic entity and rather supports the hypothesis that REAH may indeed be a benign neoplasm rather than a hamartoma [33]. Using in situ hybridization for EBER, EBV has been found sporadically in REAH epithelial cells in patients from Southern China, but the significance of this finding is limited because samples of unaffected sinonasal mucosa had similar staining distribution [41].

Differential Diagnosis

REAH must be differentiated from more aggressive sinonasal epithelial lesions to avoid unnecessary radical surgery for an otherwise benign process (see Table 4 in chapter "Epithelial Tumors"). The distinction from well-differentiated sinonasal intestinal-type adenocarcinoma is straightforward, because the appearance of neoplastic cells resembles that of the intestinal epithelia, and they are typically positive for CK20 and CDX2, a feature not seen in REAH. Sinonasal low-grade non-intestinal type adenocarcinomas may be difficult to separate from REAH, especially those showing extensive mucinous metaplasia, because they usually lack cellular atypia and invasion may not be readily apparent in small biopsy specimens. Absence of complex back-to-back glandular architecture and presence of thick eosinophilic basement membranes and of ciliated epithelium lining are features in favor of a diagnosis of REAH.

Sinonasal inverted papilloma should also be distinguished from REAH for its locally aggressive growth and propensity to recur. Markedly thickened epithelium with squamous metaplasia and mucocytes, intraepithelial mucous cysts, and presence of inflammatory cells permeating through the epithelium are findings that support the diagnosis of inverted papilloma. In addition, REAH often contains a component of residual seromucinous glands, which are usually not seen in inverted papilloma.

REAH-like changes of the sinonasal mucosa, including invagination of the surface epithelium and thickened basement membrane, can be observed in other reactive proliferations, mainly inflammatory polyps, and even in normal mucosa [43]. Thus, only polypoid lesions showing significant typical epithelial changes should be diagnosed as REAH.

Treatment and Prognosis

Complete endoscopic resection is curative [34].

Seromucinous Hamartoma

Definition

Seromucinous hamartoma (SH) is a rare benign proliferation of seromucinous glands of the nasal cavity and paranasal sinuses [30]. It is strictly related to REAH, since lesions with histologic features of both entities have been reported.

Clinical Features

SH typically arises from the posterior nasal septum or in the nasopharynx, although in some instances the lesion took origin from the lateral nasal wall or from the paranasal sinuses. It affects adult patients (mean 55 years), with a predominance of male subjects. The most common presenting symptoms are nasal obstruction and epistaxis [44]. Association with chronic sinusitis and sinonasal polyps has been reported in some patients [44].

Pathologic Features

SH appears as a polypoid firm mass measuring up to 4 cm (mean 2.8) [44]. Microscopically, the polyp is covered by ciliated respiratory epithelium, and it is composed of a combination of invaginated respiratory epithelium forming glands and cysts often surrounded by thick hyaline basement membrane, cysts lined by low cuboidal to flat epithelium, and a proliferation of small serous glands organized in clusters and lobules [44, 45] (Figs. 16, 17, and 18). These proliferating glands are intermixed with the preexisting seromucinous glands of the nasal mucosa and sometimes are in close relationship with invaginated surface gland-like structures. Myoepithelial cells are usually not present around the proliferating glands. The background stroma is edematous to fibrous with variable mixed chronic inflammatory infiltrate.

Immunohistochemical Findings

The surface and invaginated respiratory-type epithelium and the serous glandular proliferation are positive for cytokeratin 7 and CK19 and negative for CK20 [44]. The surface and invaginated respiratory epithelium presents also a basal cell layer positive for high-molecular-weight cytokeratins and p63 that is lost in the small glands [44, 46]. The serous glands are S100 positive, whereas the ciliated epithelium is negative. Myoepithelial markers are usually negative. The intervening stroma contains numerous myofibroblasts that

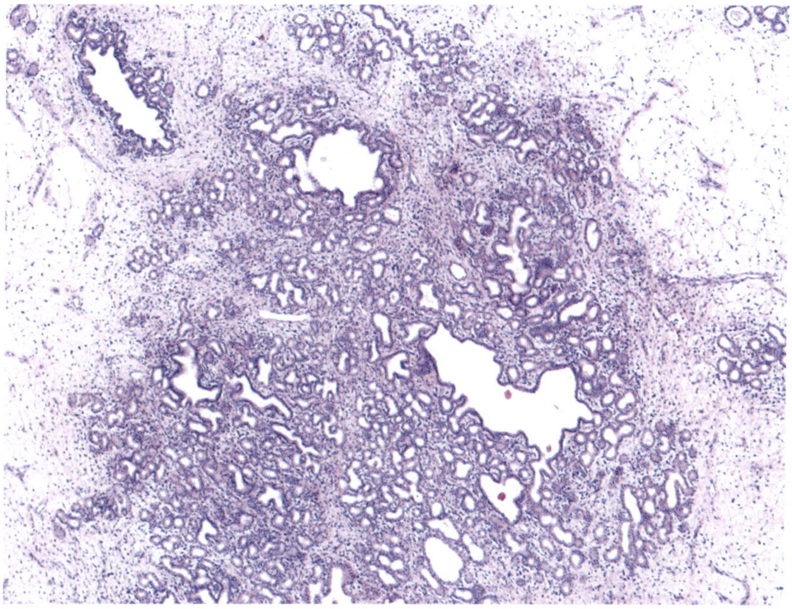

Fig. 16 Seromucinous hamartoma. Predominantly serous acinar proliferation with lobular architecture

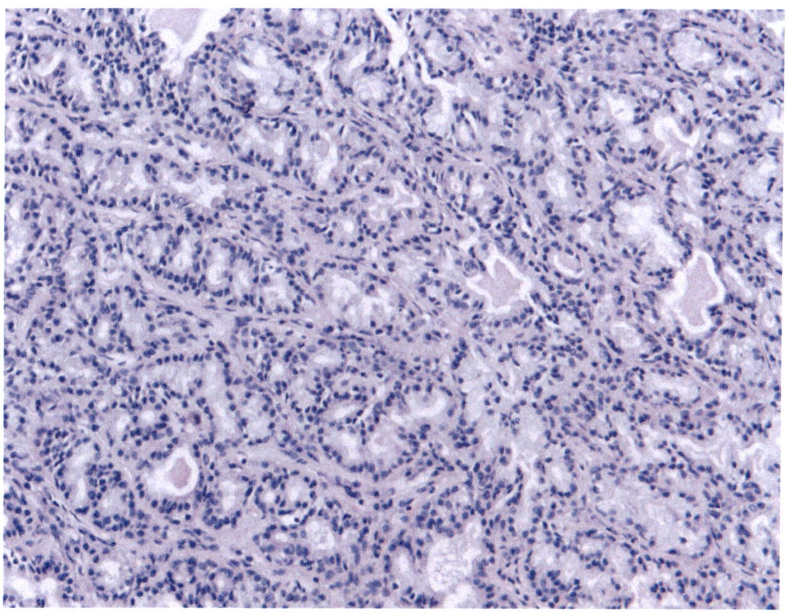

Fig. 17 Serous glands are closely packed with a back-to-back arrangement

are positive for calponin, desmin, and smooth muscle actin [46].

Molecular Features

Ambrosini-Spaltro et al. documented an increased mtDNA mutation rate, especially heteroplasmic, in the seromucinous component [46]. This is in keeping with a low cellular proliferation rate, consistent with a benign process [46].

Differential Diagnosis

The main differential diagnosis is with low-grade sinonasal adenocarcinoma (see Table 4 in chapter "Epithelial Tumors"). Presence of an organoid pattern of growth with lobular arrangement of the glands, lack of cytologic atypia and mitoses, and absence of invasion of adjacent tissues are the key features supporting the diagnosis of seromucinous hamartoma.

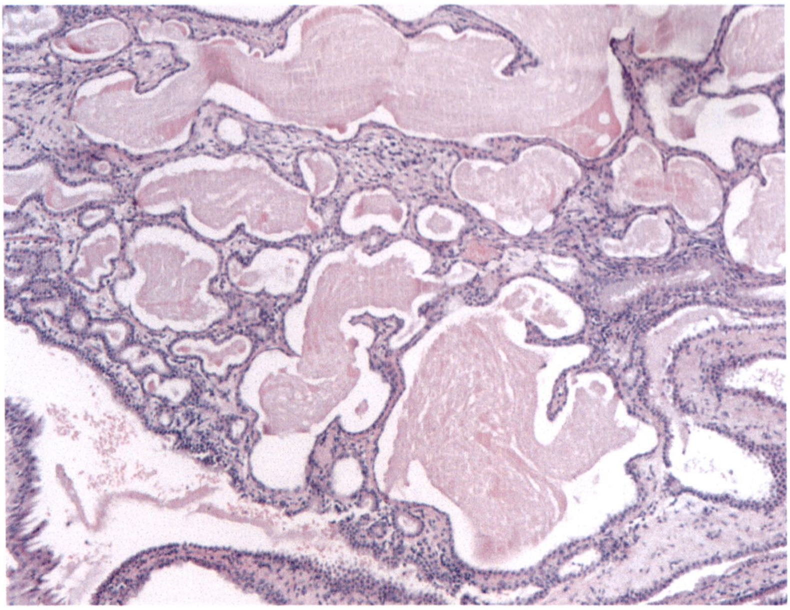

Fig. 18 Glands may be cystically dilated in seromucinous hamartoma

Treatment and Prognosis

SH is a benign lesion that is treated surgically with complete excision.

Chondromesenchymal Hamartoma

Definition

Chondromesenchymal hamartoma (CMH) is a very rare benign but locally invasive tumor-like growth composed of mixed mesenchymal elements [47].

Clinical Features

CMH occurs predominantly in male infants (median age 10 years; M:F = 2.2:1), but it has been occasionally reported in adults [48]. In 20% of the cases, there is involvement of the nasal cavity only, while in more than half of the patients the lesion involves the paranasal sinuses, with frequent intracranial or skull base extension [48]. Clinical presentations include nasal obstruction, eye signs (proptosis, hypotropia, enopthalmos, strabismus, exotropia), facial swelling, headaches or facial pain, stertor, or respiratory distress [48]. Sinonasal CMH is associated with the pleuropulmonary blastoma tumor predisposition disorder, which is due to germline or somatic mutations of the DICER gene [49].

Pathologic Features

The polypoid lesion is firm and rubbery in consistency, and the cut surface is white with blue-gray glistening nodules and areas of bone formation. It consists of variably sized lobules of hyaline cartilage, set within a variably cellular stromal component of spindle cells (Fig. 19). The cartilage nodules are usually well demarcated, but occasionally they may merge and blend with the surrounding stroma. Mitotic figures may be present in the spindle cell component. Scattered osteoclast-like, multinucleated giant cells can be detected. Bony trabeculae surround the cartilage nodules, and epithelial as well as mature adipose tissue components may also be present [47, 50]. A vascular proliferation, with both red cell-filled aneurysmal spaces and well-formed arterioles, is frequently detected. These vessels frequently have a zone of perivascular hyalinization which is often contiguous with areas of dense, keloidal collagen. Cleft-like spaces in these areas of dense collagen may produce a pseudovascular appearance that, together with hemorrhage and hemosiderin deposition, results in an appearance reminiscent of an aneurysmal bone cyst [47].

Fig. 19 Chondro-mesenchymal hamartoma. A cartilage nodule is set within hypocellular fibrous tissue with adipocytes

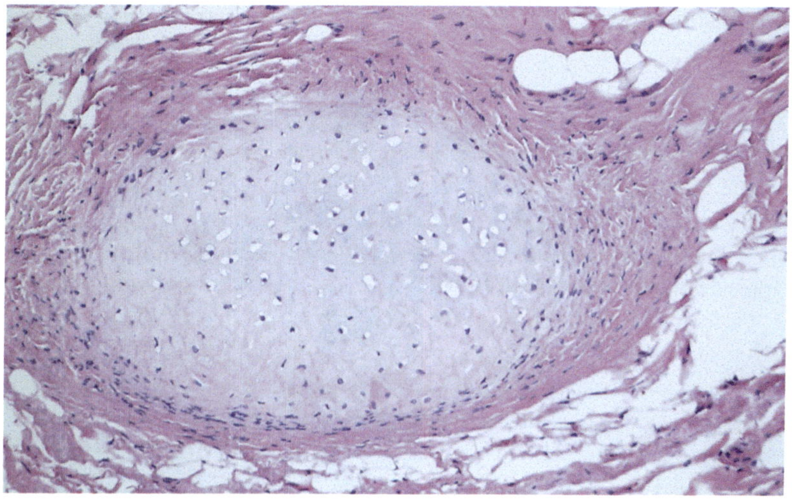

Immunohistochemical Findings

S100 is positive in the cartilaginous component, while stromal spindle cells are positive for smooth muscle actin and common muscle actin. Focal and weak staining for epithelial membrane antigen has been observed in both stromal and cartilaginous components, whereas cytokeratin is negative [50].

Molecular Features

Pathogenic somatic and germline mutations in *DICER1* have been detected in patients with CMH [49]. Cytogenetic analysis of a CMH arising in an 11-year-old boy with a past medical history of pleuropulmonary blastoma showed a novel 12;17 translocation, t(12;17)(q24.1;q21), as the sole anomaly [51].

Differential Diagnosis

The presence of cellular islands of cartilage raises the differential diagnosis with cartilaginous neoplasms, including chondroma and chondrosarcoma. However, chondrosarcoma of the craniofacial bones in the pediatric age group is very unusual. Moreover, the admixture of various mesenchymal elements seen in CMH is a distinctive feature from the various subtypes of chondrosarcoma. Other benign lesions that can be entered in the differential diagnosis of CMH are chondromyxoid fibroma, chondroblastoma, and aneurysmal bone cyst.

Treatment and Prognosis

Complete surgical resection is the treatment of choice for CMH. However, this method is not always technically feasible, especially in cases with intracranial extension, leaving the risk of recurrence as well as the possibility of continued tumor growth [48]. Disease recurrence, most likely from incomplete surgical excision, is reported to occur in approximately 15% of the patients [48]. Malignant transformation of the stromal component has been reported in an adult patient [52].

Pseudotumours

Paranasal Sinus Mucocele

Definition

Paranasal sinus mucocele (PSM) is benign cystic lesion lined by non-neoplastic epithelium that contains usually sterile mucus. It is the result of the obstruction of sinus ostia that may be due to a chronic inflammatory process (also through inflammatory polyp formation or dilation of mucous glands), a benign tumor, trauma, or prior surgery. Mucus accumulation determines the progressive enlargement of the lesion with erosion of the bony wall of the sinus and extension in adjacent anatomic structures.

Clinical Features

PSM occurs at any age, but most commonly involves patients in the third or fourth decades of life with a slight male predilection [53]. The frontal sinus is the most commonly affected, followed by the ethmoid sinuses, with 70–90% of PSM occurring in these locations. Approximately 10% arise the maxillary sinus, while the sphenoid sinus is only rarely involved [53, 54].

Presenting symptoms depend on the site of the lesion and include most commonly facial pain, maxillofacial pressure, headache, and increased nasal drainage. Ocular and periocular symptoms (palpebral swelling, orbital cellulitis, diplopia, loss of visual acuity) are common as well [54, 55]. PSM may also be an incidental finding detected during radiological or fibroscopic examinations performed for surveillance sinus disease [56].

Pathologic Features

The material received for histopathologic analysis usually consists of fragments of respiratory mucosa lined by pseudostratified ciliated columnar epithelium with variable chronic inflammatory infiltrate. Additional findings include the presence of cholesterol crystals, hemorrhage, fibrosis, and granulation tissue. In longstanding lesions, squamous metaplasia of the surface epithelium may be present. Reactive bone formation can also be observed near the cyst wall.

Differential Diagnosis

Histopathologic findings are nonspecific and not sufficient for the diagnosis that requires correlation with the clinical and radiologic findings (CT scan and MRI).

Treatment and Prognosis

Patients are treated in most cases exclusively by endonasal endoscopic surgery through marsupialization of the lesion [57]. For lateral or extensive frontal lesions, a combined approach with open surgery may be required [56]. The recurrence rate varies in different series and may be as high as 23% [56]. Lesions occurring in posterior ethmoid or sphenoid or in patients with multi-operated, chronic paranasal sinus inflammation are more prone to recur [56, 58].

Necrotizing Sialometaplasia

Definition

Necrotizing sialometaplasia (NSM) is a reactive change of seromucous glands that undergo coagulative necrosis and squamous metaplasia. Although it mainly involves the minor salivary glands of the palate, it may also occur in the sinonasal mucosa [59–63]. It is likely due to an ischemic event, and it is commonly associated with trauma or surgical procedures. It may also occur in association with sinusitis [64].

Clinical Features

NSM presents as a localized swelling that becomes ulcerated. Pain may be present.

Pathologic Features

Histologically, it is characterized by necrosis of the gland acini and squamous metaplasia of the ducts. Importantly, glandular lobular architecture is maintained (Fig. 20). Mucin spillage with inflammation may be present. The overlying epithelium can show pseudoepitheliomatous hyperplasia. However, dysplastic changes and abnormal mitotic figures are not observed.

Differential Diagnosis

The most important entities to be considered are squamous cell carcinoma squamous carcinoma and mucoepidermoid carcinoma. The presence of metaplastic squamous nest in the stroma may mimic invasive squamous carcinoma. However, the lobular architecture of the salivary gland is maintained, the squamous nest are round to oval and present a smooth contour, and there is no cytologic atypia. NSM may also be present in association with sinonasal squamous carcinoma [65].

The presence of mucin pools in association with metaplastic squamous epithelium may resemble mucoepidermoid carcinoma. In comparison, in NSM there is minimal cyst formation, there are no intermediate or clear cells, and there is true squamous differentiation, while in mucoepidermoid carcinoma, there are epidermoid cells rather than true squamous cells.

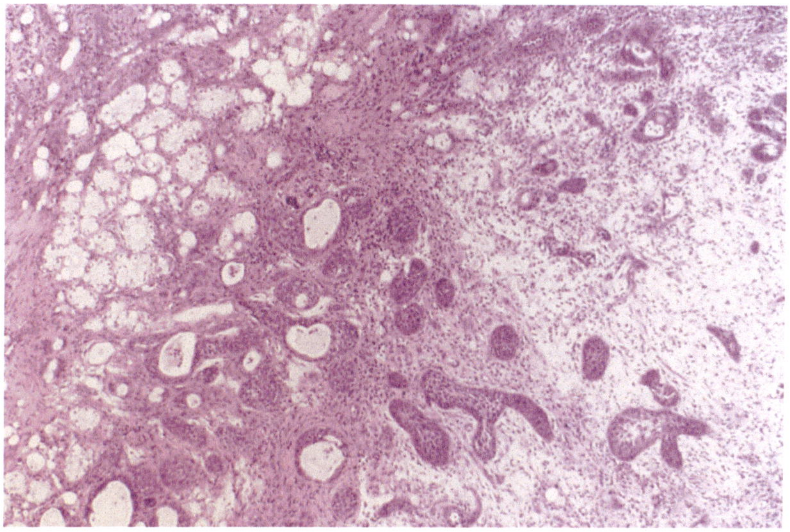

Fig. 20 Necrotizing sialometaplasia of the maxillary sinus mucosa. The squamous metaplastic component of the minor salivary gland maintains a characteristic lobular architecture

Treatment and Prognosis

Treatment is not necessary as the lesion heals spontaneously, usually within 5–6 weeks in average.

Organized Hematoma

Definition

Organized hematoma (OH) is a rare non-neoplastic lesion that causes mucosal swelling and bone destruction in the nasal cavities or in the paranasal sinuses [66]. Due to its expansive and destructive nature, it may be clinically confused with a malignant process.

Clinical Features

Patients are more frequently males with a mean age of 50 years, who present with frequent epistaxis and nasal obstruction [66–68]. Association with bleeding disorders, such as coagulation factor deficiency, end-stage renal failure, liver cirrhosis, or use of anticoagulation agents, have been well documented [67]. OH mainly originates in the maxillary sinus or nasal cavity unilaterally and presents as an expansile mass that extends into the nasal cavity. Frequently OH has an aggressive appearance on CT scans due to bone remodeling, erosion, and destruction, thus requiring differential diagnosis with a malignant tumor. However, MRI findings are usually indicative of hemorrhage and neovascularization and help in the distinction [69].

Pathologic Features

Grossly, the specimen consists more frequently of hemorrhagic fragments and clotted blood. Otherwise, the lesion may appear as a cyst with a thick fibrous wall containing clotted blood (Fig. 21). Histologically, there is abundant deposition of fibrinoid amorphous eosinophilic material, mixed with extravasated erythrocytes, fragments of dense fibrous tissue with hemosiderin deposition, and dilated vessels [70, 71].

Differential Diagnosis

The diagnosis is usually straightforward if the clinical presentation and the imaging features are known. Vascular tumors are the main differential diagnosis.

Treatment and Prognosis

Complete surgical removal is the treatment of choice [66–68]. Prior to surgery, angiography and coil embolization can be performed. A nasal endoscopic approach is usually preferred, but in patients with extensive bone destruction, the Caldwell-Luc approach has been used [66–68]. The treatment is curative and recurrence is rare.

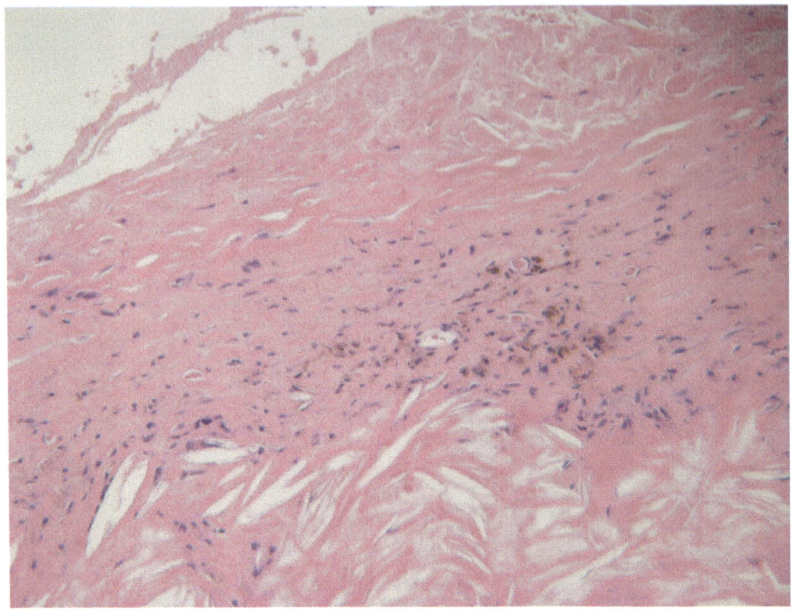

Fig. 21 Organized hematoma. The wall of the lesion consists of fibrinoid material adherent to a hyaline stroma with focal lymphohistiocytic infiltrate with cholesterol crystals

Amyloidosis

Definition

Amyloid is defined as an amorphous, eosinophilic proteinaceous deposit that shows a typical green birefringence in polarized light after staining with Congo red, the presence of non-branching linear fibrils of indefinite length with a mean diameter of 10 nm, and a distinct X-ray diffraction pattern consistent with a cross beta-fibril [72]. Amyloid deposits derive from protein precursors that differ in their primary structure and function, but they are all characterized by the ability to form aggregates under specific circumstances, which leads to the formation and deposition of amyloid [72].

Amyloidosis can be classified in acquired systemic, organ-limited, or localized forms. Moreover, amyloid deposits may be categorized according to whether they occur in association with an immunocyte dyscrasia and consist of immunoglobulin light chain deposition (AL) or with chronic infection, inflammatory diseases, or non-immunocyte neoplasia (amyloid associated—AA proteins) [73].

Clinical Features

Localized amyloid deposition in the sinonasal mucosa is very rare, with about 20 cases reported in the English literature [74–77].

Idiopathic primary sinonasal amyloidosis affects more frequently women over a wide age range, with a mean age at presentation of 34 years [76]. Nasal obstruction is the most common presenting symptom, followed in frequency by nasal discharge and epistaxis. Facial pain may also be present, and it is often associated with significant bony erosion [76]. The most common site of origin is the nasal cavity. Erosion of the bony walls of the sinonasal tract and of the skull base may mimic the clinical appearance of a malignant tumor.

Pathologic Features

Grossly, it presents either as an exophytic firm nodule or as a diffuse process with thickening of the mucosa. Histologically, there is a deposition of amorphous eosinophilic material in the stroma, around blood vessels, and around ducts of seromucous glands, which is often associated with diffuse chronic inflammation and foreign body granulomatous reaction (Fig. 22). Occasionally, amyloid deposits may appear as multiple globular eosinophilic deposits with a lamellar appearance reminiscent of corpora amylacea, which may be partially calcified [77]. Amyloid stains orange with Congo red and is typically apple-green birefringent at polarized light examination. The

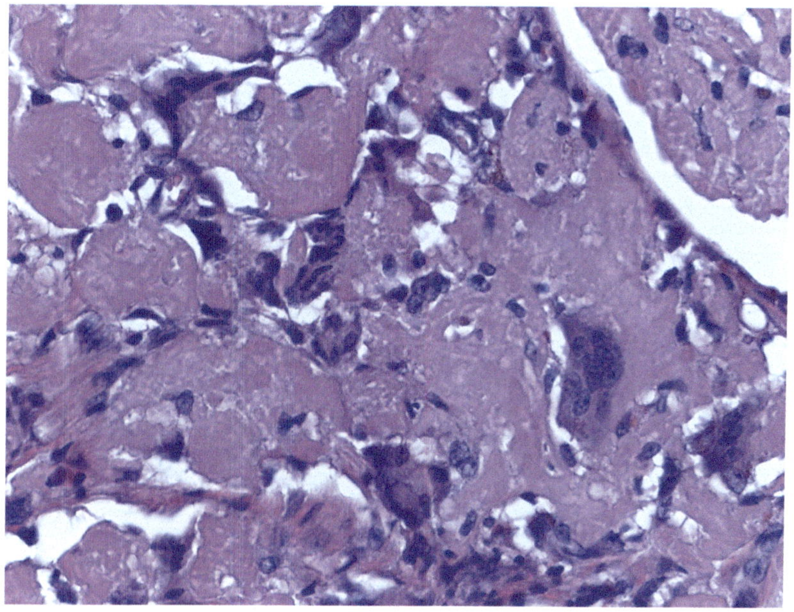

Fig. 22 Amyloid deposits consist of amorphous eosinophilic material with interspersed foreign body giant cells

Congophilia is lost after pretreatment of the tissue with potassium permanganate in cases of AA, beta 2 microglobulin, or apolipoprotein amyloid.

Immunohistochemical Features

Immunohistochemistry may help to identify the type of amyloid deposition. In the head and neck, most cases are of the primary (AL) type, and therefore they are positive for kappa or lambda light chain. Other protein constituents of systemic amyloid can be tested by immunohistochemistry [72, 78].

Differential Diagnosis

Amyloid deposits may be overlooked and/or confused with fibrosis or sclerotic changes of the mucosa.

Treatment and Prognosis

For sinonasal localized amyloidosis, conservative surgical removal relieves symptoms in most patients. However, systemic causes of amyloidosis, such as multiple myeloma, tuberculosis, and rheumatic diseases, must be excluded with appropriate tests.

Eosinophilic Angiocentric Fibrosis

Definition

Eosinophilic angiocentric fibrosis (EAF) is a rare benign lesion of unknown etiology which involves the sinonasal and upper respiratory tract mucosa. It was first reported by Holmes and Panje in 1983 as "intranasal granuloma faciale" [79], while Roberts and McCann coined the descriptive name 2 years later [80], based on the histologic appearance characterized by concentric fibrosis surrounding small-caliber arterioles, with numerous eosinophils scattered throughout the lesion. EAF is currently considered part of the spectrum of IgG4-related systemic disease [81].

Clinical Features

The most common presenting symptoms are nasal obstruction, nasal swelling, and deformities [82, 83]. The diagnosis is often delayed, with an average time from the onset of symptoms to diagnosis of 5–6 years [84, 85]. EAF is frequently associated with a prior history of sinonasal surgery or trauma [83]. Most patients are in the fourth and fifth decades, and there is no gender predilection [82, 83]. Elevated serum levels of IgG4 have been detected, in keeping with the hypothesis that EAF is a form of IgG4-related disease [81]. At clinical examination, the lesion appears as a submucosal thickening or a firm fibrotic mass, in most cases originating from the nasal septum.

Pathologic Features

The histologic picture in the early phases is dominated by a dense inflammatory infiltrate with

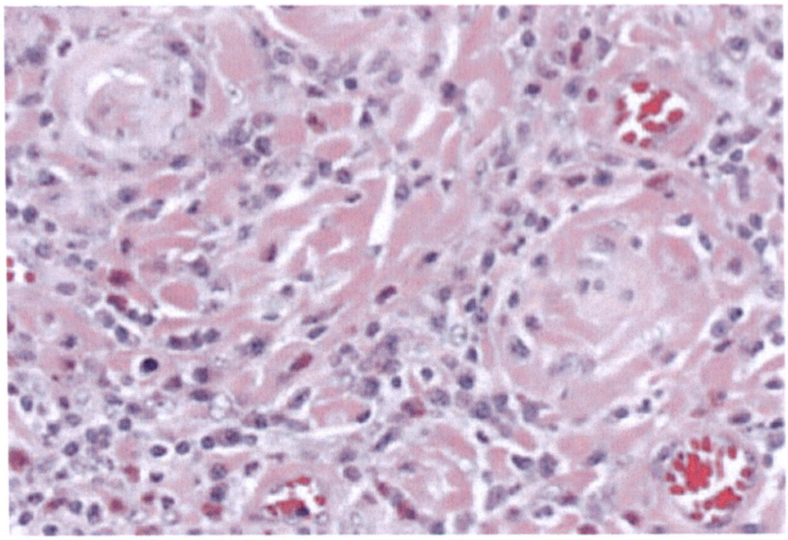

Fig. 23 Eosinophilic angiocentric fibrosis. Perivascular fibrosis with onion-skin type whorling pattern associated with an inflammatory infiltrate containing plasma cells and eosinophils (*Reproduced with permission from Jain R. et al, Head and Neck Pathol (2008) 2:309–315*)

numerous eosinophils, but lymphocytes, plasma cells, and neutrophils are present as well [81, 86]. The distinctive feature of EAF is the presence of small-caliber arterioles surrounded by concentric layers of fibrosis with an onion skinning appearance (Fig. 23). Whorled fibrosis is more prominent in the late stage, where it is associated with some degree of eosinophilic infiltration.

Immunohistochemical Findings

IgG4-positive plasma cells are identified in the majority of cases, with IgG4:IgG ratios ranging from 0.68 to 0.97 [81]. The stromal cells may show focal staining for smooth muscle actin or common muscle actin, while S100 and CD35 are negative [85, 87].

Differential Diagnosis

The differential diagnosis is broad and includes lesions with prominent inflammatory infiltrate rich in eosinophils. Nasal polyps and chronic sinusitis can be excluded based on the presence of the characteristic angiocentric fibrosis. Absence of necrosis, giant cells, and vasculitis help to distinguish EAF from Wegener granulomatosis and the Churg-Strauss syndrome. In addition, blood test positive for c-ANCA and p-ANCA supports the diagnosis of Wegener granulomatosis and Churg-Strauss syndrome, respectively [86]. Kimura disease can be excluded for the absence of dense lymphoid aggregates with prominent germinal centers. Granuloma faciale has many histologic features in common with EAF, and it is considered by some authors to represent the cutaneous manifestation of EAF [81, 88]. Patients with concurrent EAF and granuloma faciale have been reported [83].

Treatment and Prognosis

EAF is an indolent slowly progressive disease. Treatment consists of surgical resection alone or in combination with local and/or systemic corticosteroid administration. However, corticosteroid treatment does not seem to give an advantage in patient outcome over treatment with surgery alone. The recurrence rate in patients receiving only surgery is approximately 50% [83].

References

1. Walgama ES, Hwang PH. Aspirin-exacerbated respiratory disease. Otolaryngol Clin N Am. 2017;50:83–94.
2. Hellquist H. Nasal polyps update. Histopathology. Allergy Asthma Proc. 1996;17:237–42.
3. Ardehali MM, Amali A, Bakhshaee M, Madani Z, Amiri M. The comparison of histopathological characteristics of polyps in asthmatic and nonasthmatic patients. Otolaryngol Head Neck Surg. 2009;140:748–51.

4. Compagno J, Hyams VJ, Lepore ML. Nasal polyposis with stromal atypia. Review of follow-up study of 14 cases. Arch Pathol Lab Med. 1976;100:224–6.
5. Kindblom LG, Angerval L. Nasal polyps with atypical stromal cells: a pseudosarcomatous lesion: a light and electron microscopic and immunohistochemical investigation with implications on the type and nature of the mesenchymal cells. Acta Pathol Microbiol Immunol Scand. 1984;92:65–72.
6. Nakayama M, Wenig BM, Heffner DK. Atypical stromal cells in inflammatory nasal polyps: immunohistochemical and ultrastructural analysis in defining histogenesis. Laryngoscope. 1995;105:127–34.
7. Tuziak T, Kran A, Woyke S. Edematous nasal polyp with atypical stromal cells misdiagnosed cytologically as rhabdomyosarcoma. Acta Cytol. 1995;39:521–4.
8. Hadravsky L, Skalova A, Kacerovska D, et al. Angiomatoid change in polyps of the nasal and paranasal regions: an underrecognized and commonly misdiagnosed lesion. Report of 45 cases. Virchows Arch. 2012;460:203–9.
9. Heffner DK. Sinonasal angiosarcoma? Not likely (a brief description of infarcted nasal polyps). Ann Diagn Pathol. 2010;14:233–4.
10. Yfantis HG, Drachenberg CB, Gray W, Papadimitriou JC. Angiectatic nasal polyps that clinically simulate a malignant process. Report of 2 cases and a review of the literature. Arch Pathol Lab Med. 2000;124:406–10.
11. Sheahan P, Crotty PL, Hamilton S, Colreavy M, McShane D. Infarcted angiomatous polyps. Rhinology. 2004;262:225–30.
12. Southwood JE, Loehrl TA, Poetker DM. Advances in surgery: extended procedures for sinonasal polyp disease. Adv Otorhinolaryngol. 2016;79:148–57.
13. Thomas AJ, Alt JA. Oral therapeutics for rhinosinusitis with nasal polyposis. Adv Otorhinolaryngol. 2016;79:138–47.
14. Oakley GM, Harvey RJ. Topical steroids. Adv Otorhinolaryngol. 2016;79:121–30.
15. Halderman AA, Lane AP. Immunomodulators in the treatment of nasal polyposis. Adv Otorhinolaryngol. 2016;79:103–13.
16. Avdeeva K, Fokkens W. Precision medicine in chronic rhinosinusitis with nasal polyps. Curr Allergy Asthma Rep. 2018;18:25.
17. Brescia G, Zanotti C, Parrino D, Barion U, Marioni G. Nasal polyposis pathophysiology: endotype and phenotype open issues. Am J Otolaryngol. 2018;39:441–4.
18. Lee DH, Yoon TM, Lee JK, Lim SC. Difference of antrochoanal polyp between children and adults. Int J Pediatr Otorhinolaryngol. 2016;84:143–6.
19. Choudhury N, Hariri A, Saleh H, Sandison A. Diagnostic challenges of antrochoanal polyps: a review of sixty-one cases. Clin Otolaryngol. 2018;43:670–4.
20. Kelles M, Toplu Y, Yildirim I, Okur E. Antrochoanal polyp: clinical presentation and retrospective comparison of endoscopic sinus surgery and endoscopic sinus surgery plus mini-Caldwell surgical procedures. J Craniofac Surg. 2014;25:1779–81.
21. Al-Mazrou KA, Bukhari M, Al-Fayez A. Characteristics of antrochoanal polyps in the pediatric age group. Ann Thorac Med. 2009;4:133–6.
22. Behar PM, Muller S, Gerber ME, Todd NW. Heterotopic neuroglial tissue causing airway obstruction in the newborn. Arch Otolaryngol Head Neck Surg. 2001;127:997–1002.
23. Penner CR, Thompson LDR. Nasal glial heterotopia: a clinicopathologic and immunophenotypic analysis of 10 cases with a review of the literature. Ann Diagn Pathol. 2003;7:354–9.
24. Madjidi A, Couly G. Heterotopic neuroglial tissue of the face. Report of six cases and review of the literature. Oral Surg Oral Med Oral Pathol. 1993;76:284–8.
25. Adil E, Robson C, Perez-Atayde A, et al. Congenital nasal neuroglial heterotopia and encephaloceles: an update on current evaluation and management. Laryngoscope. 2016;126:2161–7.
26. Yeoh GP, Bale PM, de Silva M. Nasal cerebral heterotopia: the so-called nasal glioma or sequestered encephalocele and its variants. Pediatr Pathol. 1989;9:531–49.
27. Tetzlaff MT, Liu P, O'Malley BW Jr, LiVolsi VA, Elder D. Report of a case of sinonasal undifferentiated carcinoma arising in a background of extensive nasal gliomatosis. Head Neck. 2008;30:549–55.
28. Chan JK, Lau WH. Nasal astrocytoma or nasal glial heterotopia? Arch Pathol Lab Med. 1989;113:943–5.
29. Wenig BM, Franchi A, Ro JY. Tumours of the nasal cavity, paranasal sinuses and skull base: respiratory epithelial lesions: respiratory epithelial adenomatoid hamartoma. In: El-Naggar AK, Chan JKC, Grandis JR, Takata T, Slootweg PJ, editors. WHO classification of head and neck tumours. Lyon: IARC; 2017. p. 31–2.
30. Ro JY, Franchi A. Tumours of the nasal cavity, paranasal sinuses and skull base: respiratory epithelial lesions: seromucinous hamartoma. In: El-Naggar AK, JKC C, Grandis JR, Takata T, Slootweg PJ, editors. WHO classification of head and neck tumours. Lyon: IARC; 2017. p. 32.
31. Kossay M, El Zein S, Wassef M, et al. Olfactory epithelial hamartoma: a new subtype of sinonasal hamartoma. Am J Surg Pathol. 2018;42:9–17.
32. Wenig BM, Heffner DK. Respiratory epithelial adenomatoid hamartomas of the sinonasal tract and nasopharynx: a clinicopathologic study of 31 cases. Ann Otol Rhinol Laryngol. 1995;104:639–45.
33. Ozolek JA, Hunt JL. Tumor suppressor gene alterations in respiratory epithelial adenomatoid hamartoma (REAH): comparison to sinonasal adenocarcinoma and inflamed sinonasal mucosa. Am J Surg Pathol. 2006;30:1576–80.
34. Lee JT, Garg R, Brunworth J, Keschner DB, Thompson LD. Sinonasal respiratory epithelial adenomatoid hamartomas: series of 51 cases and literature review. Am J Rhinol Allergy. 2013;27:322–8.

35. Cao Z, Gu Z, Yang J, Jin M. Respiratory epithelial adenomatoid hamartoma of bilateral olfactory clefts associated with nasal polyposis: three cases report and literature review. Auris Nasus Larynx. 2010;37:352–6.
36. Delbrouck C, Fernandez Aguilar S, Choufani G, Hassid S. Respiratory epithelial adenomatoid hamartoma associated with nasal polyposis. Am J Otolaryngol. 2004;25:282–4.
37. Gauchotte G, Marie B, Gallet P, et al. Respiratory epithelial adenomatoid hamartoma: a poorly recognized entity with mast cell recruitment and frequently associated with nasal polyposis. Am J Surg Pathol. 2013;37:1678–85.
38. Choi E, Catalano PJ, Chang KG. Chondro-osseous respiratory epithelial hamartoma of the sinonasal tract. Otolaryngol Head Neck Surg. 2006;134:168–9.
39. Fang G, Wang C, Piao Y, Zhang L. Chondro-osseous respiratory epithelial adenomatoid hamartoma of the nasal cavity. Pediatr Int. 2016;58:229–31.
40. Jo VY, Mills SE, Cathro HP, et al. Low-grade sinonasal adenocarcinomas: the association with and distinction from respiratory epithelial adenomatoid hamartomas and other glandular lesions. Am J Surg Pathol. 2009;33:401–8.
41. Hua X, Huang X, Liao Z, Xian Q, Yu L. Clinicopathological and EBV analysis of respiratory epithelial adenomatoid hamartoma. Diagn Pathol. 2014;9:70.
42. Ozolek JA, Barnes EL, Hunt JL. Basal/myoepithelial cells in chronic sinusitis, respiratory epithelial adenomatoid hamartoma, inverted papilloma, and intestinal-type and nonintestinal-type sinonasal adenocarcinoma: an immunohistochemical study. Arch Pathol Lab Med. 2007;131:530–7.
43. Weinreb I. Low grade glandular lesions of the sinonasal tract: a focused review. Head Neck Pathol. 2010;4:77–83.
44. Weinreb I, Gnepp DR, Laver NM, et al. Seromucinous hamartomas: a clinicopathological study of a sinonasal glandular lesion lacking myoepithelial cells. Histopathology. 2009;54:205–13.
45. Khan RA, Chernock RD, Lewis JS Jr. Seromucinous hamartoma of the nasal cavity: a report of two cases and review of the literature. Head Neck Pathol. 2011;5:241–7.
46. Ambrosini-Spaltro A, Morandi L, Spagnolo DV, et al. Nasal seromucinous hamartoma (microglandular adenosis of the nose): a morphological and molecular study of five cases. Virchows Arch. 2010;457:727–34.
47. McDermott MB, Ponder TB, Dehner LP. Nasal chondromesenchymal hamartoma: an upper respiratory tract analogue of the chest wall mesenchymal hamartoma. Am J Surg Pathol. 1998;22:425–33.
48. Mason KA, Navaratnam A, Theodorakopoulou E, Chokkalingam PG. Nasal Chondromesenchymal hamartoma (NCMH): a systematic review of the literature with a new case report. J Otolaryngol Head Neck Surg. 2015;44:28.
49. Stewart DR, Messinger Y, Williams GM, et al. Nasal chondromesenchymal hamartomas arise secondary to germline and somatic mutations of DICER1 in the pleuropulmonary blastoma tumor predisposition disorder. Hum Genet. 2014;133:1443–50.
50. Ozolek JA, Carrau R, Barnes EL, Hunt JL. Nasal chondromesenchymal hamartoma in older children and adults: series and immunohistochemical analysis. Arch Pathol Lab Med. 2005;129:1444–50.
51. Behery RE, Bedrnicek J, Lazenby A, et al. Translocation t(12;17)(q24.1;q21) as the sole anomaly in a nasal chondromesenchymal hamartoma arising in a patient with pleuropulmonary blastoma. Pediatr Dev Pathol. 2012;15:249–53.
52. Li Y, Yang QX, Tian XT, Li B, Li Z. Malignant transformation of nasal chondromesenchymal hamartoma in adult: a case report and review of the literature. Histol Histopathol. 2013;28:337–44.
53. Lee TJ, Li SP, Fu CH, et al. Extensive paranasal sinus mucoceles: a 15-year review of 82 cases. Am J Otolaryngol. 2009;30:234–8.
54. Scangas GA, Gudis DA, Kennedy DW. The natural history and clinical characteristics of paranasal sinus mucoceles: a clinical review. Int Forum Allergy Rhinol. 2013;3:712–7.
55. Kim YS, Kim K, Lee JG, Yoon JH, Kim CH. Paranasal sinus mucoceles with ophthalmologic manifestations: a 17-year review of 96 cases. Am J Rhinol Allergy. 2011;25:272–5.
56. Devars du Mayne M, Moya-Plana A, Malinvaud D, Laccourreye O, Bonfils P. Sinus mucocele: natural history and long-term recurrence rate. Eur Ann Otorhinolaryngol Head Neck Dis. 2012;129:125–30.
57. Kennedy DW, Josephson JS, Zinreich SJ, et al. Endoscopic sinus surgery for mucoceles: a viable alternative. Laryngoscope. 1989;99:8858–95.
58. Loo JL, Looi AL, Seah LL. Visual outcomes in patient with paranasal mucoceles. Ophthal Plast Reconstr Surg. 2009;25:126–9.
59. Johnston WH. Necrotizing sialometaplasia involving the mucous glands of the nasal cavity. Hum Pathol. 1977;8:589–92.
60. Maisel RH, Johnston WH, Anderson HA, Cantrell RW. Necrotizing sialometaplasia involving the nasal cavity. Laryngoscope. 1977;87:429–34.
61. Chen KT. Necrotizing sialometaplasia of the nasal cavity. Am J Otolaryngol. 1982;3:444–6.
62. Close LG, Cowan DF. Recurrent necrotizing sialometaplasia of the nasal cavity. Otolaryngol Head Neck Surg. 1985;93:422–5.
63. Abrams AM. Necrotizing sialometaplasia of the nasal cavity. Otolaryngol Head Neck Surg. 1986;94:416.
64. Granich MS, Pilch BZ. Necrotizing sialometaplasia in the setting of acute and chronic sinusitis. Laryngoscope. 1981;91:1532–5.
65. Franchi A, Gallo O, Santucci M. Pathologic quiz case 1. Necrotizing sialometaplasia obscuring recurrent well-differentiated squamous cell carcinoma of the maxillary sinus. Arch Otolaryngol Head Neck Surg. 1995;121:584–6.
66. Pang W, Hu L, Wang H, et al. Organized hematoma: an analysis of 84 cases with emphasis on difficult pre-

diction and favorable management. Otolaryngol Head Neck Surg. 2016;154:626–33.
67. Choi SJ, Seo ST, Rha KS, Kim YM. Sinonasal organized hematoma: clinical features of seventeen cases and a systematic review. Laryngoscope. 2015;125:2027–33.
68. Kim JS, Oh JS, Kwon SH. The increasing incidence of paranasal organizing hematoma: a 20-year experience of 23 cases at a single center. Rhinology. 2016;54:176–82.
69. Kim EY, Kim HJ, Chung SK, et al. Sinonasal organized hematoma: CT and MR imaging findings. AJNR Am J Neuroradiol. 2008;29:1204–8.
70. Yokoi H, Arakawa A, Matsumoto F, Yokoi N, Ikeda K, Kohno N. Organized hematoma of the maxillary sinus: a clinicopathologic study of 5 cases. Ear Nose Throat J. 2014;93:E23–6.
71. Omura G, Watanabe K, Fujishiro Y, Ebihara Y, Nakao K, Asakage T. Organized hematoma in the paranasal sinus and nasal cavity—imaging diagnosis and pathological findings. Auris Nasus Larynx. 2010;37:173–7.
72. Röcken C, Sletten K. Amyloid in surgical pathology. Virchows Arch. 2003;443:3–16.
73. Glenner GG. Amyloid deposits and amyloidosis. The beta-fibrilloses. N Engl J Med. 1980;302(1283–1292):1333–43.
74. Mufarrij AA, Busaba NY, Zaytoun GM, Gallo GR, Feiner HD. Primary localized amyloidosis of the nose and paranasal sinuses. A case report with immunohistochemical observations and a review of the literature. Am J Surg Pathol. 1990;14:379–83.
75. Tsikoudas A, Martin-Hirsch DP, Woodhead CJ. Primary sinonasal amyloidosis. J Laryngol Otol. 2001;115:55–6.
76. Prasad D, Somayaji GK, Aroor R, Abdulla MN. Primary nasal amyloidosis. Internet J Otorhinolaryngol. 2009;9:2.
77. Kumar B, Pant B, Kumar V, Negi M. Sinonasal globular amyloidosis simulating malignancy: a rare presentation. Head Neck Pathol. 2016;10:379–83.
78. Schönland SO, Hegenbart U, Bochtler T, et al. Immunohistochemistry in the classification of systemic forms of amyloidosis: a systematic investigation of 117 patients. Blood. 2012;119:488–93.
79. Holmes DK, Panje WR. Intranasal granuloma faciale. Am J Otolaryngol. 1983;4:184–6.
80. Roberts PF, McCann BG. Eosinophilic angiocentric fibrosis of the upper respiratory tract: a mucosal variant of granuloma faciale? A report of three cases. Histopathology. 1985;9:1217–25.
81. Deshpande V, Khosroshahi A, Nielsen GP, Hamilos DL, Stone JH. Eosinophilic angiocentric fibrosis is a form of IgG4-related systemic disease. Am J Surg Pathol. 2011;35:701–6.
82. Heft Neal ME, Rowan NR, Willson TJ, Wang EW, Lee SE. A case report and systematic review of eosinophilic angiocentric fibrosis of the paranasal sinuses. Ann Otol Rhinol Laryngol. 2017;126:415–23.
83. Fang CH, Mady LJ, Mirani NM, Baredes S, Eloy JA. Sinonasal eosinophilic angiocentric fibrosis: a systematic review. Int Forum Allergy Rhinol. 2014;4:745–52.
84. Tabaee A, Zadeh MH, Proytcheva M, LaBruna A. Eosinophilic angiocentric fibrosis. J Laryngol Otol. 2003;117:410–3.
85. Thompson LD, Heffner DK. Sinonasal tract eosinophilic angiocentric fibrosis. A report of three cases. Am J Clin Pathol. 2001;115:243–8.
86. Jain R, Robblee JV, O'Sullivan-Mejia E, et al. Sinonasal eosinophilic angiocentric fibrosis: a report of four cases and review of literature. Head Neck Pathol. 2008;2:309–15.
87. Altemani AM, Pilch BZ, Sakano E, Altemani JM. Eosinophilic angiocentric fibrosis of the nasal cavity. Mod Pathol. 1997;10:391–3.
88. Stelini RF, Moysés MD, Cintra ML, et al. Granuloma faciale and eosinophilic angiocentric fibrosis: similar entities in different anatomic sites. Appl Immunohistochem Mol Morphol. 2017;25:213–20.

Part III

Sinonasal Tumors

Epithelial Tumors

Alessandro Franchi

Benign Epithelial Tumors

Sinonasal Papillomas

Definition

Sinonasal papillomas (SP; synonym: Schneiderian papilloma) are benign epithelial neoplasms that arise from the pseudostratified ciliated (or Schneiderian) epithelium that lines the nasal cavities and paranasal sinuses. Three major subtypes can be recognized: inverted (or endophytic), exophytic (or fungiform), and oncocytic. Each type presents distinct clinicopathologic features, and current molecular data (see below) support the hypothesis that SPs are not variants of a single entity but rather distinct subtypes [1–4].

Clinical Features

SP are rare tumors, and their estimated incidence is 1–2 cases per 100,000 inhabitants per year [5, 6]. Their salient clinicopathologic features are summarized in Table 1.

A. Franchi (✉)
Department of Translational Research and of New Technologies in Medicine and Surgery, University of Pisa, Pisa, Italy
e-mail: alessandro.franchi@unipi.it

The etiology of sinonasal papillomas remains unknown. Epidemiological studies have shown a significant relationship between industrial occupation, exposure to organic solvents, and inverted papilloma [7, 8], while cigarette smoking and alcohol consumption do not seem to be involved [9]. However, cigarette smoking is associated with increased risk of recurrence [10] and malignant transformation of ISP [11].

In addition, a role of HPV as potential etiological factor for sinonasal papillomas has been postulated in several studies (see below). Presenting symptoms are nonspecific and include unilateral nasal obstruction, epistaxis, facial pain, and purulent discharge. Usually, SPs are unilateral although they are often multifocal.

Pathologic Features

ESPs almost always originate from the nasal septum, while ISPs and OSPs characteristically arise in the lateral nasal wall and/or paranasal sinuses. Grossly, ESPs have papillary or warty appearance, whereas ISPs appear as firm, tan, or reddish polyps, with an undulating surface that, unlike inflammatory polyps (IPs), does not transilluminate [2]. OSPs are reddish-brown or tan, fleshy exophytic lesions.

The three types of SP present some common architectural and cytologic features, such as thickened epithelium (Fig. 1), presence of

A. Franchi (ed.), *Pathology of Sinonasal Tumors and Tumor-Like Lesions*,
https://doi.org/10.1007/978-3-030-29848-7_6

Table 1 Salient clinicopathologic features of sinonasal papillomas

	Exophytic	Inverted	Oncocytic
Frequency (%)	32	62	6
Age	III–V decades	V–VI decades	>50
Gender distribution (M:F)	2–10:1	3:1	1:1
Site	Nasal septum	Lateral nasal wall, paranasal sinuses	Lateral nasal wall, paranasal sinuses
Symptoms	Nasal obstruction, epistaxis	Nasal obstruction, epistaxis, rhinorrhea	Nasal obstruction, epistaxis
Etiology	HPV (mainly HPV 6/11)	*EGFR* mutations; HPV < 20%, mainly HPV6/11	*KRAS* mutations
Malignant transformation	Extremely rare	2–20%	5–15%

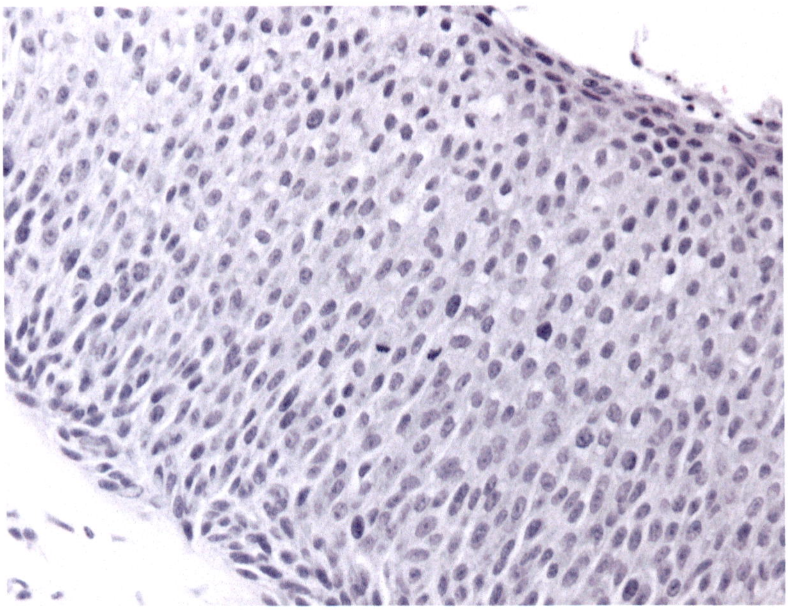

Fig. 1 The epithelium of this exophytic papilloma is thick and shows maturation. Mitotic figures are present in the middle layers

scattered mucous cells (Fig. 2), mucin-filled microcysts, and intraepithelial neutrophils, either as single transmigrating cells or forming microabscesses (Fig. 3). ESPs are composed of papillary fronds with a thin central core of fibrovascular tissue lined most often by a thick (5–20 cells) non-keratinizing squamous epithelium, but transitional and columnar-ciliated respiratory epithelia are also observed (Fig. 4). Scattered mucin-containing cells are often present. Koilocytic changes of the superficial squamous epithelium, including nuclear enlargement, hyperchromasia, multinucleation, and perinuclear "haloes," can be present. Keratinization is usually absent or scant, unless the lesion has been irritated or exposed to the drying effect of the air.

ISP is characterized by an endophytic growth pattern with multiple invaginations of the surface epithelium into the underlying stroma, although some degree of exophytic growth may be seen at the surface. In histologic sections, rounded, elongated, and anastomosing epithelial nests surrounded by an intact basement membrane grow downward in the stroma (Figs. 5 and 6), that may be edematous or show a mixed inflammatory infiltrate, with macrophages and neutrophils, but eosinophils may also be present. The lesion may involve the underlying bone, a finding that should

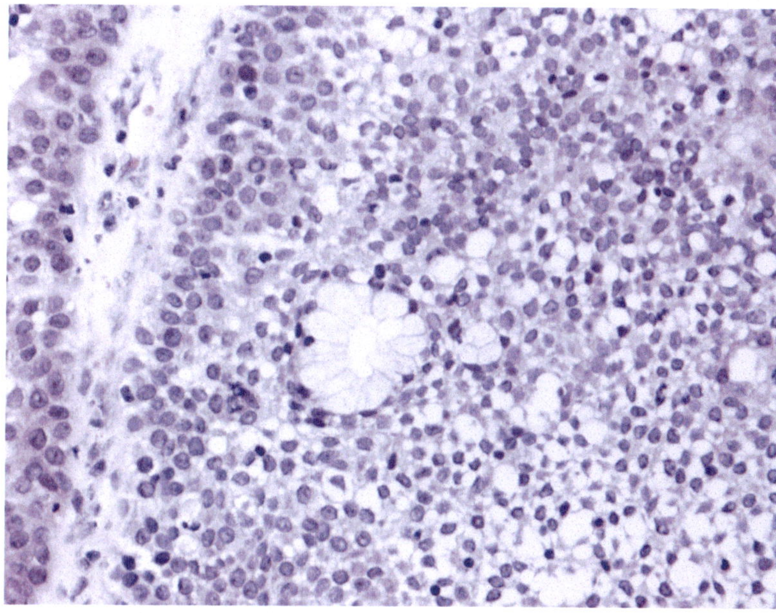

Fig. 2 Mucous cells within the epithelial lining of a sinonasal papilloma

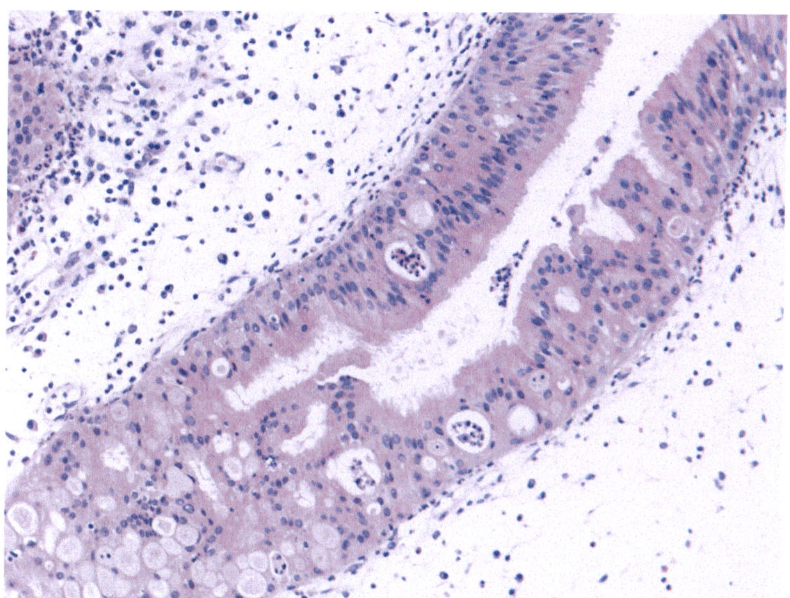

Fig. 3 Oncocytic sinonasal papilloma with intraepithelial microabscesses

not be misinterpreted as evidence of malignant transformation. The neoplastic epithelium is most often of the non-keratinizing squamous type (5–30 cells thick), but the surface of the epithelial lining may be covered by ciliated respiratory epithelium, which often merges with a transitional-type epithelium. "Transitional" cells present monotonous bland nuclei and scant eosinophilic cytoplasm. Scattered mucocytes are present. Up to 20% of ISPs may show some degree of cellular atypia, a finding that should prompt to thorough examination of the lesion. Mitotic figures may also be seen, but they are limited to the basal and parabasal layers. Typically, there are no or few adjacent submucosal seromucinous glands. ISP may also be associated with sinonasal hamartomas.

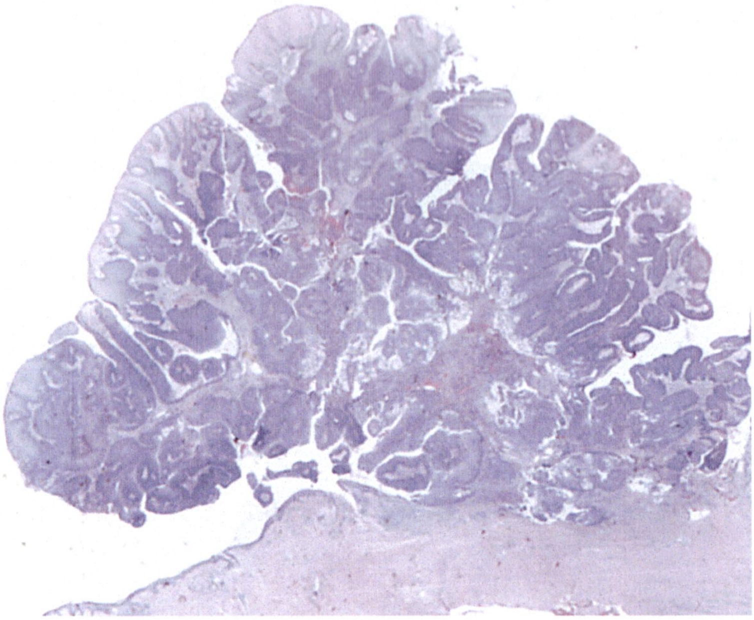

Fig. 4 Exophytic sinonasal papilloma composed of papillary fronds with a thin central core of fibrovascular tissue lined by thick non-keratinizing squamous epithelium

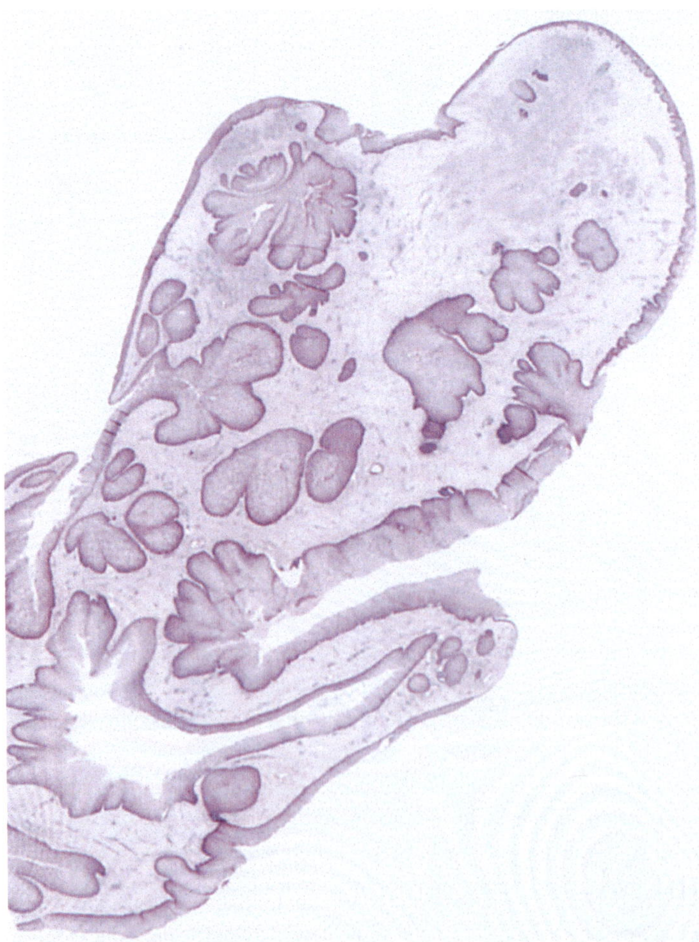

Fig. 5 Inverted sinonasal papilloma presenting an endophytic growth pattern

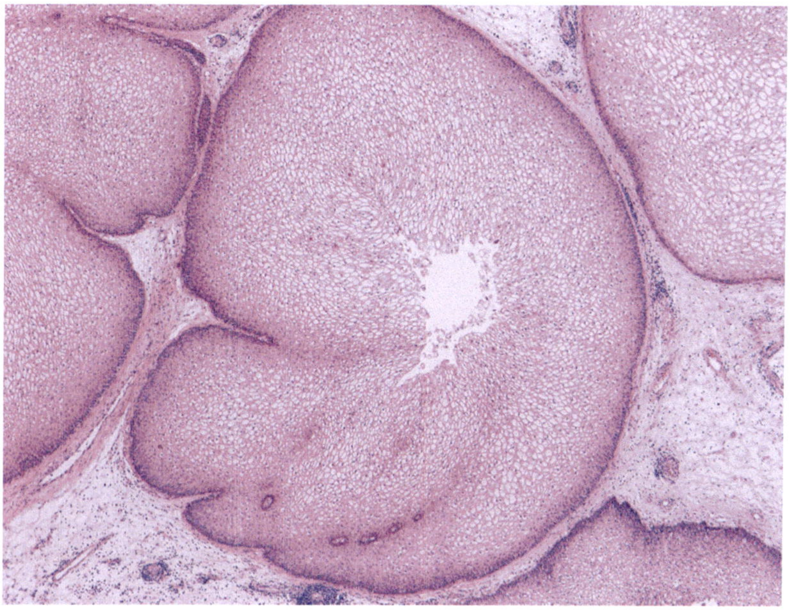

Fig. 6 The epithelial islands of inverted sinonasal papilloma present regular smooth borders and are devoid of atypia

OSP presents both exophytic and endophytic growth patterns (Fig. 7). The multilayered epithelium (2–8 cells thick) consists of tall columnar cells with oncocytic features, showing abundant finely granular eosinophilic cytoplasm and small hyperchromatic or slightly vesicular nuclei with small nucleoli. The outermost cells may present cilia in various stages of regression (Fig. 8). Intraepithelial cysts containing neutrophils and/or mucin are frequently seen. The stroma is edematous to fibrous and contains few inflammatory cells.

Almost constantly the histologic appearance of an SP allows its assignment to a specific subtype, but in rare instances it may present mixed features, with both areas of ISP and ESP or ISP and OSP [2].

Immunohistochemical Findings

ISPs are positive for cytokeratins associated with columnar and squamous differentiation while inflammatory polyps are negative for the latter [12].

Molecular Features

Recent studies have identified recurrent genetic alterations that characterize the different histologic subtypes of SP. ISP presents activating *EGFR* mutations in nearly 90% of the cases [13]. These mutations are considered to be the initiating events in ISP pathogenesis and appear to be mutually exclusive with HPV infection [14]. Identical mutations are present in squamous cell carcinomas (SCCs) arising in ISP, providing evidence of a biologic link between these tumors and supporting the use of EGFR inhibitors in the treatment of these patients [13].

Conversely, OSP does not present *EGFR* mutations, but in 100% of the cases these tumors show *KRAS* mutations that, in turn, are not present in ISP [15]. Again, identical mutations are detected in OSP and concurrent associated carcinomas supporting the role of OSP as a precursor to sinonasal carcinomas [15].

The role of HPV in the pathogenesis of SP and their progression to carcinoma remains controversial. HPV can be detected in 40% of all SP, but with significant differences according to

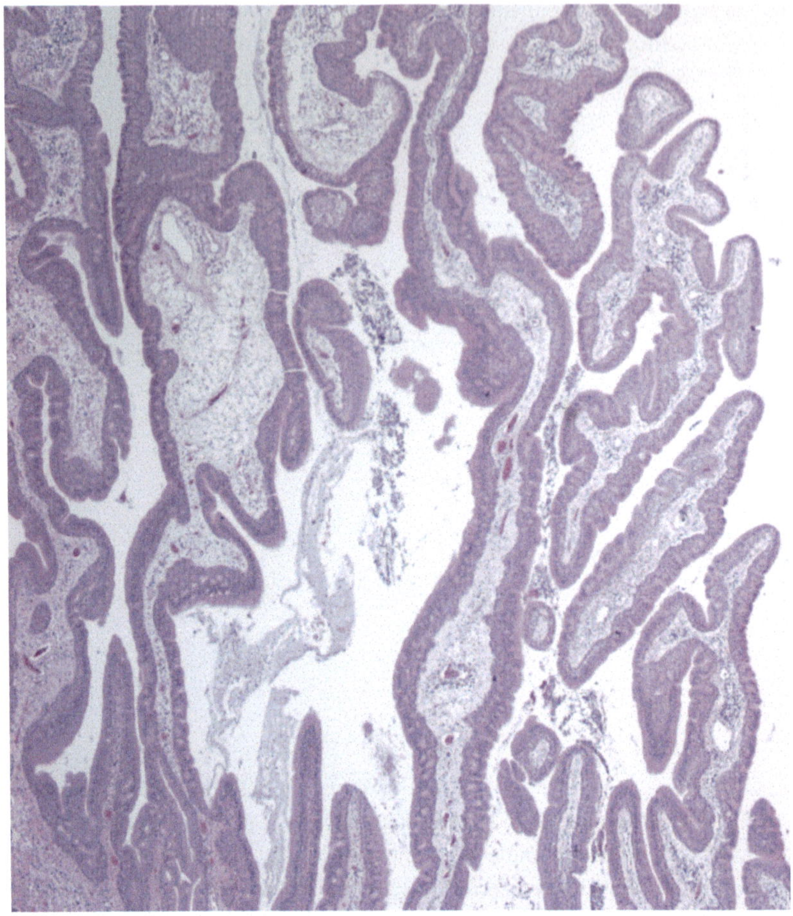

Fig. 7 Oncocytic (cylindrical cell) papilloma with an exophytic growth

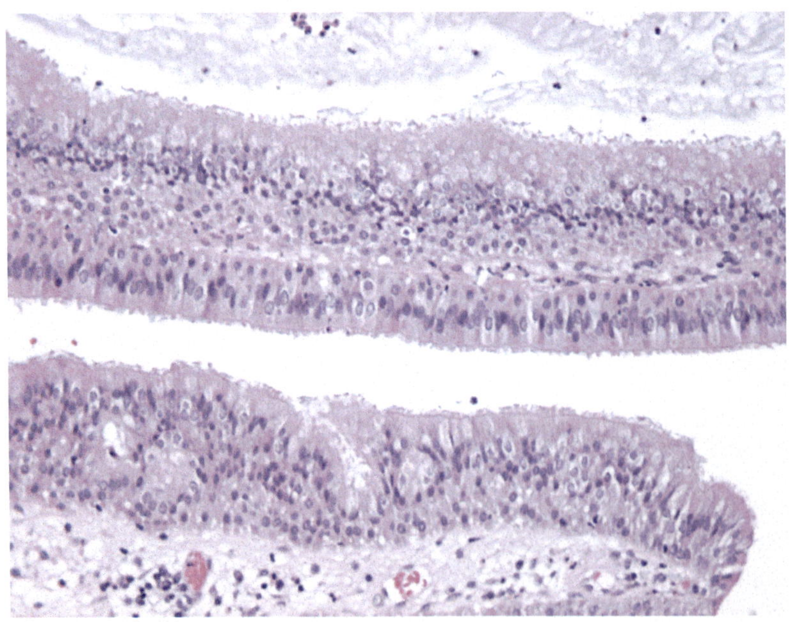

Fig. 8 The outermost epithelial cells are ciliated

the histologic types and to the methods of detection. The highest prevalence has been found in ESP (65%), followed by ISP (38%) and OSP (20%) [16]. Low-risk HPV types (6 and 11) are more frequently detected than high risk types (16, 18, and very rarely 31 and 33). However, even studies employing more recently developed methods of HPV detection that distinguish biologically active HPV from inactive, "passenger" virus, such as in situ hybridization for E6/E7 mRNA, still reported highly different prevalence of HPV infection in ISP [17, 18]. Another controversial aspect is the possible role of HPV in the transformation of ISP in carcinoma, with studies supporting a role for high-risk HPV types in the onset of dysplastic changes and invasive carcinoma [19] and others showing a very low frequency or even absence of high-risk HPV in transformed ISPs [18]. More recent data show that *EGFR* mutations and HPV infection represent mutually exclusive mechanisms in the development of ISP and carcinoma ex-ISP and that the same HPV low-risk types can be found in ISP and matched carcinoma [14].

Differential Diagnosis

SPs must be separated from several benign and malignant sinonasal lesions. ESP can be distinguished from squamous papilloma of the nasal vestibule because the latter shows a keratinizing squamous epithelium and lacks mucous cells and ciliated or transitional epithelium. Sinonasal polyps can sometimes be confused with ESP and ISP, especially if they present squamous metaplasia of the surface epithelium. Features of sinonasal polyps that are not seen in SP are thickening and hyalinization of the basement membrane, prominent seromucous glands, and presence of numerous inflammatory cells, especially eosinophils. In addition, the epithelium of sinonasal polyps lacks the transmigration of neutrophils seen in SP. Respiratory epithelial adenomatoid hamartoma (REAH) typically arises from the posterior septum and presents an inverted growth pattern that frequently causes confusion with IP. However, REAH is composed of gland-like structures lined by ciliated respiratory epithelium, which may also be seen in ISP but is usually not dominant. In addition, the basement membranes around the epithelial islands in ISP are thin and not thick and hyalinized as those seen in REAH.

Invasive squamous cell carcinoma, especially the non-keratinizing variant, can be very difficult to separate from ISP (Figs. 9 and 10). Presence of significant nuclear pleomorphism, atypical mitoses, an increased epithelium to stroma ratio, desmoplastic stromal reaction with loss of the basement membrane, and destructive invasion of cartilage and bony structures support the diagno-

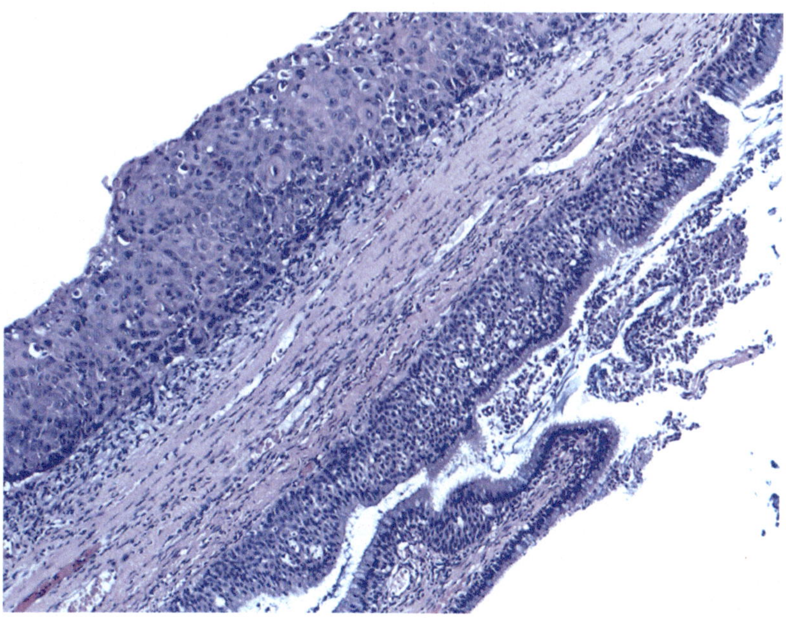

Fig. 9 Sinonasal papilloma with areas of "in situ" carcinoma. Such finding must prompt the search for areas of invasive carcinoma

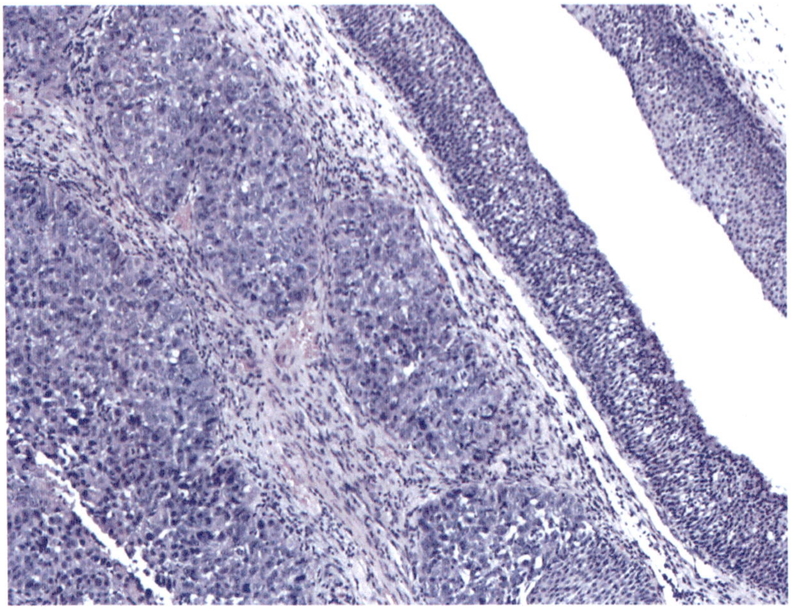

Fig. 10 Same case as in Fig. 9. Areas of invasive poorly differentiated non-keratinizing carcinoma

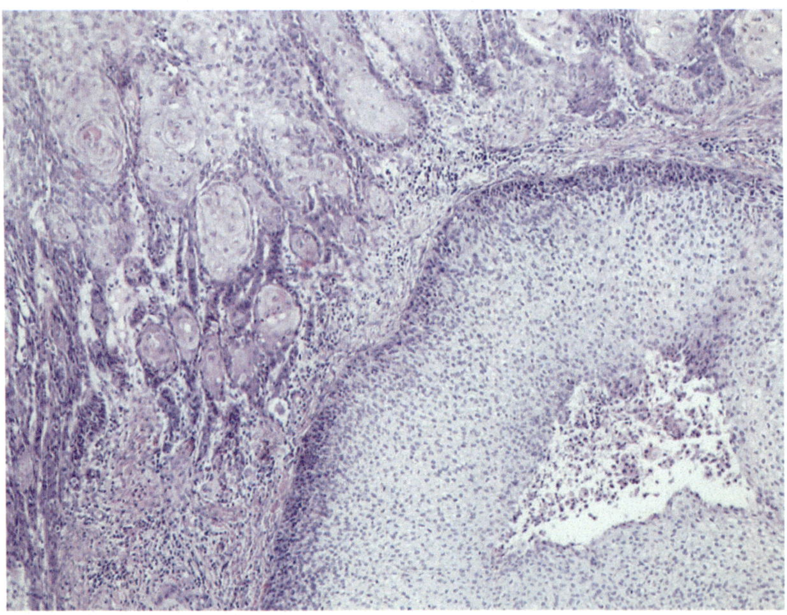

Fig. 11 Keratinizing squamous cell carcinoma arising in inverted sinonasal papilloma

sis of squamous carcinoma (Fig. 11). A couple of examples of the so-called low-grade papillary Schneiderian carcinoma"have been reported in the literature [20, 21]. Such tumors mimic quite closely the histologic appearance of SPs, presenting with papillary and inverted growth patterns of uniformly round and polygonal stratified cells, with no significant atypia and mitotic activity. However, they lack the respiratory-type columnar to squamous gradation (or "transitional" pattern) that is typical of inverted and exophytic Schneiderian papillomas and do not present intraepithelial neutrophils and mucus cells [20].

The main differential diagnosis of OSP is with low-grade adenocarcinomas of intestinal and non-intestinal type. Usually, sinonasal low-grade adenocarcinomas present a single-layered non-oncocytic epithelium. Moreover, nuclear atypia, mitotic activity, true lumen formation, presence of back-to-back glands, and stromal invasion are not features of OSP and support the diagnosis of adenocarcinoma.

Treatment and Prognosis

Surgery is the treatment of choice of SPs, and a purely trans-nasal endoscopic approach may be currently considered the gold standard in the vast majority of patients, whereas only a minority of cases require a combined or external approach [22–26]. The recurrence rate does not appear to be related to the type of surgical approach [26]. The average recurrence rate is 13% for endoscopic procedures and 14–17% for lateral rhinotomy with medial maxillectomy, but it is as high as 58% for limited endonasal procedures [27]. Most recurrences present within 24 months, but late relapses can also be observed. IP of the frontal sinus tends to show a higher rate of recurrences, in comparison with those of the maxillary sinus and naso-ethmoidal complex [26, 27].

Malignant transformation is a well-known event in SPs, with a reported frequency that varies greatly among different series (2–27%). However, this phenomenon is rare, since in a recent analysis of a large series of SPs, the frequency of malignant transformation was 1.9% [28]. Clinically, nasal bleeding, pain, bone destruction, and extent of disease on CT and MRI findings may indicate malignancy [29]. However, malignancy is only infrequently suspected before surgical removal of the lesion and histopathologic examination [29]. ISP and OSP are more prone to malignant progression, while only rare examples of carcinomas arising in ESP have been observed [28].

In general, development of an invasive carcinoma does not seem to be related to the number of recurrences of the SP. Indeed, in the majority of the cases, the patient presents synchronous SP and carcinoma, while the metachronous development of invasive carcinoma after SP recurrence is less frequent [28].

Histologically, over 80% of carcinomas ex-SP are squamous cell carcinomas (both keratinizing and non-keratinizing) (Figs. 9, 10, and 11), while only sporadic examples of mucoepidermoid carcinoma, low-grade adenocarcinoma, sinonasal undifferentiated carcinoma (SNUC), and carcinoma NOS have been reported [28, 30–32]. The majority of patients presents in advanced stage, and approximately 40% dies with local or disseminated disease, usually within 3 years from the diagnosis. Treatment consists of surgery followed by radiotherapy.

Some attempts have been made to identify histopathological features indicative of risk of recurrence and malignant transformation of SP [33, 34]. Among these, increase in hyperkeratosis, presence of squamous epithelial hyperplasia, presence of more than two mitoses per high power field, and absence of associated areas of inflammatory polyp have been related to increased risk for recurrence. The so-called dysplasia" of the epithelial lining of the papilloma has been proposed as predictive factor. However, the lack of well-defined and reproducible criteria to assess and grade "dysplasia" in SP is a significant limit to its practical use and may explain the variable results reported in the literature. Similarly, HPV status has not been clearly shown to correlate with malignant transformation of SP [18].

Salivary Gland-Type Adenomas

Definition

Salivary gland-type adenomas are benign tumors originating from the seromucous glands of the sinonasal mucosa that replicate the histologic appearance of adenomas of oral salivary gland. Overall, they are rare tumors, and pleomorphic adenoma (PA) is the most common histologic type. Other tumor types are oncocytoma, myoepithelioma, and basal cell adenoma.

Clinical Features

Sinonasal PA occurs over a wide age range (20–80 years), with a mean of 50 years, with no significant gender predilection [35, 36]. Most patients present with nasal obstruction, and a significant number shows also nasal deformity [35]. The duration of symptoms ranges between 1 month and 2 years [35]. The most common primary sites are the nasal septum and the lateral nasal wall [35, 36].

Pathologic Features

Sinonasal PAs appear as polypoid, broad-based swellings, and histologically, although similar to their counterparts of major salivary glands, they tend to be more cellular, with little or no stromal component, thus simulating more aggressive epithelial neoplasms [37]. Histologically, the tumor grows in the subepithelial tissue and is well demarcated, often with a thin collagenous capsule that separates it from the surrounding connective tissue [38] (Fig. 12). Epithelial, basal, and modified myoepithelial elements are intermixed with variable amounts of myxoid, chondroid, or hyaline stroma (Fig. 13). Cuboidal or columnar epithelial cells form ducts and small tubules or can be arranged in cribriform structures. Myoepithelial cells with various morphology (epithelioid, plasmacytoid, spindle, clear, oncocytic) are arranged in sheets, small islands, or trabeculae (Fig. 13). Foci of squamous metaplasia with keratinization can be present (Fig. 13). An unusual case of nasal PA showing bona fide skeletal muscle differentiation has been described by Lam and coworkers, raising the practical issue of possible confusion with rhabdomyosarcoma [39]. As in the oral counterparts, nuclear atypia can be present in sinonasal PA, especially in foci rich in myoepithelial cells, and it is interpreted as a degenerative change similar to the "ancient" change in schwannomas. Mitotic figures are sparse, and areas of hemorrhage and necrosis are not usually present.

Sporadic cases of sinonasal *myoepithelioma* have been described, including examples with spindle cell morphology, that require distinction from epithelial and mesenchymal tumors [40].

In sinonasal *oncocytoma*, neoplastic cells with abundant eosinophilic granular cytoplasm as a consequence of a high mitochondrial content are arranged in solid sheets, trabecular, and duct-like structures (Figs. 14 and 15). Evidence of infiltration, cellular pleomorphism and atypia, and frequent mitoses is associated with higher risk of recurrence and distant metastases. Such cases have also been reported as oncocytic carcinomas [41].

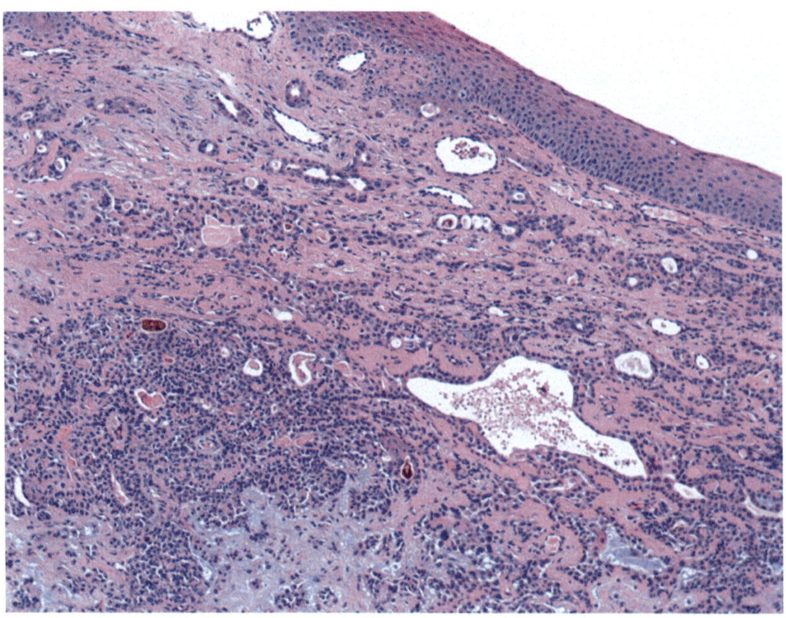

Fig. 12 Pleomorphic adenoma of the nasal septum. The tumor is not encapsulated and grows in the subepithelial space

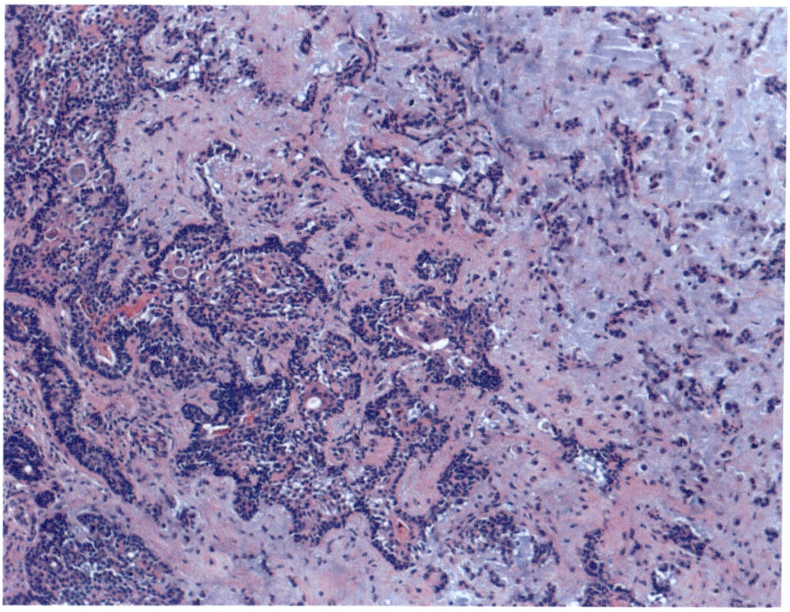

Fig. 13 Pleomorphic adenoma of the nasal septum. The tumor presents various growth patterns of epithelial and myoepithelial elements, including foci of squamous metaplasia. Tumor cells produce myxoid matrix

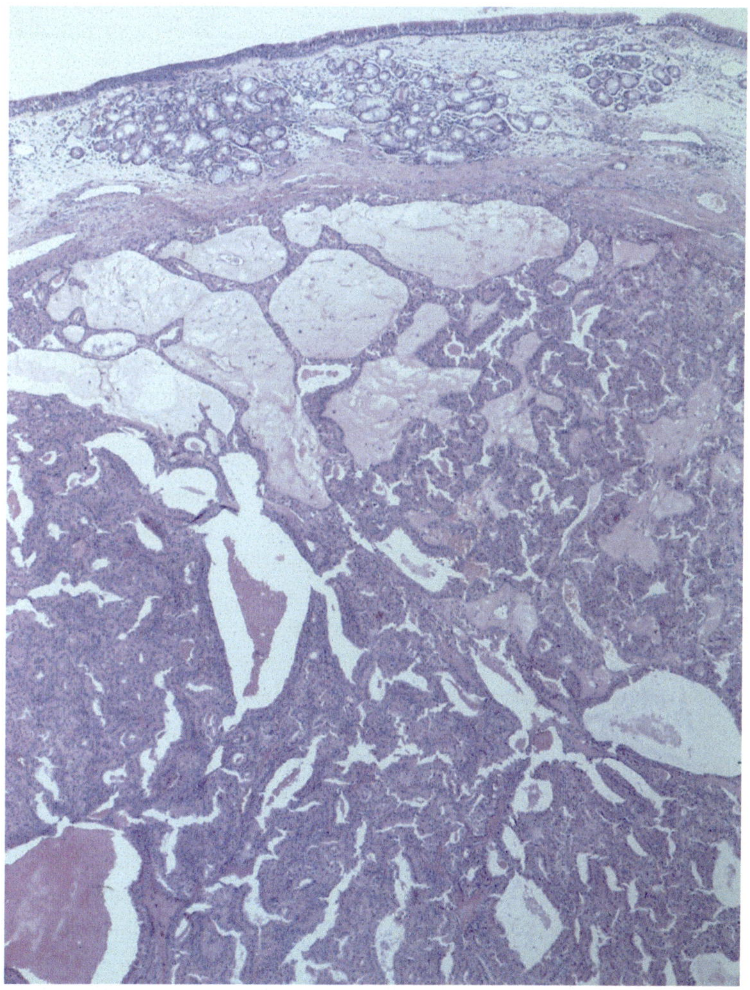

Fig. 14 Sinonasal oncocytoma. Low power view showing the tumor growing in the subepithelial space with well-circumscribed margins

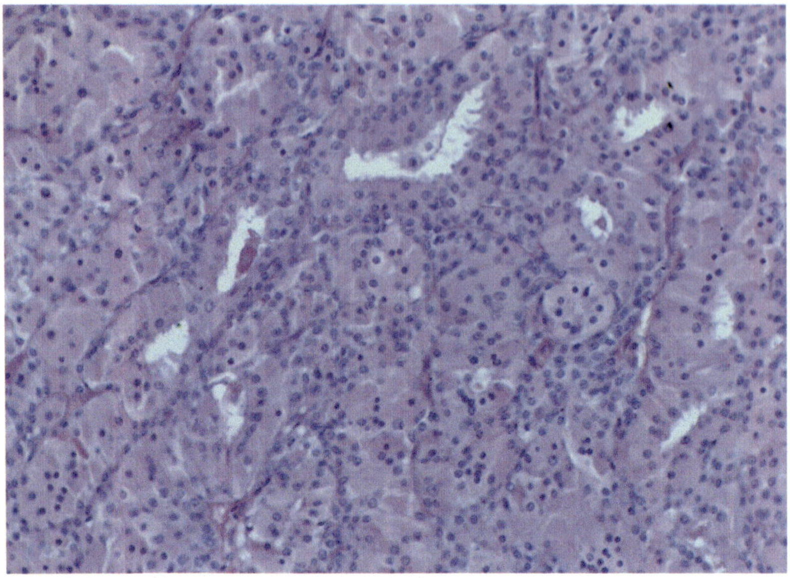

Fig. 15 Sinonasal oncocytoma. Neoplastic cells present abundant eosinophilic granular cytoplasm and are arranged in solid sheets, nests, and duct-like structures

Immunohistochemical Findings

The immunohistochemical findings are similar to those of PA of the parotid gland [38, 42]. Cytokeratins are positive in luminal cells of tubular structures and in abluminal cells and myoepithelial cells. Vimentin, GFAP, S100, calponin, and p63 are variably positive in the non-luminal or modified myoepithelial cells, whereas actins are usually negative or only focally positive.

Molecular Features

PA presents gene rearrangements that result in gene fusions involving the *PLAG* gene on chromosome 8q12. However, tumors arising in the nasal cavities have not been tested for this translocation so far.

Differential Diagnosis

PA should be distinguished from other salivary-type adenoma, including myoepithelioma and basal cell adenoma. PA with areas of squamous and mucinous metaplasia has to be distinguished from mucoepidermoid carcinoma, while the presence of cribriform epithelial areas requires distinction from adenoid cystic carcinoma.

Treatment and Prognosis

The mainstay of sinonasal PA treatment is complete surgical excision with clear margins, and the majority of cases may be surgically accessed through an endonasal, endoscopic approach [36]. Local recurrence occurs in approximately 20% of patients [36].

One example of metastasizing PA to a submandibular lymph node, in a patient with recurrent septal PA, has been reported [43]. Development of a carcinoma ex-PA is a rare but well-recognized possibility [44–47].

Ameloblastoma

Definition

Ameloblastoma is a benign locally aggressive epithelial odontogenic tumor that usually originates from the mandible or the maxilla. True primary sinonasal ameloblastoma (SA) without connection to gnathic sites is an uncommon tumor [48–50]. To explain its origin, it has been hypothesized that due to the contiguity of the nasal and oral cavities during the embryonic development, the sinonasal tract mucosa may either incorporate odontogenic epithelium or acquire cells capable of odontogenesis during development [48].

Clinical Features

SA affects adult patients (mean age 60 years), with a male predilection of 4:1 [48]. The patients present with a mass lesion, nasal obstruction, epistaxis, facial swelling, dizziness, and headaches [48]. The tumor may originate from the nasal cavity (nasal septum or lateral wall), the paranasal sinuses (maxillary, frontal, ethmoid, sphenoid), or both.

Pathologic Features

The tumor tissue is solid and polypoid in appearance, firm to rubbery in consistency. Histologically, the plexiform pattern predominates in the majority of the cases [48]. The tumor strands present a characteristic peripheral palisading of the columnar epithelium, which shows reverse polarized nuclei due to a subnuclear cytoplasmic vacuolization that displaces the nucleus away from the basement membrane (Fig. 16). The stellate reticulum cell component occupies the central core and consists of loosely arranged angulated cells (Fig. 17). Squamous metaplasia and keratinization are occasionally present in the central portion of the epithelial islands (acanthomatous pattern). The follicular pattern, characterized by islands of neoplastic epithelium that resemble the epithelial component of the enamel organ, is rarely seen [48]. The neoplastic epithelium is in direct continuity with intact sinonasal surface mucosal epithelium in the majority of the cases.

Immunohistochemical Profile

Neoplastic cells exhibit strong immunoreactivity for cytokeratins (AE1/AE3, CK 5, 14, and 19), and calretinin is positive in 90% of the cases [51].

Molecular Features

In a study of 29 gnathic osseous and peripheral head and neck ameloblastomas, low-risk HPV was detected in a peripheral tumor from an HIV-positive patient [52]. This tumor originated from the maxillary sinus and had recurred several times to the adjacent skin and soft tissue [52]. This finding was interpreted to represent more likely a coincidental secondary infection by HPV in the setting of HIV-related immunosuppression [52]. No case showed positivity for high-risk HPV in this series [52].

Gnathic ameloblastomas present mutations in genes of the MAPK pathway, with *BRAF* V600E being the most commonly observed. However, molecular studies of SA are currently lacking.

Differential Diagnosis

Before making a diagnosis of SA, an extension of a gnathic tumor in the nasal cavities should be excluded by reviewing the imaging features of

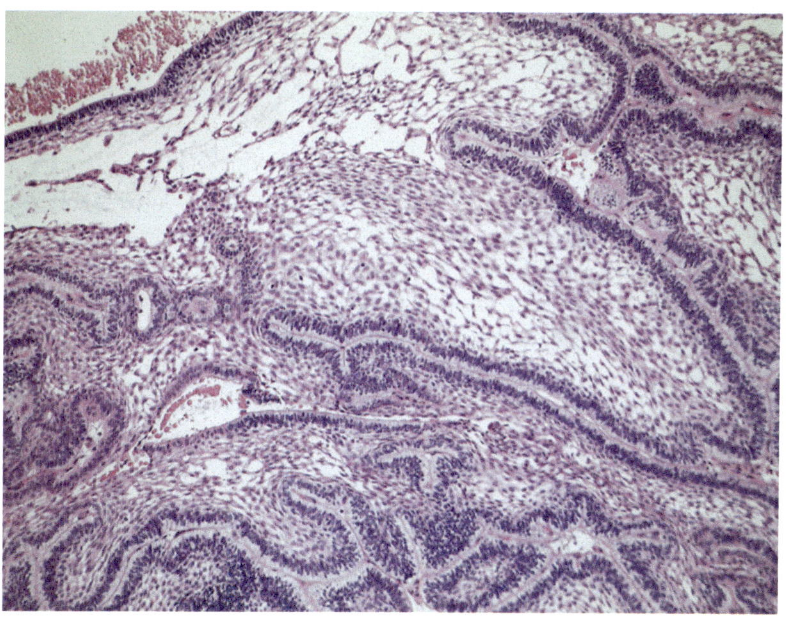

Fig. 16 Ameloblastoma of the maxillary sinus. The tumor islands beneath the respiratory-type surface epithelium present a characteristic peripheral palisading of the columnar epithelium

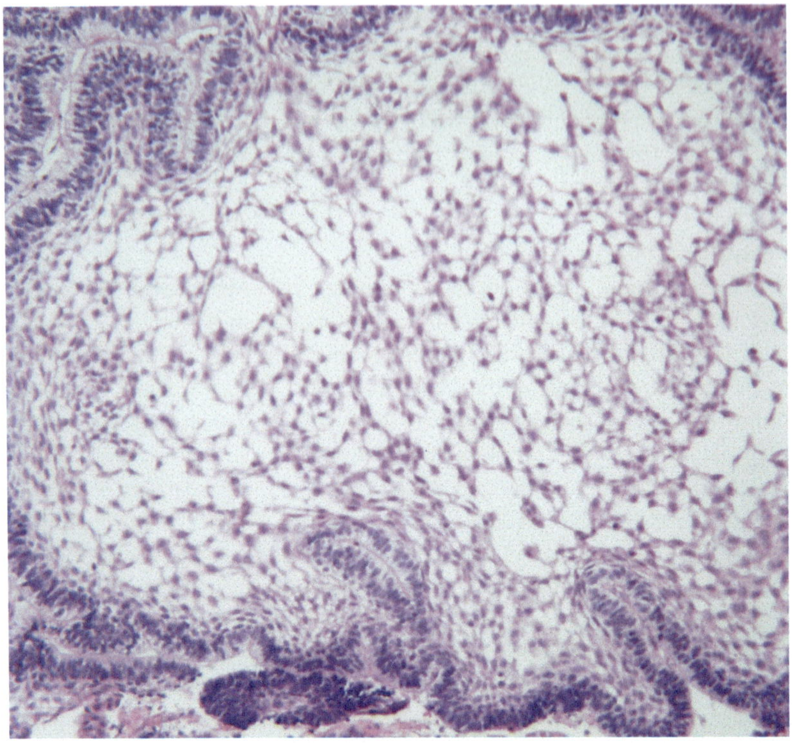

Fig. 17 Ameloblastoma of the maxillary sinus. The stellate reticulum cell component occupies the central core and consists of loosely arranged angulated cells

the tumor. The main histologic differential diagnosis of SA is with basaloid squamous cell carcinoma. The typical peripheral palisading with reverse polarization of ameloblastoma is not present in basaloid squamous cell carcinoma, which in addition usually presents areas of necrosis, brisk mitotic activity, and cellular atypia.

Treatment and Prognosis

The treatment of choice is complete surgical resection that can be accomplished with conservative endoscopic approaches in most cases. No distant metastases or tumor-related deaths have been documented. Local recurrence may occur in incompletely resected tumors, usually within 2–3 years of the initial treatment [48].

Malignant Epithelial Tumors

Squamous Cell Carcinoma

Definition

Squamous cell carcinoma (SCC) is a malignant epithelial tumor arising from the surface epithelium of the sinonasal tract showing squamous differentiation.

Clinical Features

SCC is by far the most frequent sinonasal malignant tumor, representing up to 75% of sinonasal neoplasms [52]. The overall average incidence from 1973 to 2009 was 0.36 cases per 100,000 patients, and a significant decrease has been noted in the last 30 years [52]. There is a clear predominance of the male gender (1.81:1 male-to-female prevalence ratio), with 80% of cases reported in patients older than 55 [52]. Some industrial work exposure and cigarette smoking have been associated with development of sinonasal SCC (see Part I). In addition, SCC may arise from a pre-existing sinonasal papilloma. The primary tumor site is the nasal cavity in 45% of the cases and the paranasal sinuses (mainly the maxillary sinus) in 55%. Presenting symptoms are nonspecific and include nasal obstruction, epistaxis and rhinorrhea, while facial pain, proptosis, and diplopia are present in advanced stage tumors.

Pathologic Features

Grossly, the lesion is white and friable, with areas hemorrhage and necrosis. The growth pattern may be mainly exophytic or with diffuse invasion and destruction of adjacent structures. The surface is often ulcerated.

Histologically, several subtypes can be recognized.

- *Keratinizing SCC*. This type of SCC is the most common, and its histologic features are identical to those of SCC arising at other mucosal sites of the upper aerodigestive tract. It consists of irregular nests and cords of neoplastic cells showing variable degrees of squamous differentiation and keratinization and often associated with desmoplastic reaction of the surrounding stroma. It can be graded in well (G1), moderately (G2) and poorly differentiated (G3) forms. Most cases of SCC arising in the maxillary sinus are moderately or poorly differentiated [53] (Figs. 18 and 19). It is thought to originate from areas of squamous metaplasia of the respiratory epithelium, but dysplastic changes of the surface epithelium are uncommonly seen.
- *Non-keratinizing SCC* (synonyms: Schneiderian carcinoma, transitional cell carcinoma, cylindrical cell carcinoma). This SCC variant lacks keratin formation, although small foci of keratinization may be occasionally present, and consists of ribbons and interlacing cords of atypical squamous epithelial cells with a high nuclear to cytoplasm ratio (Figs. 20 and 21). Basal cells tend to show nuclear palisading. The tumor often shows a well-delineated pushing invasion front, without accompanying stromal desmoplasia, and invasion can be difficult to demonstrate, especially in biopsy material (Fig. 22).
- *Spindle cell carcinoma* (synonym: sarcomatoid carcinoma) is a biphasic tumor characterized by a conventional SCC component and a predominant population of spindle and pleomorphic cells derived from the squamous epithelium by epithelial-to-mesenchymal transition mechanisms (Fig. 23). The conventional squamous cell carcinoma component is often difficult to demonstrate and limited to few elements in the superficial portion of the tumor in association with dysplasia or carcinoma in situ of the surface epithelium. The sarcomatous component more frequently has a nonspecific appearance, being composed by atypical spindle and pleomorphic cells, sometimes dispersed in myxoid matrix, or organized in intersecting fascicles. Only occasionally a specific line of differentiation (leiomyosarcomatous, rhabdomyosarcoma-

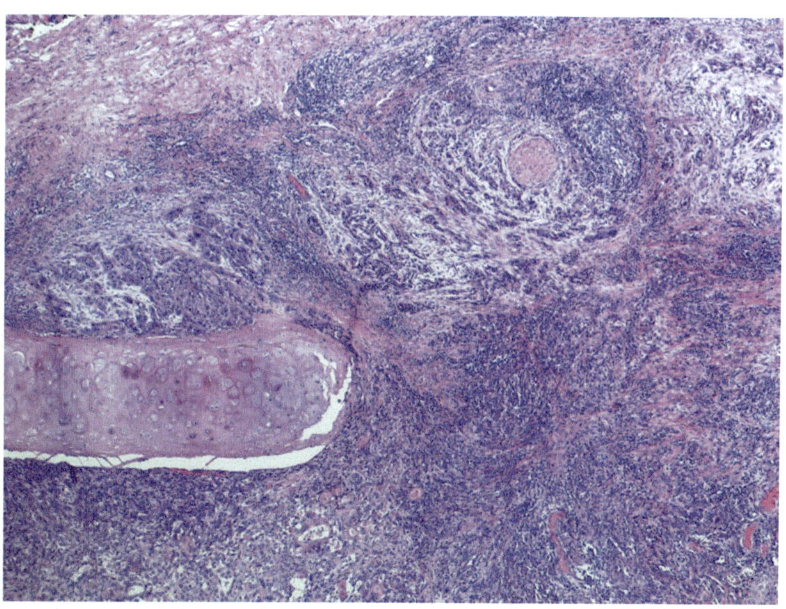

Fig. 18 Poorly differentiated keratinizing squamous cell carcinoma. The tumor destroys the cartilage and shows perineurial spread

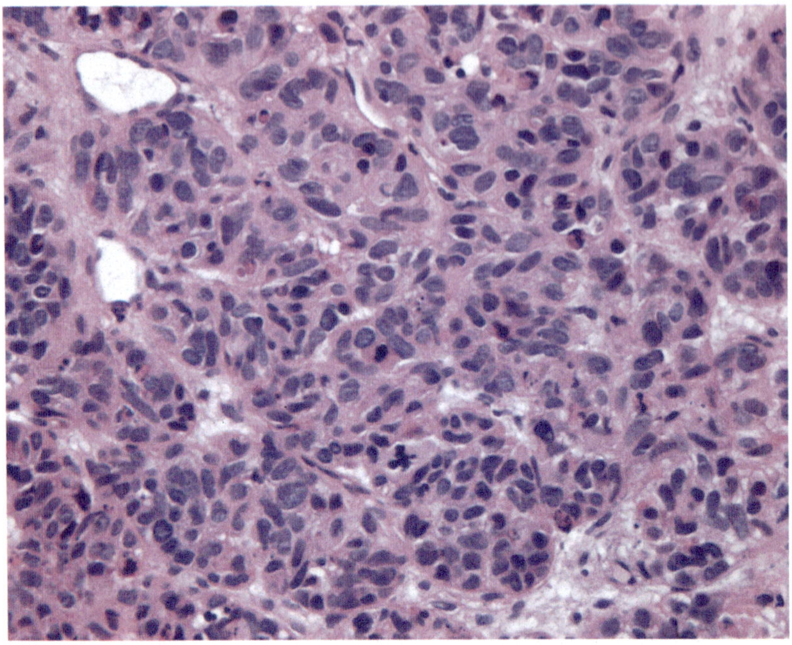

Fig. 19 Poorly differentiated keratinizing squamous cell carcinoma of the maxillary sinus. There is marked cellular pleomorphism. Atypical mitotic figures are present

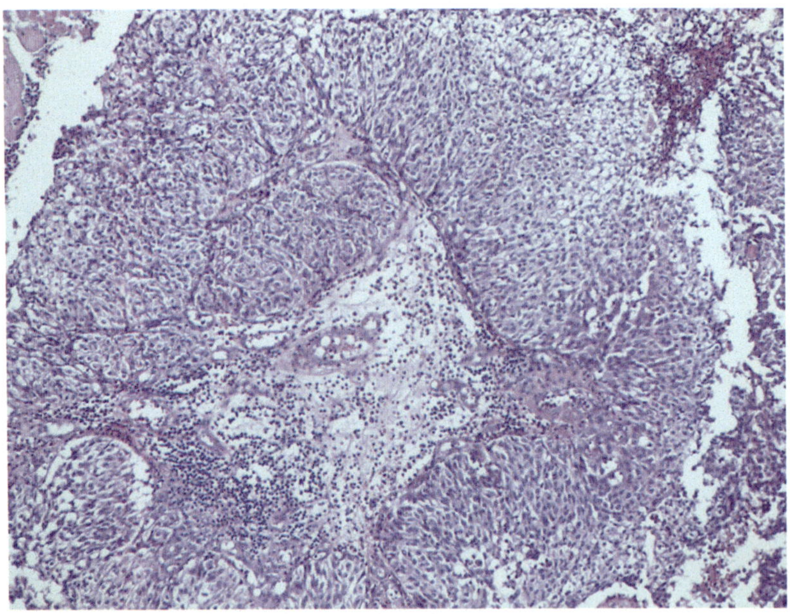

Fig. 20 Non-keratinizing squamous cell carcinoma. The tumor consists of interconnecting ribbons of atypical cells

tous, etc.) or production of osteoid or cartilage matrix can be identified.

- *Basaloid SCC* is characterized by a usually minor component of conventional SCC associated with irregular nests formed by closely packed cells with round hyperchromatic nuclei and scant cytoplasm, with peripheral palisading (Fig. 24). Central comedonecrosis is present in larger nests. Neoplastic cells are closely packed or separated by hyaline stroma formation (Fig. 25). Gland-like spaces with collection of mucinous material are frequently

Fig. 21 Non-keratinizing squamous cell carcinoma. The tumor nests show a smooth contour

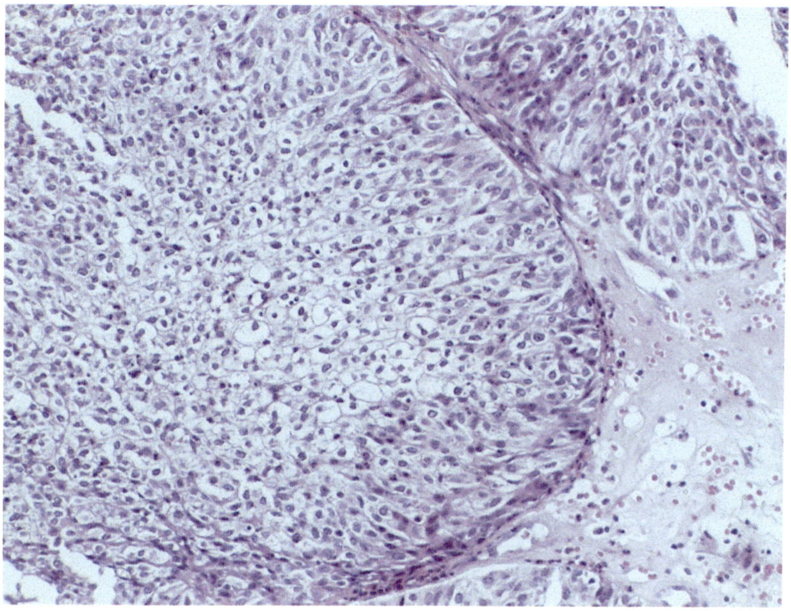

Fig. 22 Non-keratinizing squamous cell carcinoma. The tumor invades with pushing borders

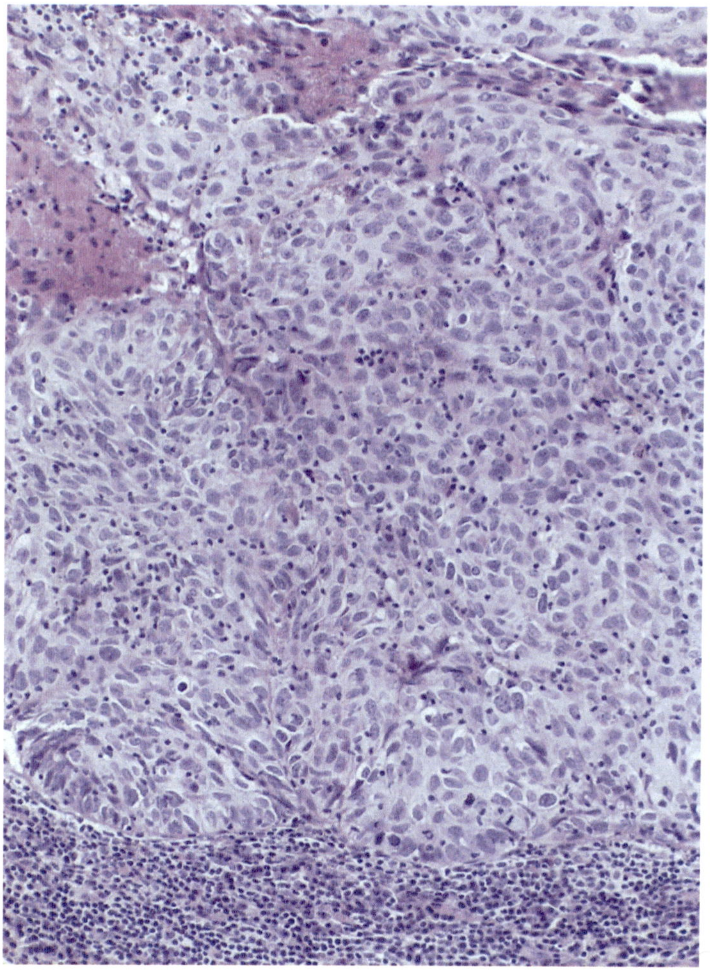

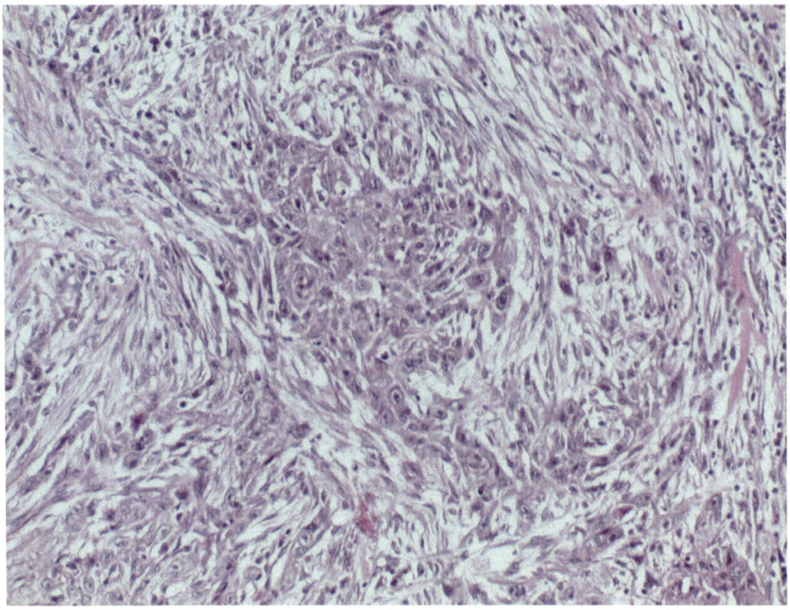

Fig. 23 Spindle cell (sarcomatoid carcinoma) showing a biphasic appearance

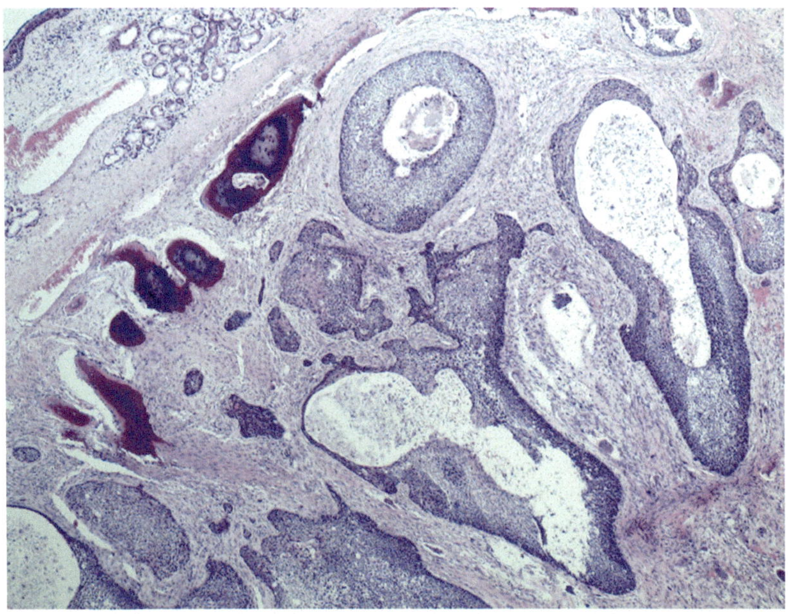

Fig. 24 Basaloid squamous cell carcinoma infiltrating the sinonasal mucosa and the bone. The tumor is composed by discrete tumor islands of basaloid cells with central areas of comedonecrosis

seen. The conventional SCC component consists of nests of neoplastic cells with evidence of keratinization, but abrupt keratinization of the basaloid component and dysplasia of the surface epithelium can also be present.

- *Adenosquamous carcinoma* is only rarely observed in the sinonasal region, and it is composed by a mixture of a SCC and adenocarcinoma. The overlying squamous epithelium is often dysplastic confirming the origin from the surface epithelium. The two components are strictly associated: the SCC shows evidence of keratinization and the adenocarcinoma consists of gland-like structures with mucin production or of cribriform areas (Figs. 26 and 27). Thus, the overall appearance may mimic quite closely that of adenoid cystic carcinoma.
- *Papillary SCC* is a rare variant characterized by an exophytic growth pattern. It *consists* of

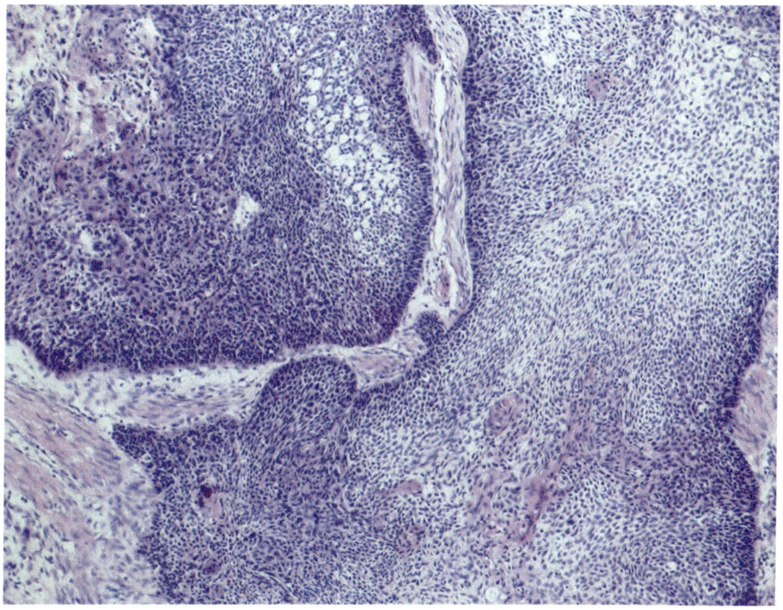

Fig. 25 Tumor cells have a basaloid morphology, with focal areas of keratinization

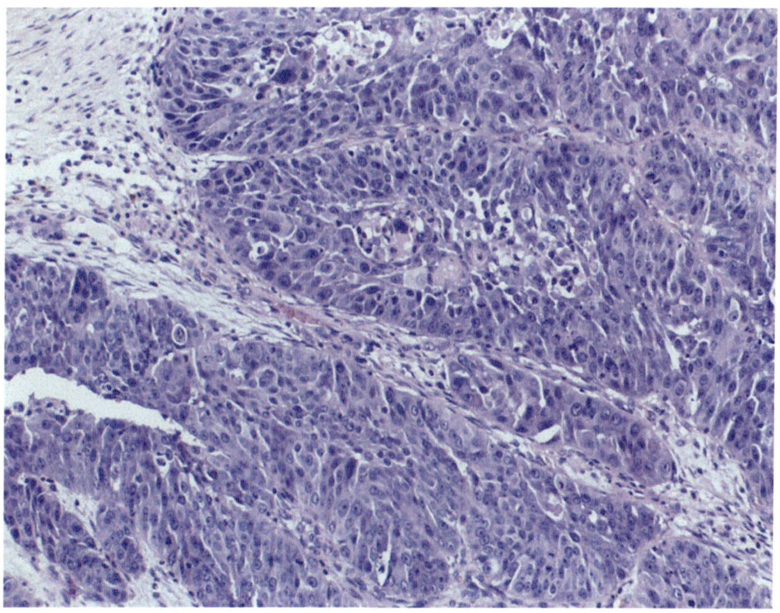

Fig. 26 Adenosquamous carcinoma consisting of areas keratinizing squamous cell carcinoma and small gland-like spaces

thin projections with a central fibrovascular core covered by atypical squamous cells either without evidence of keratinization or with surface maturation and keratinization (Figs. 28 and 29). Invasion may be difficult to demonstrate, and the papillary pattern may be retained or lost in the invasive component. Lewis and coworkers reported a unique case of low-grade papillary carcinoma of the sinonasal tract with bland histologic features that closely mimicked the histologic appearance of a sinonasal papilloma [20]. However, the tumor progressively invaded deep soft tissues and, over an 18-year period of progressive disease recurrence with lymph node metastases, resulted in patient death. Another example has been subsequently reported [21].

- *Verrucous carcinoma* is only rarely reported in the sinonasal cavities [54, 55]. It typically shows an exophytic growth and a broad

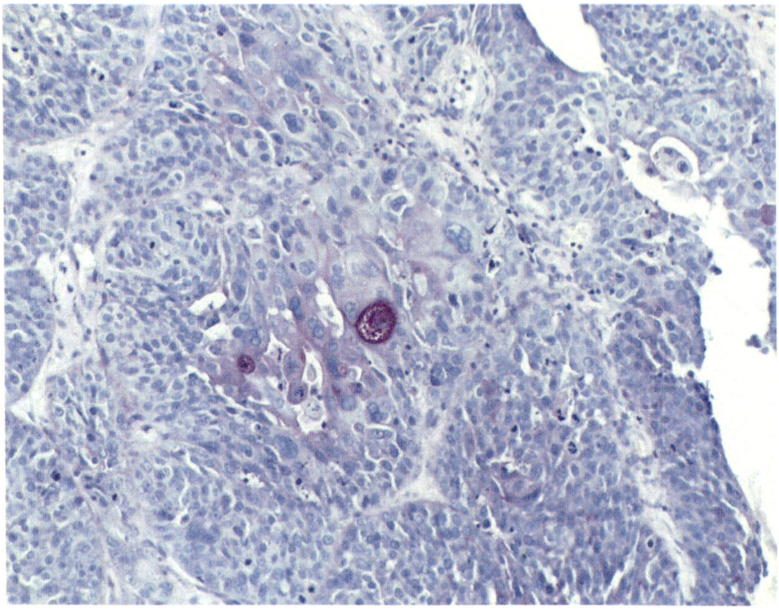

Fig. 27 Mucin production is documented by PAS diastase staining

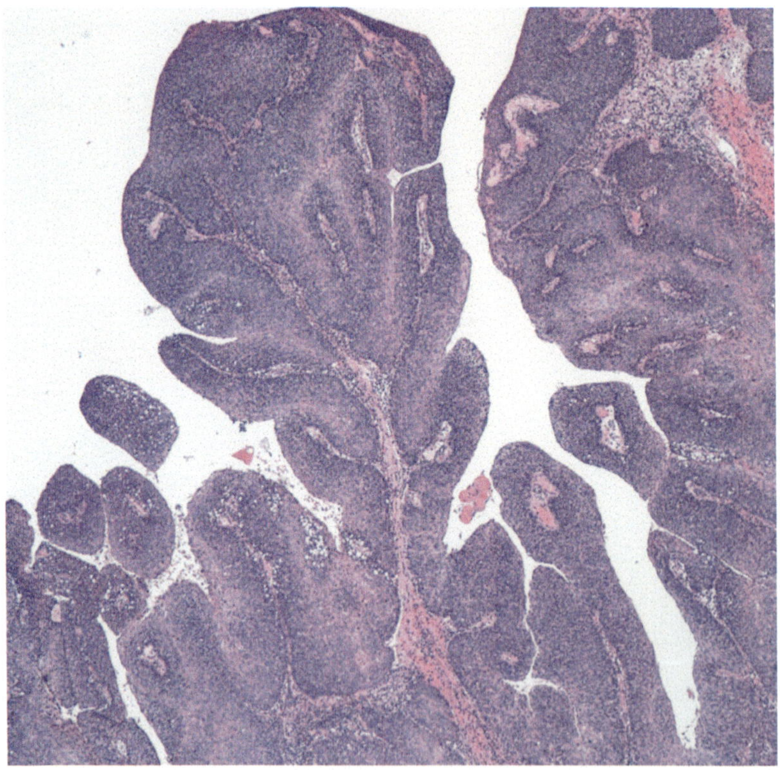

Fig. 28 Papillary squamous cell carcinoma has a complex exophytic architecture

implant base and consists of well-*differentiated* thick keratinizing squamous epithelium, forming projections and invaginations (Fig. 30). The tumor invades the stroma with a pushing border, and a dense inflammatory infiltrate is usually present at the interface. The keratinizing squamous epithelium does not present significant atypia, and only few mitotic figures can be detected in the basal layers (Fig. 31). If areas of invasive conventional SCC are

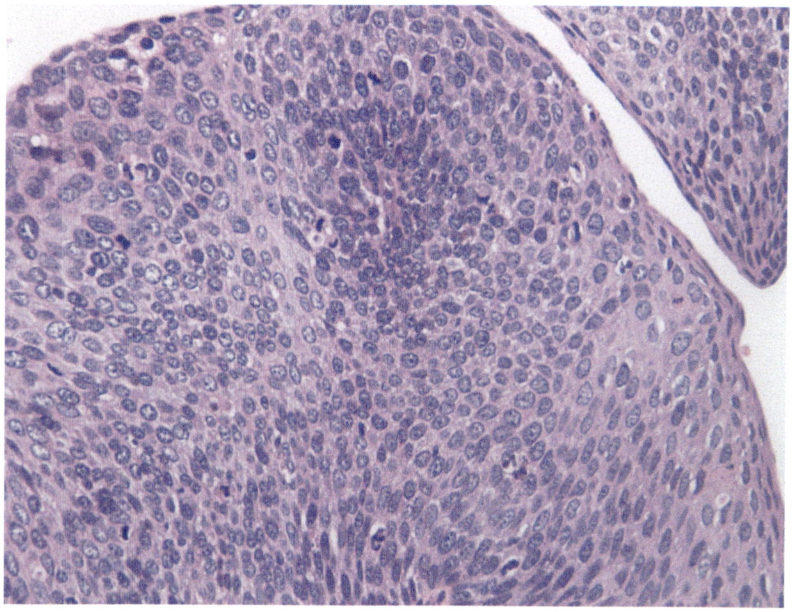

Fig. 29 The papillae of papillary squamous cell carcinoma lack keratinization and are composed of atypical neoplastic cells. Numerous mitotic figures are visible in this microscopic field

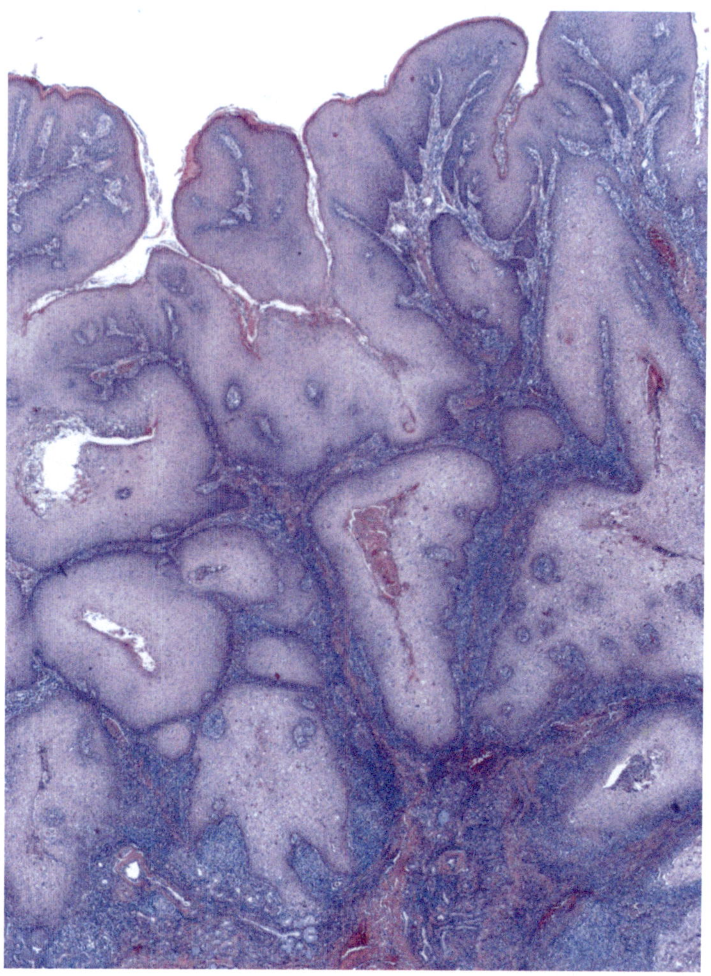

Fig. 30 Verrucous carcinoma of the maxillary sinus. The tumor shows an exophytic growth pattern and consists of well-differentiated keratinizing nests. The squamous nests of the deep portion of the tumor are sharply demarcated and surrounded by intense inflammatory infiltrate

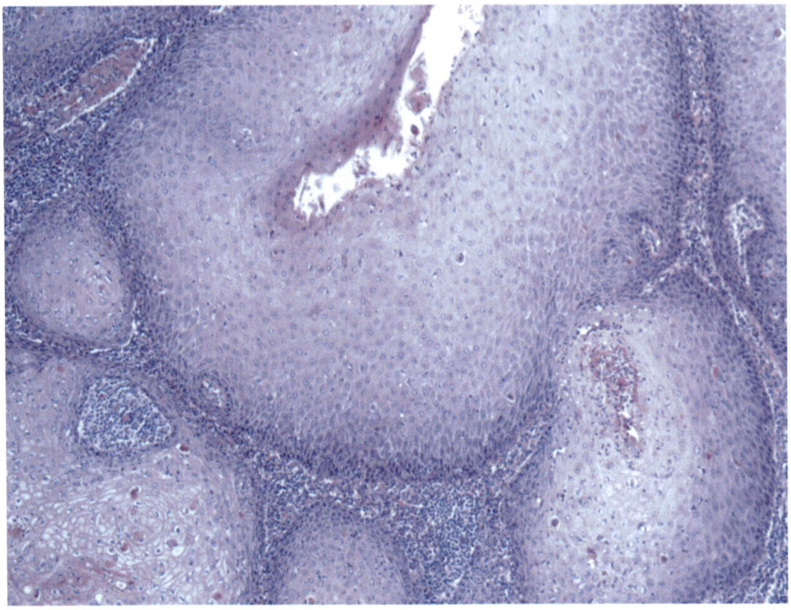

Fig. 31 The well-differentiated squamous cells lack significant atypia

present, then the tumor is designated as hybrid carcinoma.

Immunohistochemical Profile

SCC is typically positive for cytokeratins of various molecular weights, including cytokeratin 5/6, EMA, p63, and p40. Poorly differentiated SCC tends to lose the expression of high molecular weight cytokeratins and to acquire the expression of low molecular weight cytokeratins. In spindle cell SCC, the epithelial markers are often not expressed in the sarcoma-like component, which in turn is positive for vimentin and often also for actins. In adenosquamous carcinoma, the glandular component is positive for cytokeratin 7 and CAM5.2, while cytokeratin 20 is negative.

High-Risk Human Papilloma Virus (HPV) in Sinonasal Squamous Cell Carcinoma

A significant proportion (25–30%) of sinonasal SCCs harbors transcriptionally active HPV, mainly the type 16 [56–61]. The majority of HPV-positive sinonasal SCC occurs in the group of non-keratinizing SCC (35–50%), while keratinizing SCC is less frequently associated with HPV (0–20%). Other subtypes frequently showing HPV positivity are the papillary SCC (80%), the adenosquamous (83%), and the basaloid (50%) variants, while sinonasal spindle cell SCC appears not to be HPV related [59, 61].

As for other anatomic sites, HPV-positive tumors exhibit intense and diffuse p16 expression [56–59].

Conflicting data have been reported regarding the clinical significance and the prognostic impact of HPV positivity in sinonasal SCC [56–59]. However, in a recent analysis of 770 cases of sinonasal SCC with known HPV status conducted on the National Cancer Database, 31.7% of the cases were HPV positive [62]. As in other studies, non-keratinizing, basaloid, and papillary subtypes were more frequently associated with HPV than conventional keratinizing SCC. HPV-positive tumors had a significantly higher 5-year overall survival than HPV-negative tumors (68.1% vs. 51.5%) and on multivariate analyses, HPV positivity remained a favorable prognostic factor [62].

Molecular Features

The pattern of DNA copy number abnormalities observed in sinonasal SCC is similar to that of other head and neck sites, despite possible differences in the etiology [63, 64]. Copy number losses most frequently included genes at 9p21,

13q14, 17p13, 17q21, and 18q11, while gains were more frequently observed on 8q24, 11q13, 17q12, 19p13, and 20q11–q13 [64]. The genes involved in regions of losses include *BRCA1*, *CDH2*, *CRK*, *STCH*, *RB1*, *CDKN2A*, and *IL18*, while gains involve *EMS1* and *BCL2L1*, *RECQL4*, *RELA*, *ERBB2*, *CCND1*, *PTPN1*, and *MYC* [64].

Although the number of cases studied is low, it seems that, similar to other head and neck sites, the molecular profile of sinonasal SCC also depends on the HPV status of the tumor: *TP53* and *CDKN2A/B* genes are frequently altered in HPV-negative tumors, whereas *PIK3CA* and *PTEN* are the most commonly altered genes in HPV-positive tumors [65].

In addition, SCCs arising from sinonasal-inverted papillomas present activating, somatic *EGFR* exon 19 and 20 mutations. The same mutation is present in the papilloma and the paired SCC, establishing a clonal relationship between the two tumors [13]. Interestingly, the presence of *EGFR* mutation is mutually exclusive with the presence of HPV infection [14].

Differential Diagnosis

Well-differentiated conventional *keratinizing SCC* has to be distinguished from benign reactive lesions, such as necrotizing sialometaplasia and pseudoepitheliomatous hyperplasia, that do not present cellular atypia and the atypical mitotic figures seen in SCC. In addition, necrotizing sialometaplasia maintains a characteristic lobular architecture, which is not found in SCC. Well-differentiated SCC can be separated from v*errucous carcinoma* for the presence of cellular atypia and atypical mitotic figures. Poorly differentiated keratinizing SCC may be difficult to distinguish from *non-keratinizing SCC*. Histologic features that may help in the distinction are the presence of pushing borders, lack of stromal reaction, and ribbony nesting pattern in non-keratinizing SCC. The differential diagnosis of poorly differentiated SCC includes also NUT carcinoma, which however presents a characteristic abrupt keratinization and shows nuclear positivity for NUT.

The main differential diagnosis of *non-keratinizing SCC* is with sinonasal papillomas, particularly with the inverted and oncocytic types. The epithelium of papillomas however lacks the atypia of non-keratinizing SCC and presents signs of maturation. When a SCC develops in a sinonasal papilloma, the two components are usually well demarcated one from the other.

For *spindle cell carcinoma*, the differential diagnosis is with spindle cell and pleomorphic sarcomas. Most spindle cell carcinomas are biphasic tumors and present at least focal areas of conventional SCC, either invasive or in situ. In addition, although spindle cell carcinomas resembles true sarcomas histologically, most lack any definable sarcoma pattern such as leiomyosarcoma, rhabdomyosarcoma, or osteosarcoma, a feature that may help in the differential diagnosis. In addition, immunohistochemical expression of p63, p40, and/or cytokeratins in neoplastic cells supports the diagnosis of spindle cell carcinoma.

The differential diagnosis of *basaloid SCC* includes other poorly differentiated carcinomas like SNUC, SMARCB1-deficient carcinoma, NUT carcinoma, solid adenoid cystic carcinoma, and HPV-related multiphenotypic sinonasal carcinoma. Basaloid SCC is diffusely positive for squamous carcinoma immunohistochemical markers (p63, p40, and cytokeratin 5/6), and this is helpful in the distinction from SNUC, adenoid cystic carcinoma, and HPV-related multiphenotypic sinonasal carcinoma, that are negative or only partially positive. SMARCB1 can be separated from basaloid SCC by demonstrating loss of INI1 expression by neoplastic cells, while NUT carcinoma is positive for NUT. Finally, neuroendocrine carcinomas (NECs) are positive for neuroendocrine markers, which is not a feature of basaloid SCC.

The obvious cellular atypia and mitotic activity allow the distinction of *papillary SCC* from exophytic sinonasal papillomas and also from verrucous carcinoma.

Adenosquamous carcinoma can be distinguished from mucoepidermoid carcinoma for the presence of dysplasia of the surface epithelium, for the prevalent distribution of the glandular component in the deeper part of the lesion and adjacent to the squamous component, and for the absence of *MAML2* rearrangements.

Verrucous carcinoma is frequently misdiagnosed as a benign lesion in small biopsies, due to the lack of obvious features of malignancy. Therefore, it is important to correlate the histologic findings with the clinical appearance of the lesion, which is often indicative of malignancy, and to obtain a full thickness biopsy. The differential diagnosis with exophytic sinonasal papilloma is based on the presence of non-keratinizing squamous epithelium, admixed with ciliated respiratory epithelium that contains interspersed mucin-secreting cells, in the latter.

Treatment and Prognosis

The treatment of sinonasal SCC is based on surgery, either open or endoscopic, followed by radiotherapy or chemoradiotherapy [66, 67]. Elective irradiation of the neck can be considered in advanced T stage tumors (T3 and T4), because of the higher frequency of lymph node metastases [67]. Surgery is followed by chemo-/radiotherapy in case of positive margins or if histologic evidence of perineurial and/or vascular invasion is available [67].

Induction chemotherapy protocols has been employed in poorly differentiated SCC in T3–T4 stage and has shown encouraging results [68].

The majority of patients presents with advanced stage disease. Lymph node metastases are relatively uncommon (10–20%), and distant metastases are rare (5–10%). The presence of lymph node metastases is associated with poorer prognosis [69].

The 5-year survival rate for sinonasal SCC ranges between 50 and 60% and has not significantly improved in the recent past [52], while the rates for paranasal sinus carcinomas is lower (25–30%) [53, 70].

Considering prognostic histologic parameters, perineurial invasion has been documented in 22% of sinonasal SCC, and it was associated with a higher frequency of positive margins, but not with a worst survival rate [71].

There are some relevant differences in the clinical aggressiveness of the SCC variants, as highlighted in a recent large population-based study [72], which however do not seem to reflect entirely data from other head and neck sites like larynx and oral cavity. In particular, sinonasal verrucous carcinoma, papillary SCC, and basaloid SCC have a better prognosis than conventional SCC, while spindle cell SCC and adenosquamous carcinoma have a prognosis similar to conventional SCC [72]. Finally, HPV-positive tumors have a better prognosis than HPV-negative tumors [62].

Sinonasal Undifferentiated Carcinoma

Definition

Sinonasal undifferentiated carcinoma (SNUC) is a high-grade carcinoma with no evidence of glandular or squamous differentiation and not otherwise classifiable.

Clinical Features

SNUC is a rare tumor that occurs in both sexes over a wide age range, with a median in the sixth decade of life [73]. It frequently originates from the ethmoid region as a large mass with invasion of adjacent sinonasal structures, as well as the orbit, skull base, and the brain. Patients present with various symptoms, including nasal obstruction, epistaxis, proptosis, visual disturbances, facial pain, and signs of cranial nerve involvement. Typically, symptoms have a relatively short duration (weeks to months).

Pathologic Features

SNUCs are large tumors, often with a fungating appearance, that invade the adjacent structures, including the bone.

Microscopically, SNUC is composed of sheets, nests, lobules, or ribbons of small to medium-sized cells, lacking evidence of squamous or glandular differentiation [74] (Fig. 32). These cells are polygonal in shape, showing round to ovoid, hyperchromatic or vesicular nuclei, with either inconspicuous or slightly prominent nucleoli, and moderate amount of eosinophilic cytoplasm (Fig. 33). Numerous mitotic figures are available, and necrosis and vascular invasion are frequently present, while desmoplastic reaction is absent.

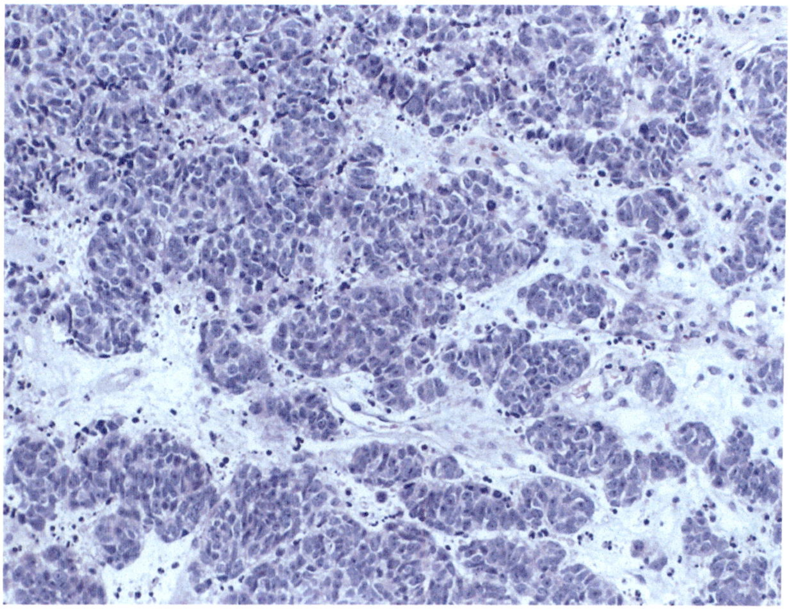

Fig. 32 Sinonasal undifferentiated carcinoma. The tumor consists of nests and ribbons of medium-sized cells, with no evidence of specific differentiation

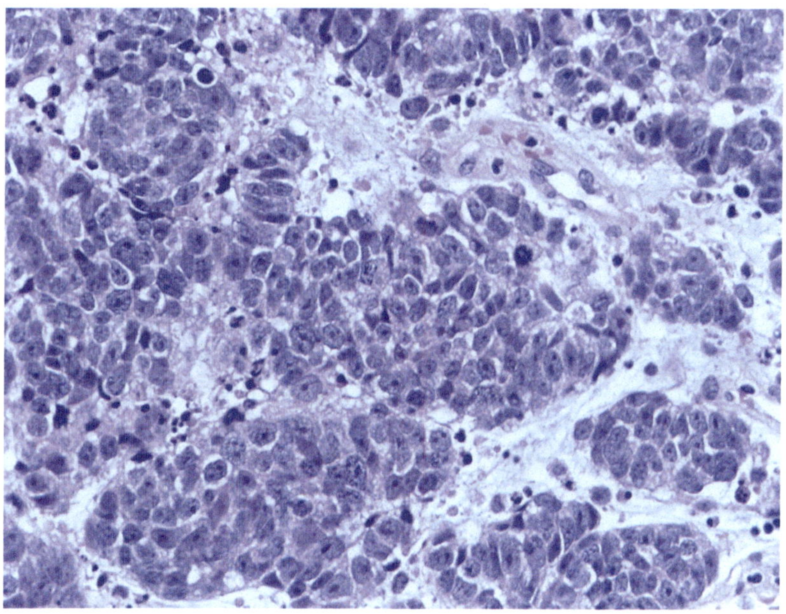

Fig. 33 Sinonasal undifferentiated carcinoma. Neoplastic cells show polygonal shape, ovoid nuclei with slightly prominent nucleoli, and moderate amount of eosinophilic cytoplasm. Mitotic figures and apoptotic bodies are easily appreciated

Immunohistochemical Features

SNUC is positive for pan-cytokeratins, simple keratins, and EMA, while CK4, CK5/6, and CK14 are negative [75]. Variable, generally low, immunoreactivity can be seen with neuron-specific enolase (NSE), chromogranin, and synaptophysin. SNUC usually shows only limited positivity for p63 and p40 [76–78], and it is typically negative for Epstein–Barr virus (EBV) [79, 80]. Association with high risk HPV has been reported with variable frequency [81, 82].

Molecular Features

The majority of SNUCs present an IDH2 R172 mutation that is also present in other high-grade carcinomas of the sinonasal tract [83, 84]. Other recurrent alterations involve the *TP53*, *CDKN2A/2B*, *MYC*, *SETD2*, and *SPEN* genes [84].

Differential Diagnosis

SNUC is a diagnosis of exclusion, requiring separation from several other epithelial and non-epithelial high-grade sinonasal malignancies (Table 2). The main differential diagnosis of SNUC is with high-grade olfactory neuroblastoma, and this diagnosis is clinically relevant because SNUC has a much worse prognosis than olfactory neuroblastoma. Both entities share clinical and light microscopic features, but SNUC is consistently cytokeratin positive and lacks the typical S100 positive cells around tumor nests as seen in olfactory neuroblastoma. Conversely, olfactory neuroblastoma is only occasionally and focally positive for cytokeratins, and it is consistently positive for neural markers.

In addition, SNUC needs to be distinguished from other primary poorly differentiated sinonasal carcinomas, such as small cell neuroendocrine carcinoma, NUT carcinoma, SMARCB1 (INI1)-deficient carcinoma, solid adenoid cystic carcinoma, and nasopharyngeal-type undifferentiated carcinoma, as well as from malignant melanoma. Neuroendocrine carcinoma can be separated from SNUC for its diffuse positivity for neuroendocrine markers, while NUT carcinoma is recognized by nuclear speckled immunoreactivity for NUT or by the identification of the recurrent t(15;19). Loss of INI1 nuclear expression by tumor cells allows the distinction of SMARCB1-deficient carcinoma from SNUC. P63 and p40 are useful to separate SNUC from poorly differentiated SCC and lymphoepithelioma (which is also EBV positive), while negativity for myoepithelial markers and CD117 helps in the distinction from adenoid cystic carcinoma.

Treatment and Prognosis

SNUC is a highly aggressive tumor that is generally treated with combined surgery and radiotherapy or chemoradiation [85, 86]. Patients with SNUC typically present with locally advanced disease (60% are in AJCC stage III or IV) and have a poor prognosis due to high rates of locoregional recurrence and distant metastasis. The long-term survival rates are in the range of 20–40% [85, 87].

NUT Carcinoma

Definition

NUT carcinoma is an aggressive poorly differentiated carcinoma, often with evidence of squamous differentiation, which is genetically defined by rearrangement of the nuclear protein in testis (*NUTM1*) gene on chromosome 15q14. Initially, it was designated as NUT midline carcinoma, to indicate that it affects organs in the midline of the body (mediastinum, sinonasal tract), and was thought to arise primarily children. Subsequently, it became apparent that it involves also pair organs and affects also young adults and adults.

Clinical Features

NUT carcinoma is a rare tumor (approximately 2% of all sinonasal carcinomas) that affects patients of all ages with a predilection for young adults [88, 89]. It may arise in other anatomic sites of the head and neck region, but the nasal cavity and the paranasal sinuses are most commonly involved [88]. It is a rapidly growing tumor, and usually patients present with a short history of nasal obstruction and bleeding, facial pain, and ocular symptoms. The tumor is locally advanced at presentation, with invasion and destruction of adjacent structures, and although lymph node and distant metastases may not be initially evident, they often develop shortly after diagnosis.

Pathologic Features

Histologically, NUT carcinoma is a high-grade poorly differentiated carcinoma with "round blue cell" morphology that consists of sheets, nests, and cords of cells with moderate amount of eosinophilic to amphophilic cytoplasm, oval nuclei with one or more prominent nucleoli (Fig. 34). Notably, despite the high-grade features, the neoplastic population is uniform with no significant pleomorphism. Squamous differentiation is identified in a minority of cases and frequently consists of keratinized squamous cells adjacent to undifferentiated cells (the so-called abrupt keratinization) or has a more conventional histologic appearance. Mitotic activity is brisk, and apoptosis and areas of necrosis are usually

Table 2 Summary of the diagnostic features of sinonasal poorly differentiated/undifferentiated carcinomas

	Histologic features	CK[a]	P63	P40	S100	Syn	HPV	EBV	Diagnostic gene alterations
SNUC	Sheets, nests, or ribbons of small- to medium-sized cells, no evidence of squamous or glandular differentiation	7+; 5/6-	–	–	–	–	– (+ in rare cases)	–	*IDH* mutations
Lymphoepithelial carcinoma	Syncytial growth pattern, prominent lymphoid infiltrate	5/6+, 13+	+	+	–	–	–	+	ND
NUT carcinoma	Sheets of monotonous undifferentiated round cells, foci of mature keratinized squamous cells occasionally seen	5/6+, 7+, 20+ in rare cases	+	+	–	–	–	–	t(15;19) NUT + by immunohistochemistry
Neuroendocrine carcinoma	Closely packed small cells with scant cytoplasm, extensive necrosis, and brisk mitotic activity; in large cell NEC, cytoplasm is abundant, nuclei are vesicular with prominent nucleoli, moderate pleomorphism is present	5/6 rarely +	–/+	–	–	+	–	–	ND
Basaloid squamous cell carcinoma	Nests of basaloid cells, peripheral palisading, comedonecrosis, foci of squamous differentiation	5/6+,34βE12+	+	+	–	–	+	–	ND
Solid adenoid cystic carcinoma	Solid nests of basaloid cells	5/6+, 7+, 34βE12+, 20-	+	–/+	+	–	–	–	t(6;9)(q22–23;p23–24)
HPV-related multiphenotypic sinonasal carcinoma	Similar to adenoid cystic carcinoma; myoepithelial, ductal, and squamous differentiation	AE1/AE3	+	+	+	–	+	–	ND
SMARCB1 (INI-1)-deficient sinonasal carcinoma	Nests of basaloid cells with peripheral palisading and variable amounts of rhabdoid cells	5+	+	+		Focal+	–	–	*SMARCB1* gene alterations; SMARCB1 negative by immunohistochemistry

CK cytokeratin, *Syn* synaptophysin, *ND* not determined

[a]All carcinomas are positive for pan-cytokeratins; only specific classes are reported

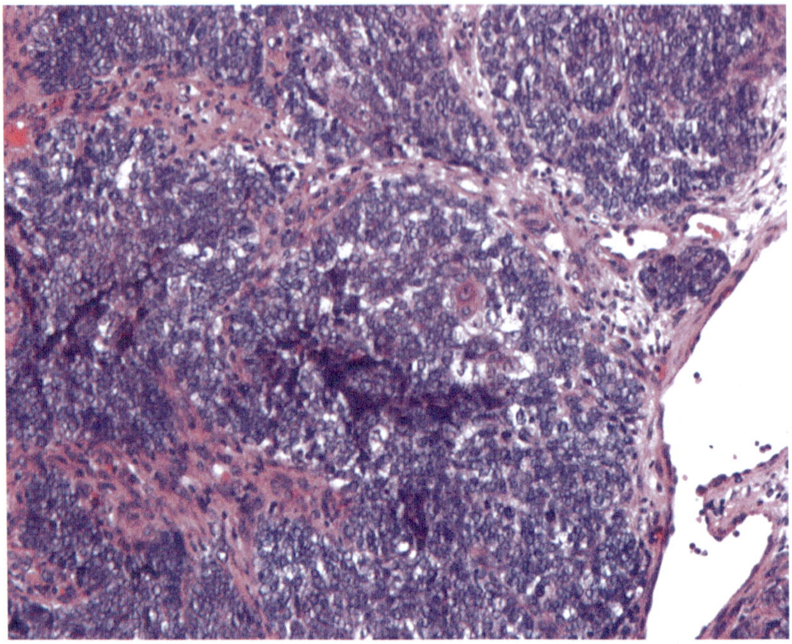

Fig. 34 NUT carcinoma consists of a uniform population of round cells with few squamous elements with larger eosinophilic cytoplasm

present. Bone infiltration and lymphovascular invasion are also frequently recognized. The surface epithelium is frequently ulcerated or intact without evidence of dysplasia.

Immunohistochemical Profile

NUT carcinoma is always positive for cytokeratins (including cytokeratins 7 and less frequently 5/6) and often positive for p63 and p40, while it is negative for chromogranin, synaptophysin, S100, HMB45, desmin, myoglobin, smooth muscle actin, common muscle actin, CD45, placental alkaline phosphatase, alpha-fetoprotein, neuron-specific enolase, CD57, and CD99 [90]. CD34 is positive in approximately half of the cases. Diffuse (>50%) nuclear staining for NUT, usually with a granular or "speckled" pattern, is considered sensitive and specific enough to support the diagnosis of NUT carcinoma [91].

Molecular Features

The most common translocation found in NUT carcinoma is the t(15;19) (q13;p13.1). In this translocation, the *NUTM1* gene on chromosome 15 is fused to the *BRD4* (bromodomain- containing protein 4) gene on chromosome 19 [92]. Less frequently, the *NUTM1* gene is fused to a different partner gene, the *BRD3* gene at 9q34.2 or *WHSC1L1* at 8p11.23 [93]. The fusion protein interferes with cellular differentiation inducing decreased expression of several genes through decreased histone acetylation [94]. When siRNA is used to knock down the expression of BRD3-NUT or BRD4-NUT in NUT carcinoma cell lines, this process results in irreversible squamous differentiation and growth arrest [95].

NUT carcinoma is negative for HPV and EBV [96].

Differential Diagnosis

NUT carcinoma is likely to be confused with other poorly differentiated and undifferentiated sinonasal carcinomas (Table 1). Before its description, most cases were diagnosed as sinonasal undifferentiated carcinoma (SNUC) or poorly differentiated squamous cell carcinoma [88, 96]. Other entities to be excluded are the recently described SMARCB1-deficient carcinoma and the adamantinoma-like Ewing sarcoma. The recognition of areas of squamous differentiation and the expression of immunohistochemical markers of squamous cell carcinoma rule out SNUC. However, the diagnosis of NUT carcinoma ultimately relies on the demonstration of the *NUT* rearrangement by FISH or other molecular methods or in the presence of diffuse (>50%) immunoreactivity for NUT using the commercially available C52 monoclonal antibody [91].

Treatment and Prognosis

NUT carcinoma has a poor prognosis, with a mean survival <1 year (6.7 months in average) [97]. Protocols including aggressive initial surgical resection with postoperative radiotherapy or chemoradiotherapy have been associated with enhanced survival [98]. Clinical trials of bromodomain and extra-terminal motif (BET) inhibitors are currently underway, and preliminary results are promising [99].

SMARCB1 (INI1)-Deficient Carcinoma

Definition

This variant is an undifferentiated carcinoma with rhabdoid histologic features and loss of SMARCB1(INI1) nuclear expression [100–104].

Clinical Features

SMARCB1 (INI1)-deficient carcinoma affects both sexes equally and occurs over a wide age range, with a mean of 50 years [100–104]. The most common symptoms are nasal obstruction, pain, and ocular symptoms. At presentation, the tumor is usually in advanced local stage with involvement of the nasal cavities, paranasal sinuses (most often the ethmoid sinus), and skull base.

Pathologic Features

Grossly, the tumor presents infiltrative margins and variable exophytic papillary surface [103]. Histologically, it consists in most cases of a relatively monomorphic population of basaloid undifferentiated cells with round nuclei containing dispersed chromatin, variably prominent nucleoli, and indistinctive cytoplasmic borders (Fig. 35). Neoplastic cells are organized in solid sheets and nests, often with peripheral palisading, surrounded by desmoplastic stroma. An inverted growth pattern reminiscent of sinonasal papilloma or carcinoma arising in sinonasal papilloma can be occasionally present. A second population of singly dispersed rhabdoid/plasmacytoid cells, with abundant eosinophilic cytoplasm and eccentrically placed nucleus, can usually be identified through a careful search. Mitotic activity is brisk, and necrosis is commonly found. No evi-

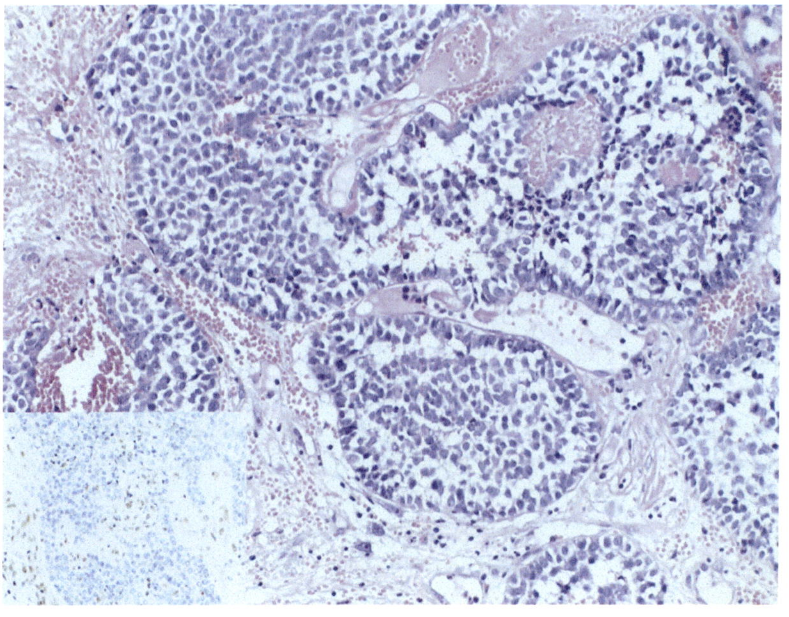

Fig. 35 This SMARCB1-deficient carcinoma consists of nests of cells with basaloid morphology. INI1 expression is lost in neoplastic cells, and it is maintained in stromal cells

dence of squamous differentiation and no signs of dysplasia of the surface epithelium are available. In approximately one third of the cases, the tumor consists predominantly of rhabdoid/plasmacytoid cells, sometimes resembling an oncocytic carcinoma or proximal-type epithelioid sarcoma. True glandular differentiation with mucous production is detected in rare cases.

Immunohistochemical Profile

By definition neoplastic cells present loss of nuclear expression of SMARCB1 (INI1), while the staining is retained in stromal fibroblasts, endothelial cells, and inflammatory infiltrate. In addition, SMARCB1-deficient carcinomas are consistently positive for cytokeratins, while p63 is expressed in approximately half of the cases. Focal positivity for neuroendocrine markers, including CD56, synaptophysin, and chromogranin A has been noted. In addition, p16 may be occasionally positive, but high-risk HPV testing has always been negative [103].

Molecular Features

By FISH, the majority of tumors shows homozygous deletion of the *SMARCB1* gene locus, while heterozygous (monoallelic) deletion is less frequently detected [103]. However, other mechanisms of *SMARCB1* inactivation (small deletions, mutations, epigenetic silencing) are likely to occur in minority of cases [103].

Differential Diagnosis

SMARCB1-deficient carcinoma may be difficult to distinguish from sinonasal non-keratinizing and basaloid squamous cell carcinomas because of the histologic and immunophenotypic similarities (positivity for cytokeratins and p63). However, SMARCB1-deficient sinonasal carcinoma does not show squamous differentiation or surface squamous dysplasia, and HPV testing is negative, while INI1 immunostaining is consistently negative. SNUC has also to be considered in the differential diagnosis, but here neoplastic cells are more pleomorphic and also positive for INI1 (Table 1).

Treatment and Prognosis

SMARCB1 (INI1)-deficient carcinomas are aggressive tumors with a poor prognosis. Patients have been treated with surgery alone, surgery plus radiotherapy and chemotherapy, or radio- and chemotherapy. Locoregional recurrence occurs in approximately 30% of the patients, while distant metastases develop in 35% [103]. In the largest series published so far, only 30% of the patients were alive without evidence of disease at last follow-up (median 26 months) [103].

Lymphoepithelial Carcinoma

Definition

Sinonasal lymphoepithelial carcinoma (LEC) is a squamous cell carcinoma variant histologically similar to the undifferentiated subtype of non-keratinizing nasopharyngeal carcinoma.

Clinical Features

LEC with exclusive sinonasal involvement is rare, representing less than 10% of all non-nasopharyngeal LECs in the United States [105]. It affects mainly adult male patients in the fifth to seventh decades of life [106, 107]. Most cases have occurred in patients from Asia [108]. The presenting symptoms include nasal obstruction, epistaxis, proptosis, and cranial nerve palsy [106, 107].

Pathologic Features

Overall, the tumor growth has a syncytial appearance and consists of sheets, islands, cords, or lobules of neoplastic cells with indistinct cytoplasmic borders, abundant lightly eosinophilic or amphophilic cytoplasm, and large oval or round nucleus with vesicular chromatin and prominent nucleoli (Fig. 36). Usually, there is no desmoplastic stromal reaction, and the lymphoplasmacytic infiltrate is often less prominent than in the nasopharyngeal counterpart. Foci of comedo-type necrosis can be present.

Immunohistochemical Profile

Neoplastic cells are positive for cytokeratins, including cytokeratin 5/6, and for p63 and p40.

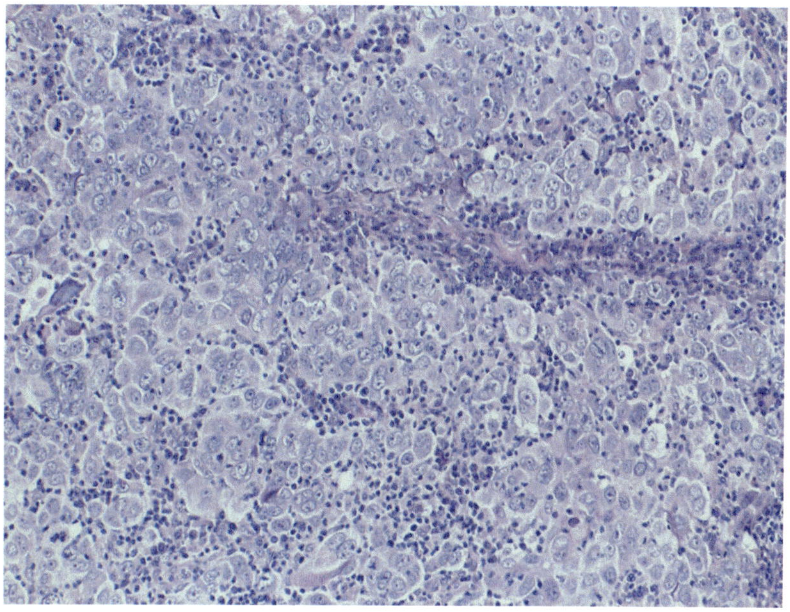

Fig. 36 Sinonasal lymphoepithelial carcinoma consists of sheets of malignant cells with indistinct cytoplasmic borders, abundant lightly eosinophilic or amphophilic cytoplasm, large oval or round nucleus with vesicular chromatin and prominent nucleoli

Molecular Features

Most but not all cases are associated with Epstein Barr virus (EBV). Thus, in situ hybridization for EBV-encoded small RNA (EBER) is usually positive.

Differential Diagnosis

Sinonasal LEC must be distinguished from SNUC, which is EBER-negative and lacks CK5/6 and p63 expression. Other potential mimics are lymphoma and melanoma. In particular, NK/T cell sinonasal lymphoma is also EBV positive, but absence of cytokeratin expression and positivity for CD3, CD56, and cytotoxic granule markers help in the distinction.

Treatment and Prognosis

The treatment includes surgery with radiotherapy or chemoradiotherapy [105, 106]. The 5-year disease-specific survival rate of sinonasal LEC is approximately 50% [105]. An improved survival is noted in patients with localized disease, with age <60 years, and of Caucasian ethnicity [105]. Metastases to neck lymph nodes are less frequent than the nasopharyngeal counterpart [106].

Neuroendocrine Carcinoma

Definition

NEC is an epithelial neoplasm showing neuroendocrine differentiation, with variable histologic grade. The current terminology used for NECs involving the head and neck region is summarized in Table 3, in comparison with alternative classifications. The vast majority of sinonasal NECs falls in the group of poorly differentiated NECs (PDNEC), which represent 30% of all NEC of the head and neck [109]. Moderately differentiated NEC (MDNEC) is significantly less frequent [110], while only isolated cases of well-differentiated NEC have been reported [111–113].

Clinical Features

Sinonasal PDNEC is a rare neoplasm with an estimated average incidence of 0.015 cases per 100,000 [114]. Nasal obstruction, epistaxis, facial swelling, and pain are the most common presenting symptoms [115]. There are few reports of sinonasal NECs with associated paraneoplastic endocrine syndromes, including syndrome of inappropriate secretion of antidiuretic hormone (SIADH), ectopic production of serotonin, and parathyroid hormone [116–118]. The nasal cavities are the most commonly involved sites, followed by the ethmoid sinus and the maxillary sinus [114, 115]. The majority of patients presents with locally advanced disease (AJCC stage IV). The peak age is in the sixth decade, with a mean of 55 years [114], and there is no significant gender predilection.

Table 3 Terminology of neuroendocrine carcinomas

WHO classification, IV edition, 2017	Alternative terminologies
Well-differentiated neuroendocrine carcinoma	Carcinoid; neuroendocrine carcinoma grade 1
Moderately differentiated neuroendocrine carcinoma	Atypical carcinoid; neuroendocrine carcinoma grade 2
Poorly differentiated neuroendocrine carcinoma Small cell neuroendocrine carcinoma Large cell neuroendocrine carcinoma	Small cell carcinoma; neuroendocrine carcinoma grade 3
	Mixed neuroendocrine carcinoma with non-neuroendocrine carcinoma

PDNEC may occur after irradiation for nasopharyngeal carcinoma, tonsillar lymphoma, or neck metastases [119]. High-risk HPV has also been detected in some cases [120, 121].

Pathological Features

In *WDNEC*, neoplastic cells are arranged in cords or nests with glandular or rosette-like structures. They present uniform round nuclei with stippled chromatin and clear or eosinophilic cytoplasm. Oncocytic change can also occur [122]. Mitotic activity is <2/10 HPF, and necrosis is absent.

In *MDNEC*, neoplastic cells are larger than those of *WDNEC* and are arranged in trabecular, glandular, acinar, nested, and organoid formations. The cytoplasm is eosinophilic, and the nucleus contains speckled chromatin with small nucleoli. Mitotic activity ranges between 2 and 10/10 HPF, and necrosis is present.

Small cell NEC consists of sheets and ribbons of small- to intermediate-sized cells with high nucleus-to-cytoplasm ratio, hyperchromatic chromatin, nuclear molding, and brisk mitotic activity (>11 mitoses/10HPF) (Fig. 37). Apoptotic bodies and areas of necrosis are easily identified. In *large cell NEC*, the cells are larger with more abundant cytoplasm, and the nucleus contains

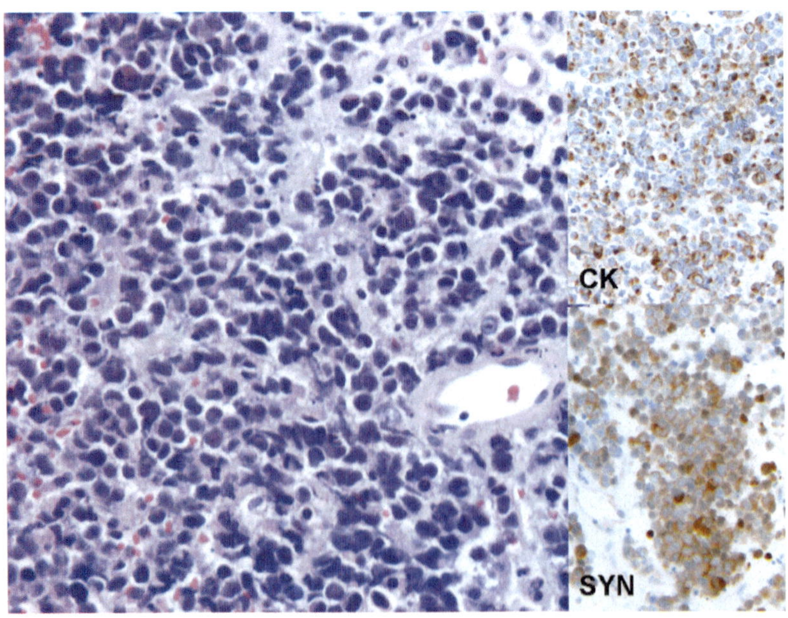

Fig. 37 In sinonasal small cell neuroendocrine carcinoma, neoplastic cells present high nucleus-to-cytoplasm ratio and hyperchromatic nuclei. Immunohistochemical positivity for pancytokeratin (right upper image) and synaptophysin (right lower panel). Abbreviations: *CK* cytokeratin, *SYN* synaptophysin

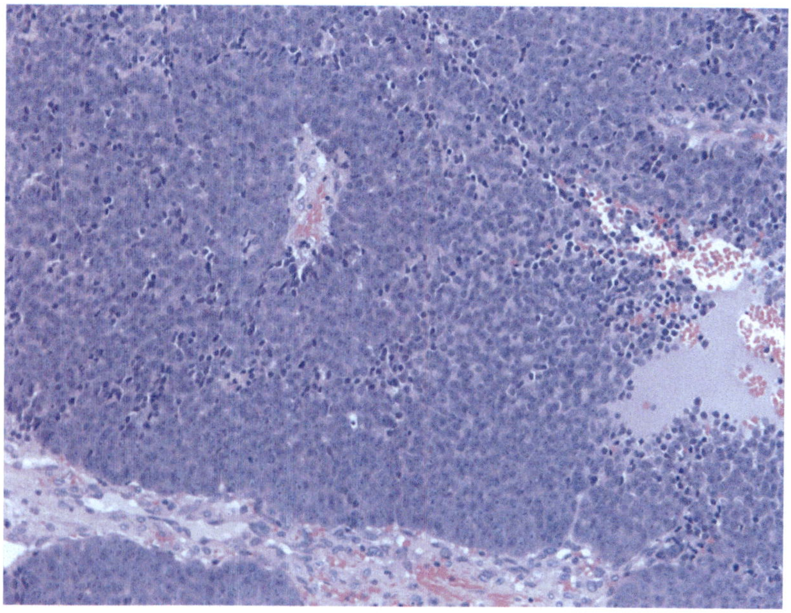

Fig. 38 In large cell neuroendocrine carcinoma, the cells are larger with more abundant cytoplasm, and the nucleus contains vesicular chromatin and prominent nucleoli

vesicular chromatin and prominent nucleoli (Fig. 38). They are organized in nests, trabeculae, and rosettes, often with peripheral palisading of nuclei. Mitotic activity is >11/10 HPF, and necrosis is present [123].

In the *mixed or combined NEC*, the NEC component (either small cell or large cell) comprises at least 30% of the lesion, and it is intermixed with a non-neuroendocrine component represented either by squamous cell carcinoma or intestinal-type adenocarcinoma [124–126].

Immunohistochemical Profile

The immunohistochemical profile of sinonasal NEC includes strong positivity for cytokeratins (AE1/AE3, 8/18, pancytokeratin), often with a dot-like paranuclear pattern, and the neuroendocrine markers synaptophysin, chromogranin and neuron-specific enolase (NSE). TTF-1 is negative [124]. P63 and cytokeratin 5/6 may be expressed, but usually the staining is limited [121, 127]. The Ki67 proliferative index is >20% in NEC and approximately 10% in carcinoid [124]. High-grade sinonasal NECs frequently show diffuse and intense p16 positivity, but they are infrequently related to HPV infection [121, 128].

Molecular Features

Only few cases of sinonasal SNEC have been analyzed at the genetic level. *TP53* and *RB1* mutations along with *BCL2* and *MYC* amplifications have been detected [84]. Similar changes are frequently observed in pulmonary small cell carcinomas supporting a common genetic background.

Differential Diagnosis

The most important differential diagnosis is with olfactory neuroblastoma, because PDNEC has a significantly worst outcome. High-grade olfactory neuroblastoma has a significant histologic overlap with PDNEC and shares the expression of neuroendocrine markers, but lacks the diffuse positivity for cytokeratins of PDNEC. The distinction of LCNEC from atypical carcinoid is mainly based on mitotic activity, that is, >10 mitoses/10 HPFs in the former versus 2–10 mitoses/10HPFs in the latter.

Ectopic pituitary adenoma can be confused with sinonasal NECs, particularly with WDNEC and MDNEC, both for the histologic overlap and the positivity for cytokeratins, chromogranin, and synaptophysin. Pituitary adenomas are usually centered in the sphenoid sinus, do not show significant pleomorphism and destructive growth, and are positive for pituitary hormones (mainly prolactin) in the majority of the cases.

Sinonasal undifferentiated carcinoma can be distinguished from PDNEC because it shows only limited expression of neuroendocrine markers.

Finally, among nonepithelial tumors, alveolar rhabdomyosarcoma and melanoma may be considered in the differential diagnosis because they occasionally show aberrant expression of cytokeratins and neuroendocrine markers.

Treatment and Prognosis

Sinonasal NEC is a highly aggressive neoplasm with dismal prognosis, often presenting in advanced stage with early systemic metastases (liver, lung, brain, bone, kidney, and pancreas) and frequent locoregional recurrences [115, 124]. The overall survival at 5 years ranges between 35 and 50% [114, 115, 124]. No significant differences in survival have been observed between small and large cell NECs [124]. Tumors involving the nasal cavities have a better prognosis than those arising in the ethmoid or maxillary sinuses [114]. In a small series of patients, the local control rates for MDNEC and PDNEC were comparable [110].

The most commonly used therapy for SNEC has been surgery, radiotherapy, or a combination of these two modalities [114]. In a recent study, the use of induction chemotherapy in NEC improved overall and disease-free survival [124].

Although the number of cases studied is small, sinonasal WDNET (carcinoid) seems to have a better prognosis than NEC [124].

HPV-Related Multiphenotypic Sinonasal Carcinoma

Definition

This is an HPV-positive carcinoma characterized by areas that closely resemble solid adenoid cystic carcinoma, that had been originally designated as "HPV-related carcinoma with adenoid cystic-like features" [129]. Because the tumor includes lines of myoepithelial, ductal, and squamous differentiation, the entity has been subsequently renamed HPV-related multiphenotypic sinonasal carcinoma (HMSC) [130].

Clinical Features

So far, the tumor appears to arise only in the sinonasal region, with the majority of the cases involving the nasal cavities (57%), and the remaining arising in the nasal cavity and paranasal sinuses (33%), or in a paranasal sinus (10%) [130]. There is a slight female predominance and the age ranges between 28 and 90 years, with a median of 54 years [130]. The presenting symptoms include nasal obstruction, epistaxis, nasal drainage/discharge, pain, and ocular symptoms.

Pathologic Features

The tumor is formed by basaloid cells mainly organized in solid lobules and sheets separated by thin fibrous bands (Fig. 39). A second pattern observed is a cribriform architecture, with neoplastic cells surrounding cylindromatous microcystic spaces filled with mucoid material (Fig. 40), while a tubular pattern is less frequent. Besides the predominant basaloid cell type, that frequently exhibits myoepithelial features, such as cytoplasmic clearing, focal spindling, plasmacytoid morphology, and focal matrix production, there is a second population of ductal cells with eosinophilic more abundant cytoplasm (Fig. 41). Areas of tumor necrosis are frequently present, and the mitotic is usually high. Bone invasion can be detected in 20% of the cases, whereas perineural invasion can be identified only rarely. The surface squamous epithelium shows signs of dysplasia/carcinoma in situ (Fig. 42), suggesting that the tumor originates from the surface epithelium, rather than from glands. Other histologic features include the presence of scattered foci of squamous

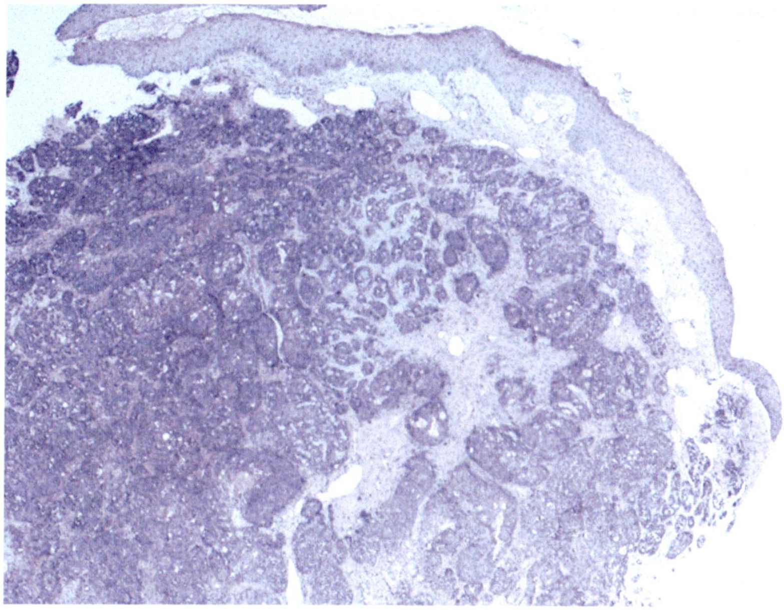

Fig. 39 HPV-related multiphenotypic sinonasal carcinoma. At low power, the tumor shows a multinodular growth pattern

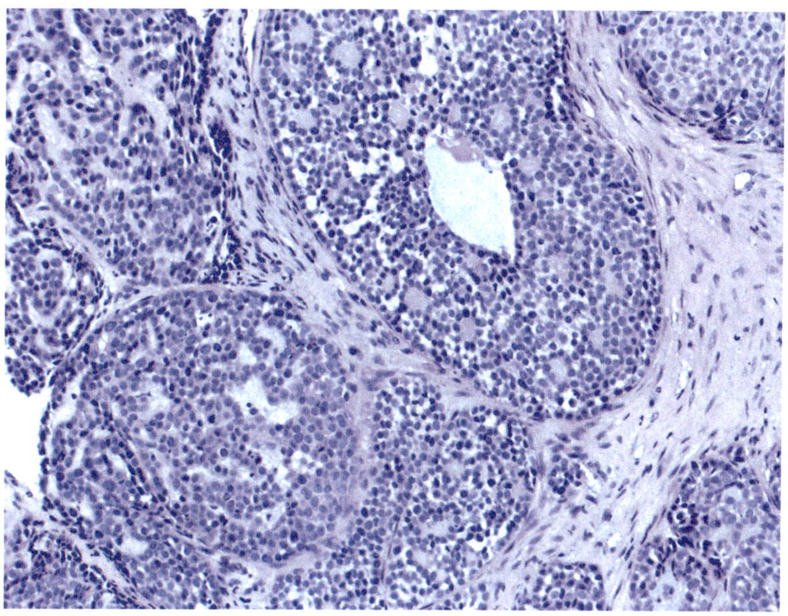

Fig. 40 This area shows a cribriform growth pattern, with neoplastic cells organized around microcystic spaces and hyaline extracellular material

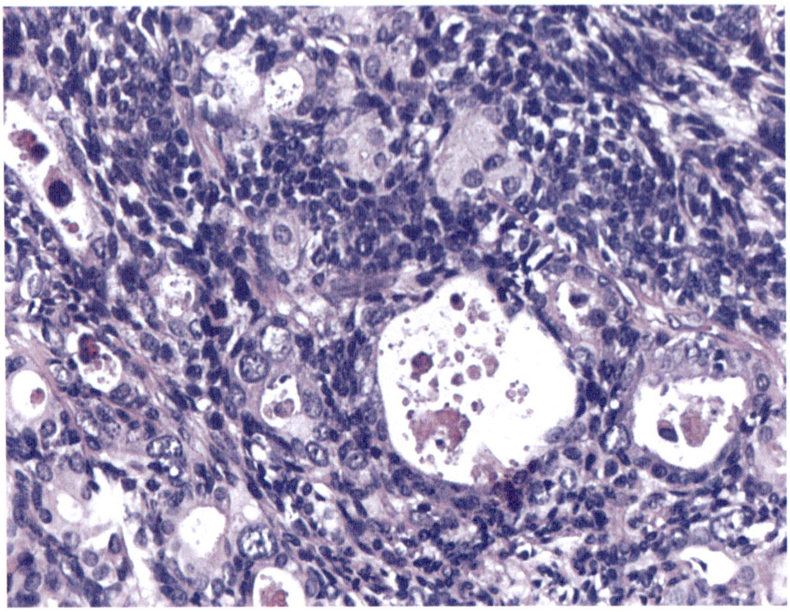

Fig. 41 In this high-power field, part of the neoplastic cells is larger, more atypical and organized to form duct-like structures

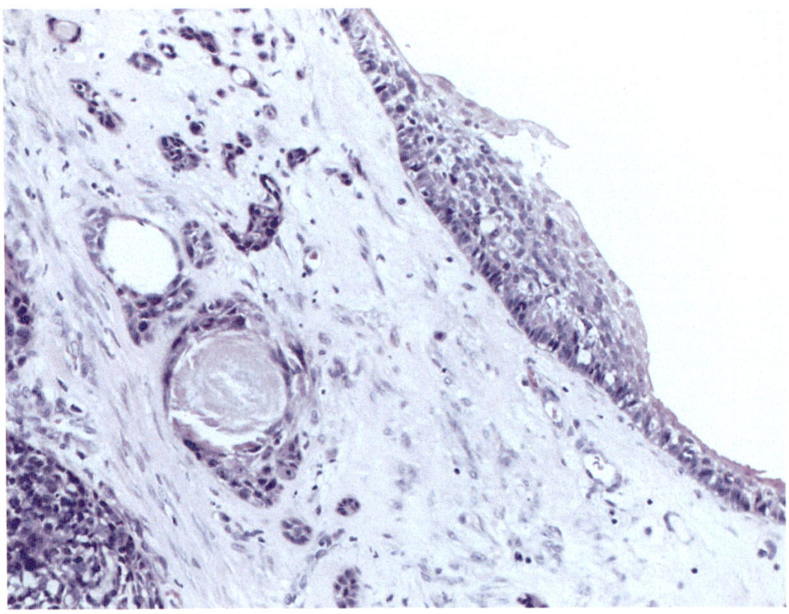

Fig. 42 The surface squamous epithelium shows severe dysplasia. Squamous differentiation is also recognized in the superficial nests of this tumor

differentiation, the presence of anaplastic giant cells randomly scattered in the invasive tumor, tumor areas resembling epithelial-myoepithelial carcinoma, a minor component of sarcomatoid differentiation with undifferentiated malignant spindled cells, and areas with chondroid or osseous differentiation.

Immunohistochemical Profile

The tumor is diffusely positive for cytokeratins. With the cytokeratin cocktail AE1/AE3, the staining is biphasic, with strong staining in the ductal cells and weaker staining in the abluminal basaloid cells (Fig. 43a). Calponin, actins, p40, and p63 are positive, mainly with an abluminal pattern. S100 (Fig. 43b) and c-kit are also frequently positive. Strong and diffuse staining for p16 is present in all cases (Fig. 43c), including also the atypical surface epithelium.

Molecular Features

High-risk HPV can be detected in all cases by in situ hybridization techniques (Fig. 43d) or by PCR-based methods. HPV 33 is the most frequent type detected, followed by HPV 35,

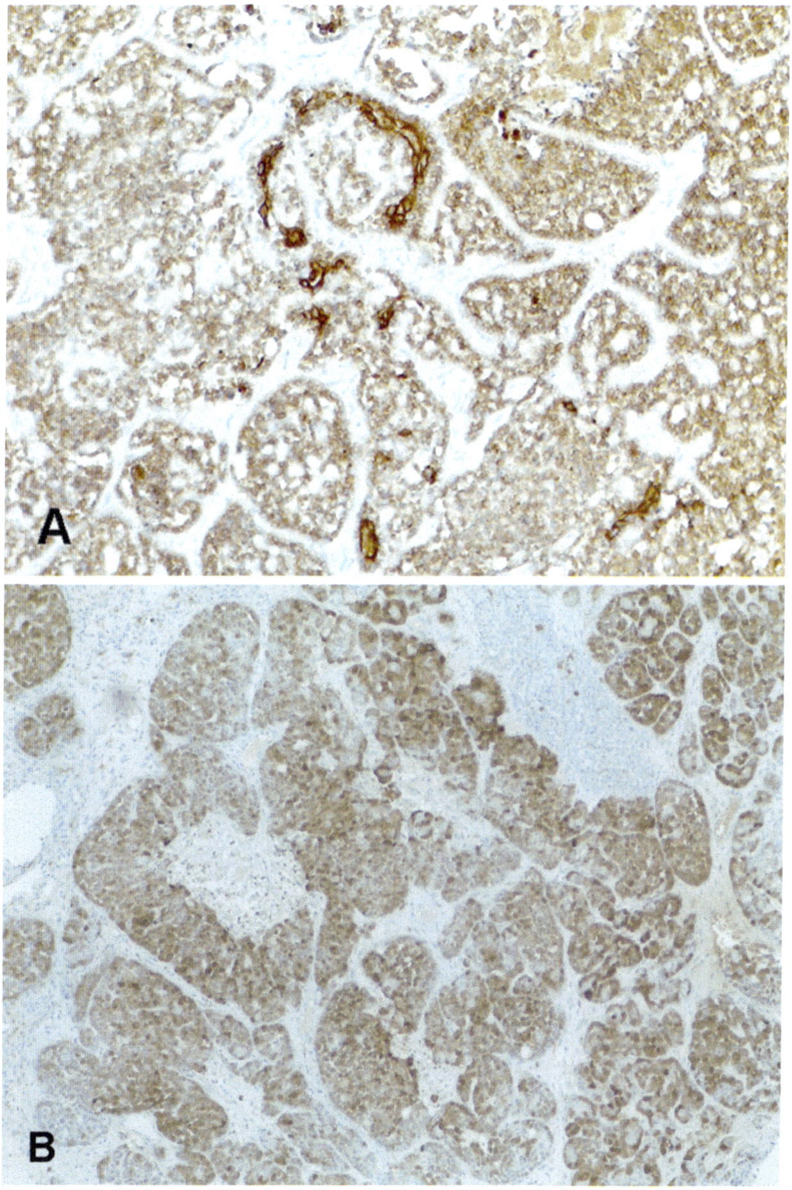

Fig. 43 HPV-related multiphenotypic sinonasal carcinoma. Immunohistochemical staining for cytokeratin AE1/AE3 (**a**) highlights two types of cells, those showing ductal differentiation in the central areas are more intensely stained, whereas the myoepithelial cells show a weaker staining. Diffuse positivity for S100 is illustrated in (**b**). P16 is intensely and diffusely positive (**c**). In situ hybridization for high-risk HPV is shown in (**d**)

Fig. 43 (continued)

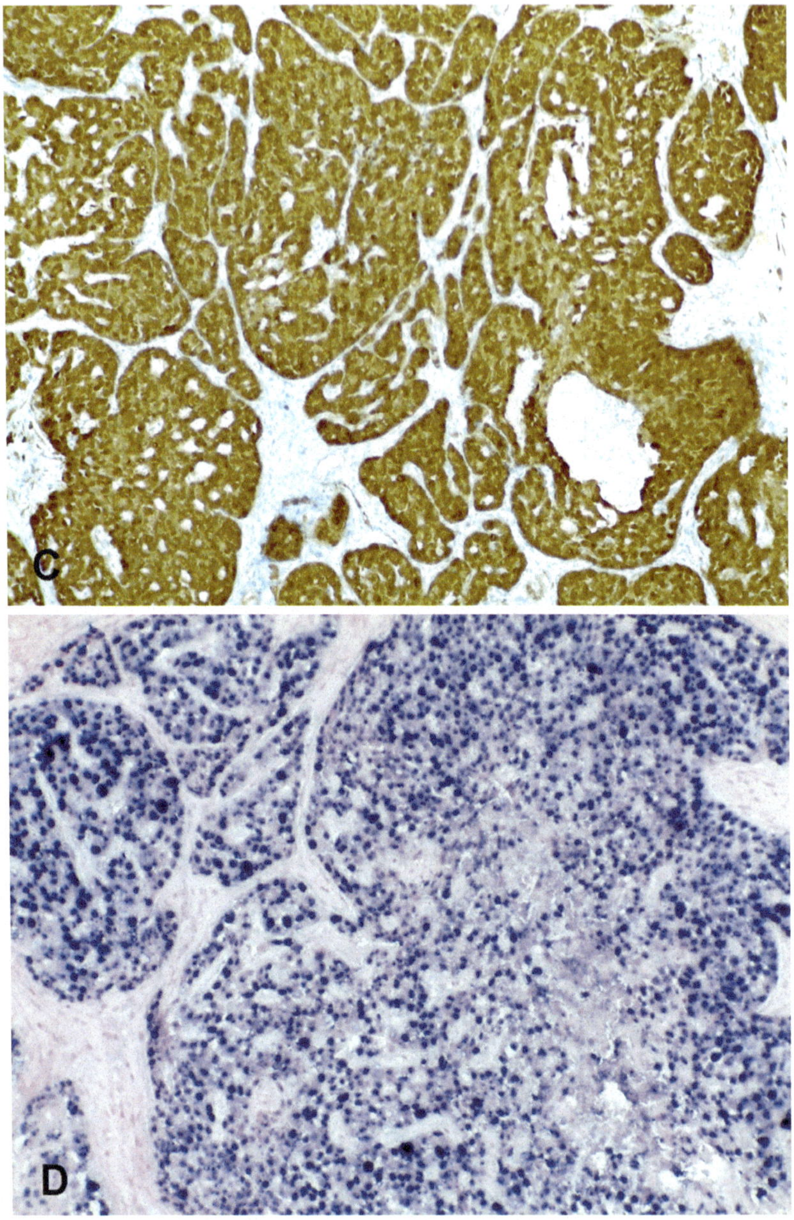

whereas HPV type 16 is only rarely present [130–132]. Rearrangements of *MYB*, *MYBL1*, and *NFIB* genes have not been detected [130–132].

Differential Diagnosis

HMSC has a strict morphologic similarity with adenoid cystic carcinoma, including the presence of solid and cribriform architecture, a dual population of ductal cells and basaloid cells, and the presence of a myoepithelial phenotype. The distinction between the two can be based on the presence of HPV and on the absence of the *MYB-NFIB* gene fusion in HSMC. In addition, the presence of squamous dysplasia of the surface epithelium is against a diagnosis of adenoid cystic carcinoma. Other salivary-type carcinomas that can be entered in the differential diagnosis are epithelial-myoepithelial carcinoma and basal cell adenocarcinoma. Both these tumor types are not related to HPV infection and are not associated with dysplastic changes of the surface epithelium.

Treatment and Prognosis

Although often presents at high tumor stage and with a high-grade histologic appearance, it tends to behave in a relatively indolent manner with frequent local recurrences but only rare metastases and no reported tumor-related deaths [130].

Intestinal-Type Adenocarcinoma

Definition

Sinonasal intestinal-type adenocarcinoma (ITAC) is a tumor that histologically resembles colorectal adenoma or adenocarcinoma. It is thought to develop through intestinal metaplasia of the surface respiratory epithelium.

Clinical Features

ITAC is a rare tumor, and its incidence varies significantly in different countries, being significantly higher in European countries than in the United States. There is a well-known association with occupational exposures to wood and leather dusts (see chapter "Epidemiology of Sinonasal Cancer") and a clear male predominance [133]. The peak age of incidence is in the sixth and seventh decades. The most common presenting symptoms are unilateral nasal obstruction, epistaxis, presence of a visible tumor, rhinorrhea, and pain, while in exophthalmos and diplopia are present in advanced stage tumors [134]. The majority of patients present with stage T3 and T4 tumors, often with multiple sites of involvement [133] and invasion of skull base and orbit. The ethmoid region, particularly the olfactory cleft, is the site of origin in the majority of the cases [133, 135].

Pathologic Features

Grossly, ITAC appears as an exophytic, friable, often ulcerated and hemorrhagic mass. Less frequently, it shows a gelatinous or mucoid consistency.

Histologically, the morphologic spectrum of ITAC closely resembles that of adenocarcinomas or adenomas of intestinal origin, or it may even mimic the appearance of normal intestinal mucosa, including the presence of Paneth cells, argentaffin cells, goblet cells, and resorptive cells, forming villi with an underlying muscularis mucosae [136, 137]. Typically, ITAC consists of a proliferation of dysplastic columnar cells with interspersed goblet cells, forming papillae and glands. Areas of intestinal metaplasia can be present in the adjacent respiratory mucosa [138, 139].

According to the architectural and cytologic features, a number of ITAC subtypes can be identified. Barnes recognized five categories: papillary, colonic, solid, mucinous, and mixed [136]. Kleinsasser and Schroeder divided ITACs into papillary-tubular cylindrical cell type (including to papillary, colonic, and solid types), alveolar goblet cell type, signet-ring cell type (corresponding to mucinous type), and transitional cell type (corresponding to mixed type) [140]. These histologic subtypes show different clinical behavior: well-differentiated papillary tumors have a relatively indolent course, while poorly differentiated/solid and mucinous subtypes show a significantly worst prognosis [136, 140, 141].

The well-differentiated papillary ITACs (15–20%) consist of elongated outgrowths lined by stratified columnar mildly atypical intestinal-type cells with interspersed goblet cells (Fig. 44). The moderately differentiated colonic type (35–40%) consists of glandular and tubular structures arranged back to back and resembles quite closely a conventional colorectal adenocarcinoma (Fig. 45). The glands are formed by atypical columnar cells, and intra- and extracellular mucin and few goblet cells may be present. Mitotic figures, including atypical forms, are easily identified, and areas of necrosis can be present. The solid/poorly differentiated pattern (10–15%) consists of cubical and cylindrical cells, with moderate to marked nuclear pleomorphism, showing only partial or focal gland formation

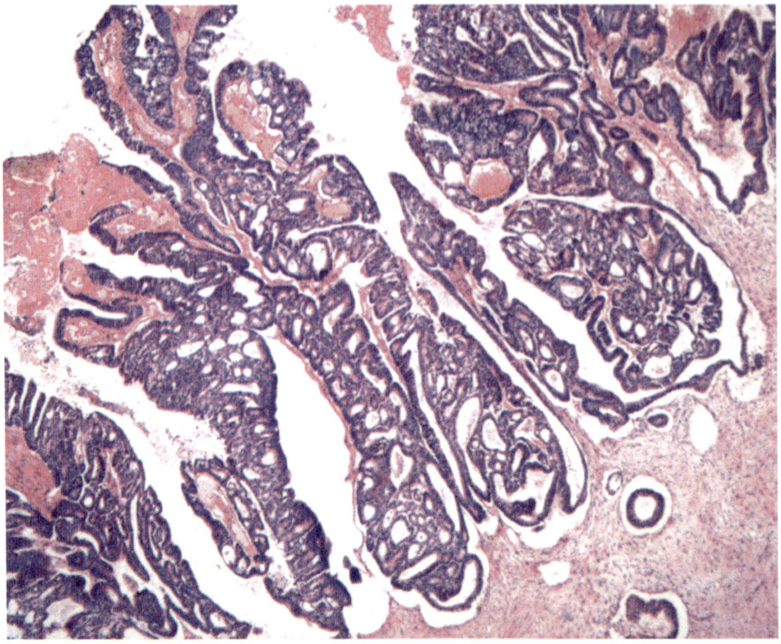

Fig. 44 Well-differentiated (G1) intestinal-type adenocarcinoma with a predominant exophytic papillary growth pattern

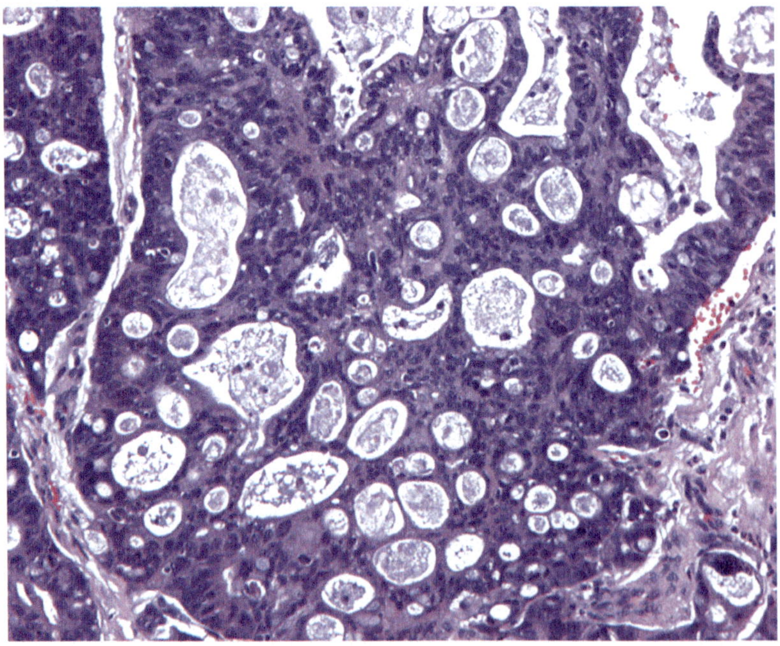

Fig. 45 Moderately differentiated (G2) intestinal-type adenocarcinoma

(Fig. 46). Approximately 20–25% of ITACs show abundant mucous production and mainly consist of dilated mucin-filled glands lined by cubical or cylindrical mucous-producing cells. Strips of neoplastic cells may be present within the extracellular mucous pools (Fig. 47). In a minority of cases, neoplastic cells show intracellular accumulation of mucin, resulting in a signet-ring appearance (Fig. 48).

The histologic spectrum of sinonasal ITAC includes also rare examples of true mixed exocrine- NEC [142, 143]. Such cases consisted of

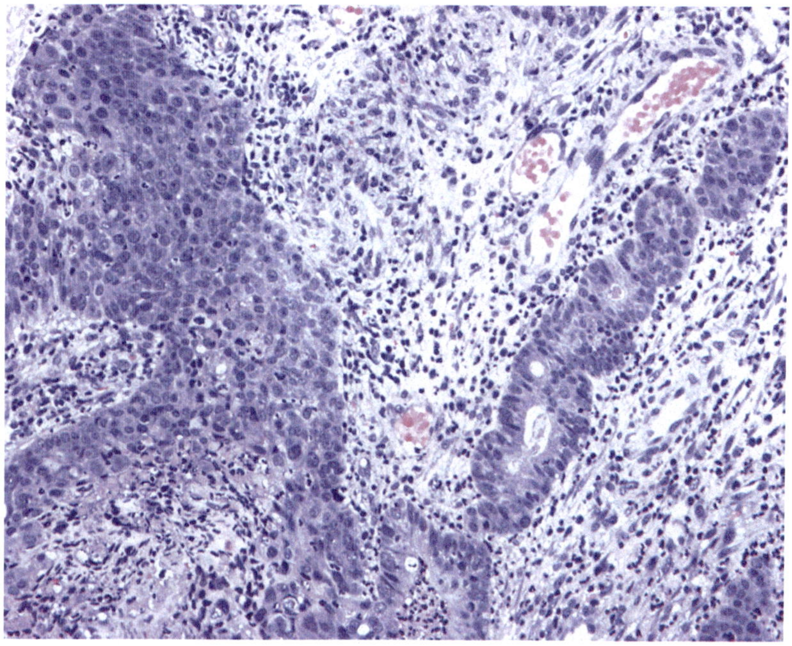

Fig. 46 Poorly differentiated intestinal-type adenocarcinoma with a predominantly solid growth pattern

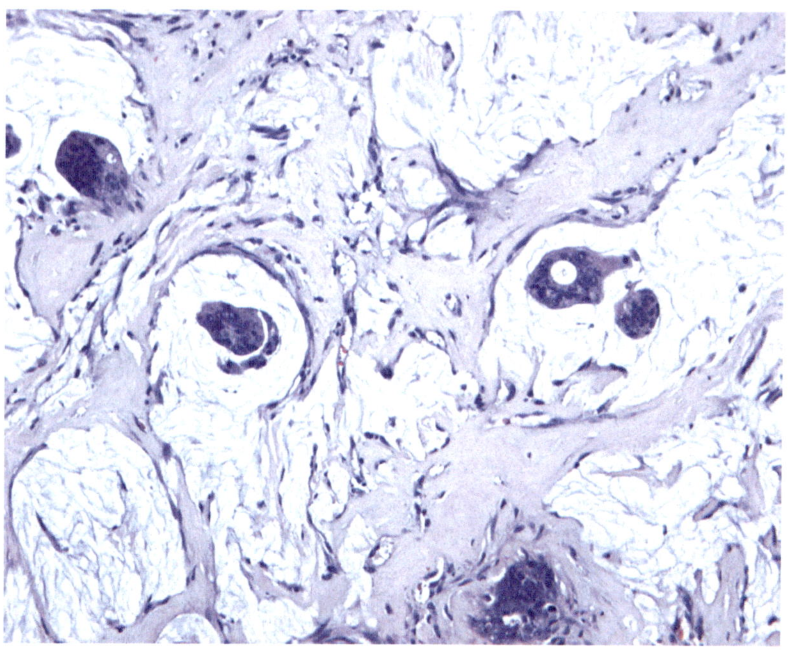

Fig. 47 Intestinal-type adenocarcinoma with abundant extracellular mucous production

a conventional ITAC component (well differentiated/papillary in one instance and poorly differentiated/mucinous in two) and a poorly differentiated NEC component.

Immunohistochemical Profile

ITACs are typically positive for pancytokeratins and EMA, while CEA is positive only infrequently. Markers of intestinal differentiation,

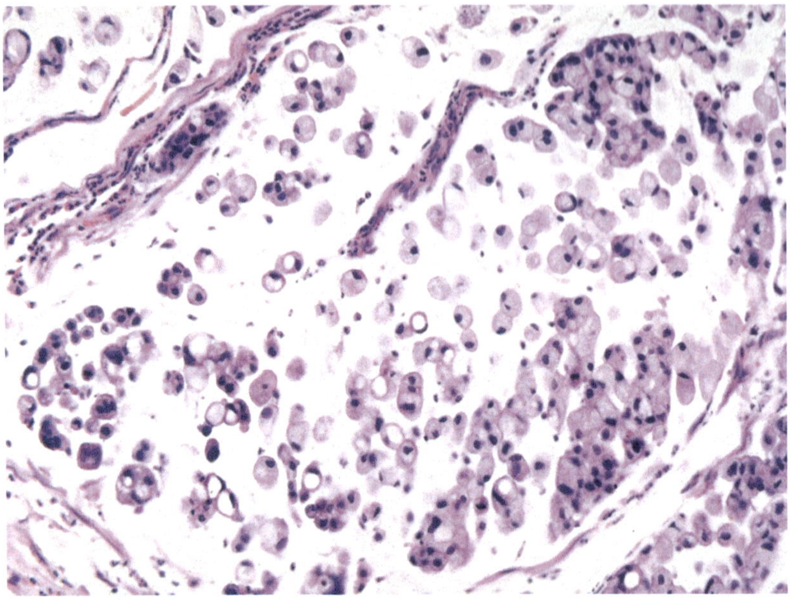

Fig. 48 Intestinal-type adenocarcinoma with signet ring morphology

including cytokeratin 20, CDX2, villin, and SATB2, are expressed in most cases [144–146], although their sensitivity and specificity are variable [147]. It is therefore advisable to use them in combination to demonstrate intestinal differentiation. Scattered cells or small groups of cells may be positive for neuroendocrine markers, including chromogranin and synaptophysin.

Genetic Profile

The genetic anomalies found in ITAC are considerably different from those observed in other sinonasal carcinomas and are only partially similar to those reported in colorectal adenocarcinoma [148]. Genome-wide studies performed with comparative genomic hybridization (CGH) and microarray CGH have shown that ITACs harbor complex karyotypes with copy number alterations involving all chromosomes. Hotspot gains have been found at 5p, 7p, 8q, 12p, and 20q, and losses at 4q, 5q, 8p, 17p, and 18q [149]. Some recurrent copy number alterations are associated with unfavorable prognosis [149].

TP53 is the most frequently mutated gene (40–50%) [150, 151], and p53 overexpression is observed at similar rates with immunohistochemistry [152]. High levels of EGFR expression and gene amplification have been detected in a subset of ITAC [153, 154], while activating mutations of *K-RAS* and *BRAF* are rare [155–157]. This scenario suggests possibilities for anti-EGFR-targeted treatments in some patients affected by ITAC.

Differential Diagnosis

ITAC can be separated from non-intestinal-type adenocarcinomas based on morphology and with the help of immunohistochemical markers of intestinal differentiation (Table 4). The distinction between mucinous ITAC and mucocele is based on the presence of cytologic atypia, brisk mitotic activity, and necrosis. Mucoepidermoid and adenosquamous carcinomas can be ruled out for the lack of squamous differentiation in ITAC.

Various attempts have been made to search for markers to separate sinonasal ITAC from metastatic gastric and colorectal adenocarcinoma, but none resulted specific and sensitive to allow a distinction [158]. Thus, exclusion of a colorectal primitive tumor has to be made on clinical grounds.

Treatment and Prognosis

Surgical resection represents the gold standard for the treatment of ITAC. Different options are currently available, which can be chosen according to the site and extension of the tumor and on the experience of the surgeon. Endoscopic

Table 4 Differential features of selected glandular lesions of the sinonasal tract

Lesion	Clinical features	Salient histopathologic features	Immunohistochemistry	Molecular changes
Respiratory epithelial adenomatoid hamartoma (REAH)	Polypoid lesion; posterior nasal septum, ethmoid sinus, nasopharynx; wide age range, male predominance	Back-to-back glands lined by ciliated columnar cells, periglandular hyalinization; occasional mucinous change of proliferating epithelium	CK7+, CK20-, CDX2-, p63+ in the basal compartment, S100-	NA
Seromucous hamartoma	Polypoid lesion; posterior nasal septum, nasopharynx; wide age range, slight male predominance	Lobular growth of small serous glands, uncommon mucinous glands; areas resembling REAH occasionally seen	S100+, CK7+, CK20-, CDX2-, myoepithelial markers-	NA
Intestinal-type adenocarcinoma (ITAC)	Exophytic lesions, often with necrotic-hemorrhagic or mucoid appearance; ethmoid sinus, nasal cavity; adult subjects, male predominance; association with wood-working and leather-working	Columnar cells, goblet cells, signet ring cells; papillary, glandular, solid, and alveolar-mucinous architecture	CK20+, CK7 variably positive, CDX2+	*TP53* frequently mutated; activating mutations of *K-RAS* and *BRAF* rarely seen; EGFR amplification in a subset of cases
Low-grade non-ITAC	Papillary/exophytic lesions; nasal cavities and ethmoid sinus; wide age range, predominantly adult patients, no gender predilection	Different growth patterns, more frequently tubulo-papillary, cribriform, clear cell; back-to-back glands, mild atypia, low mitotic activity, infiltration of mucosa and bone	CK7+, CK20-, CDX2-; myoepithelial markers, DOG1, and SOX10 + in some cases; CAIX + in sinonasal renal cell-like adenocarcinoma	*ETV6* gene rearrangements in a subset of cases
High-grade non-ITAC	Large destructive lesions, with exophytic appearance; hemorrhage and necrosis often present; nasal cavities and maxillary sinus; adult patients	Predominantly solid growth pattern, poorly formed glands, marked atypia, pleomorphism, necrosis, brisk mitotic activity	CK7+, CK20-, CDX2-	NA

approaches have been increasingly used for the treatment of sinonasal adenocarcinomas, as they show comparable outcomes to open approaches, but with a significantly lower incidence of complications [158]. Surgery is followed by postoperative radiotherapy when the lesion is locally advanced, when margins are involved or close, or when histologic features of aggressiveness, such as high grade (mucinous or G3), vascular invasion, or perineural growth, are detected in the resection specimen [159, 160]. In patients with locally advanced tumors (T3–T4) treatment may also consist of neoadjuvant chemotherapy protocols, followed by surgery and radiotherapy [161]. This approach is more effective in presence of tumors with intact p53 protein [162].

In general, ITAC can be considered a high-grade malignancy because the majority of patients develop tumor relapses. Local recurrence occurs in 30–60%, while lymph node metastases and distant metastases are infrequently detected, as they develop in 1–5% and 5–10% of the patients, respectively [133, 134, 158, 160]. The median time to recurrence is 25–30 months [133, 134]. The 5-year survival rate is 50–60%, and the 10-year survival rate is 45–50% [133, 134, 160].

Tumor extension is an important prognostic factor, as evidenced in several studies. In particular, involvement of the orbit, dura, brain, or sphenoid is associated with worst prognosis [134, 163]. Other important negative prognostic factors are local recurrence and the occurrence of distant metastasis [133, 134, 160]. The histologic features are also correlated with the clinical course, because well-differentiated papillary ITAC tends to have an indolent behavior, while mucinous and poorly differentiated variants behave more aggressively.

Non-Intestinal-Type Adenocarcinomas

Definition

Sinonasal non-intestinal-type adenocarcinomas (non-ITAC) are a heterogenous group of rare tumors defined by exclusion as glandular malignancies that do not show signs of intestinal differentiation and do not resemble any salivary gland tumor type. They can be further distinguished in low- and high-grade subtypes.

Clinical Features

Non-ITACs differ significantly from ITAC in their clinical presentation. Men are affected more frequently than females, and patients are distributed over a wide age range, with a median of 60 years [164, 165]. The nasal cavities and the maxillary sinus are the main site of origin, while the ethmoid region is less frequently involved [164]. There is no known association with occupational exposures.

Pathological Features

Macroscopically, non-ITACs tend to have an exophytic appearance. High-grade tumors are large, necrotic, ulcerated, and destructive lesions, whereas low-grade non-ITACs are smaller and relatively well-circumscribed lesions.

The histologic features of *high-grade non-ITAC* are quite variable, and several growth patterns have been described [164]. The majority shows a predominantly solid architecture, with interspersed rosette-like glands (Fig. 49). Neoplastic cells are

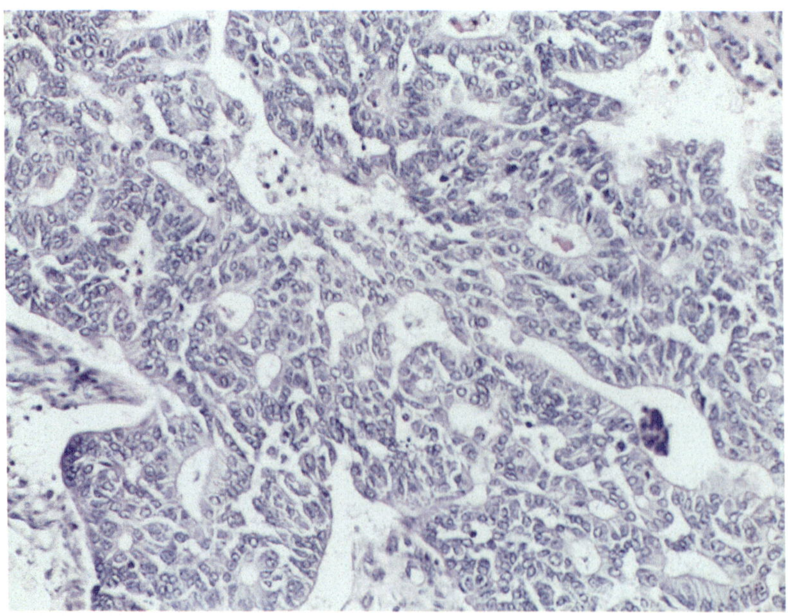

Fig. 49 High-grade non-intestinal-type sinonasal adenocarcinoma composed of poorly formed glands in a solid background

small- to medium-sized and have scant lightly eosinophilic cytoplasm. The overall appearance is similar to the "blastomatous" components of teratocarcinosarcoma. Other adenocarcinomas present predominately a poorly differentiated solid growth pattern and show only occasional micropapillary or gland-like structures (Fig. 50). Other lesions consist of infiltrating islands and glands formed by larger cells, with abundant eosinophilic cytoplasm and somewhat apocrine features, resembling ductal carcinoma of the breast or high-grade salivary duct carcinoma. Less frequently, high-grade non-ITAC consists of oncocytic cells sometimes mixed with mucinous cells and abundant extracellular mucus. Such tumors may arise in association with oncocytic papilloma.

Low-grade non-ITACs predominately show a papillary exophytic architecture (Fig. 51), with

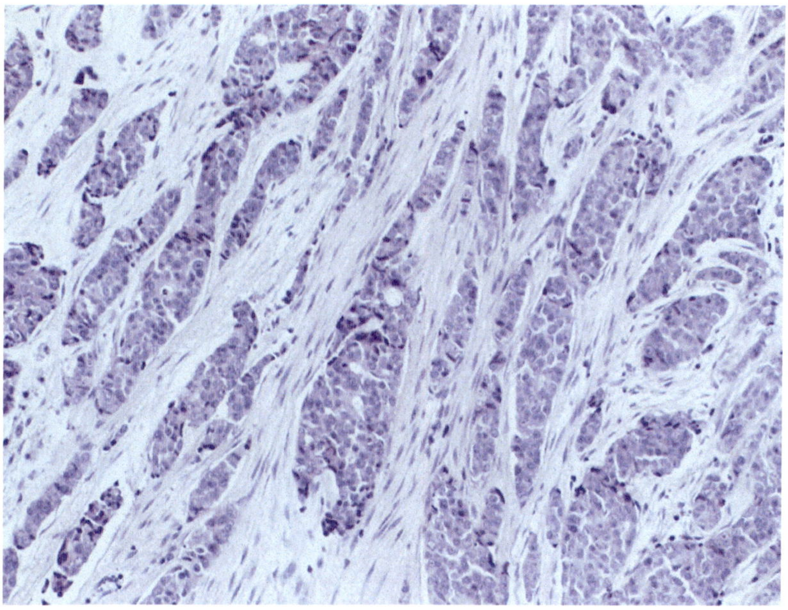

Fig. 50 This high-grade non-intestinal-type sinonasal adenocarcinoma consists of elongated tumor islands with focal glandular differentiation

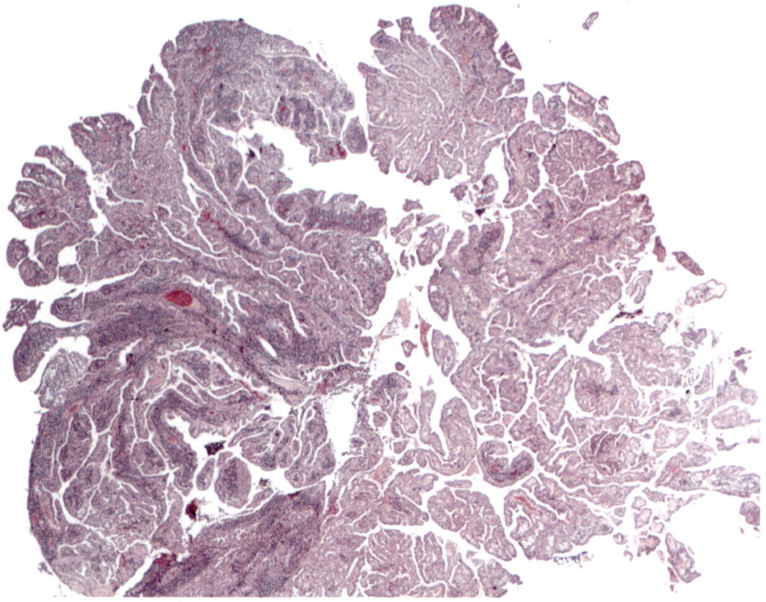

Fig. 51 Most low-grade non-intestinal-type adenocarcinomas present with an exophytic papillary architecture

fibrovascular cores lined by columnar or cuboidal cells, with absent to slight atypia.

In other instances, the core of the tumor consists of small tubules and trabeculae lined by a single layer of cuboidal to columnar cells with slightly eosinophilic cytoplasm (Figs. 52 and 53). The tubules are arranged "back-to-back" and may be fused in some areas (Fig. 54). Mucin-producing cells and microcysts filled with mucin can be present, while oncocytic and more solid appearing areas are seldom found. Focal areas of squamoid or morular metaplasia have been noted in a subset of cases [165]. Infiltration of nasal mucosa and bone is more easily identified than in papillary exophytic forms. In general, histologic signs of aggressiveness, such as perineural

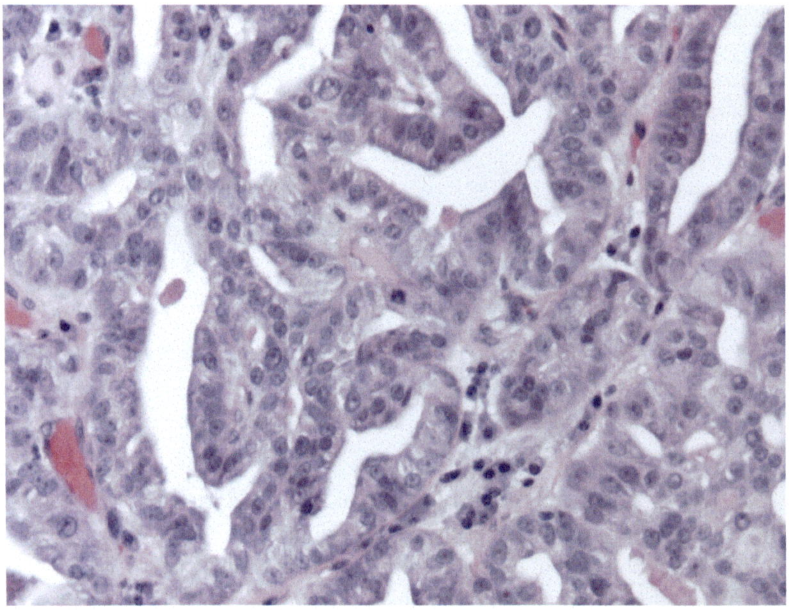

Fig. 52 Neoplastic papillae are lined by a single layer of cuboidal to columnar cells with slightly eosinophilic cytoplasm

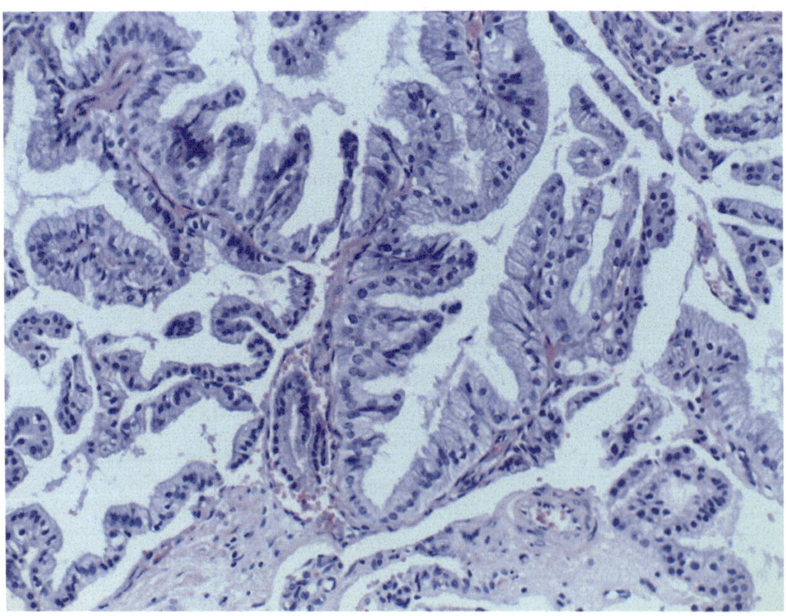

Fig. 53 This low-grade adenocarcinoma is composed of columnar cells with clear cytoplasm

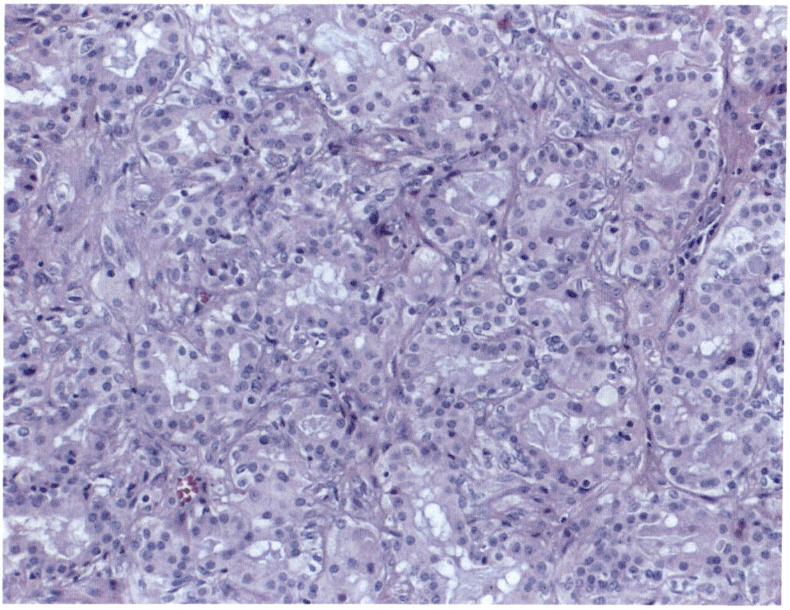

Fig. 54 Back-to-back glands composed of moderately atypical neoplastic cells

invasion, lymphovascular invasion, brisk mitotic activity, and necrosis, are absent. Low-grade non-ITAC may arise in association with benign lesions, such as sinonasal papillomas and REAHrespiratory epithelial adenomatoid hamartomas [31, 166]. A subset of low-grade non-ITAC consists of a uniform population of cuboidal to columnar cells with glycogen-rich clear cytoplasm without mucin production. These tumors resemble quite closely metastatic renal carcinoma and have been designated as *sinonasal renal cell-like adenocarcinoma* [167–169].

Immunohistochemical Profile

Non-ITAC are positive for cytokeratin cocktails and cytokeratin 7, while cytokeratin 20, CDX2, and villin are generally negative. However, CDX2 expression has been noted in areas of squamous modular metaplasia in both high-grade and low-grade non-ITAC [165] and in other high-grade sinonasal carcinomas [147]. Markers of seromucinous differentiation, including S100, DOG1, and SOX10, are expressed to varying degrees in the majority of non-ITAC while are essentially absent in ITAC. A myoepithelial/basal component can be identified as well [170]. The neoplastic cells of sinonasal renal cell-like adenocarcinoma are strongly positive for cytokeratin 7 and CAIX, but negative with PAX-8 and RCC.

Molecular Features

There are only few reports of genetic analysis in sinonasal non-ITAC. A subset of low-grade tumors presents *ETV6* gene rearrangements, usually with *ETV6-NTRK3* gene fusions [171]. In an analysis of two cases, *TP53* coding regions (exons 4–9) were not mutated [170].

Differential Diagnosis

High-grade non-ITAC can be distinguished from low-grade non-ITAC for the presence of prominent cytologic atypia, brisk mitotic activity, and/or necrosis (Table 4). ITAC can be ruled out based on the morphological resemblance to colorectal adenocarcinoma and for the positivity to intestinal markers, such as cytokeratin 20, CDX2, and villin (Table 4). In addition, ITAC differs in its clinical presentation with involvement of the ethmoid region and the frequent association with occupational exposures. Other poorly differentiated high-grade neoplasms to be considered in the differential diagnosis with high-grade non-ITAC include salivary duct carcinoma, mucoepidermoid carcinoma, adenosquamous carcinoma, and teratocarcinosarcoma.

The distinction between low-grade non-ITAC and benign lesions like REAH and seromucinous hamartoma (SH) can be challenging, especially in small biopsies (Table 4). In REAH, the gland-like structures are connected to the surface, lined by respiratory-type epithelium and surrounded by periglandular hyalinization. In SH, there is characteristic lobular arrangement that is not present in adenocarcinomas, and infiltrative growth is not present.

The renal cell-like adenocarcinoma is negative for vimentin, PAX8, and RCC, all markers expressed by renal cell carcinoma.

Salivary-Type Adenocarcinomas

Definition

Sinonasal salivary-type adenocarcinomas are a group of tumors derived from the seromucous glands of the Schneiderian mucosa histologically identical to those deriving from salivary glands of the oral cavity. Overall, they represent 5–10% of sinonasal adenocarcinomas [172]. Although a wide range of histologic types have been reported, adenoid cystic carcinoma (ACC) and mucoepidermoid carcinoma (MEC) are by far the most frequent. Thus, only the clinical findings of these entities will be discussed. Other tumor types are mentioned in the section "Pathologic features."

Clinical Features

ACC arises mainly from the maxillary sinus, followed by the nasal cavity and the ethmoid sinus. Over 85% of patients have >40 years of age at diagnosis (mean 55–60 years), and there is a slight female predominance. Most sinonasal ACC present with advanced stage disease, with low rates of nodal or distant metastasis [173].

Sinonasal MEC occurs over a wider age range, involving also young adults (mean age 55 years) with no significant gender predilection [174]. The nasal cavity is the most commonly affected site, together with the maxillary sinus, and the involvement of multiple sites [174]. Most patients present with low-stage disease [174].

Pathologic Features

Histologically, sinonasal ACC is identical to that arising at other head and neck sites. The overlying epithelium is intact, of respiratory or squamous metaplastic type, or ulcerated. Over 50% present a cribriform growth pattern, followed by tubular and solid growths (Fig. 55) [175, 176]. In the *cribriform pattern*, islands of neoplastic cells contain round pseudo-cystic structures that impart a Swiss cheese-like

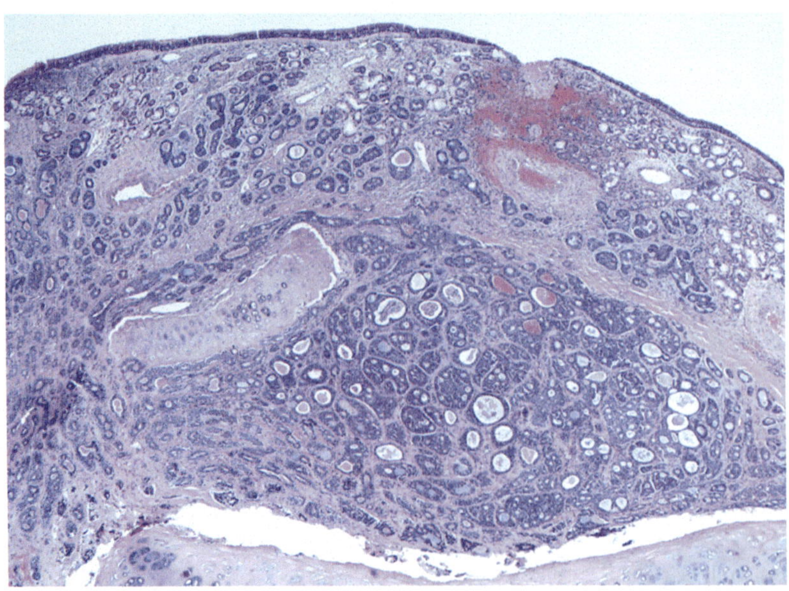

Fig. 55 Sinonasal adenoid cystic carcinoma. The tumor infiltrates the mucosa and the cartilage and presents tubular and cribriform architecture

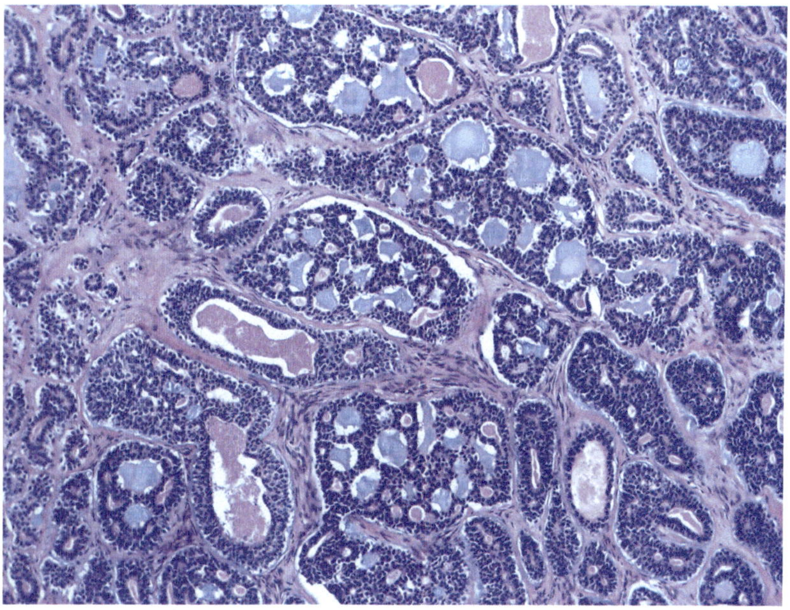

Fig. 56 In this area, the cribriform pattern predominates

appearance to the tumor (Fig. 56). These spaces are contiguous with the collagenous stroma of the tumor and contain either a basophilic substance that represents an accumulation of glycosaminoglycans or eosinophilic hyalinized material due to excessive production of basal lamina. Neoplastic cells have uniform dark nuclei and scant eosinophilic to amphophilic or clear cytoplasm. These cells are of abluminal or myoepithelial phenotype. Small foci of ductal cells are scattered among the basaloid myoepithelial cells. They have a more abundant eosinophilic cytoplasm with uniform round nuclei and surround small lumina. The same cell types are found in the *tubular pattern*. Myoepithelial cells with clear cytoplasm and irregular nuclei surround duct-type cells with eosinophilic cytoplasm. The center of the tubular neoplastic structures consists of hyaline eosinophilic or basophilic stroma, that is, in continuity with the connective tissue stroma. In the *solid pattern* of ACC, cells tend to be larger than those of the cribriform and tubular structures, with more prominent pleomorphism, and are predominantly of the basaloid myoepithelial type. Mitotic figures are more numerous, and comedo-type necrosis can be present in the center of tumor nests.

Infiltration of the bone, nerves, and of lymphovascular spaces is a frequent finding. In rare instances, sinonasal ACC may arise in a preexisting PA [44, 45]. Examples of so-called dedifferentiated ACC have also been reported in the sinonasal region [177]. These tumors consist of a conventional low-grade ACC component, with tubular or cribriform architecture, clearly separated from a high-grade undifferentiated or poorly differentiated adenocarcinoma component. However, it is not clear whether these tumors may indeed represent examples of HPV-related multiphenotypic carcinomas, and careful differential diagnosis is required.

MEC is composed of varying proportions of epidermoid cells, mucous secreting cells, clear cells, and intermediate cells (Fig. 57). True squamous differentiation with keratinization is generally not a feature of MEC, and the term epidermoid only refers to a squamous-like appearance. Epidermoid cells are large, with eosinophilic cytoplasm, whereas intermediate cells are small, have a basal-cell-like appearance with dark staining nuclei. Both these cell types may present also with clear cytoplasm (clear cells). Mucous cells are cuboidal or columnar, goblet-like-shaped cell with peripherally located nucleus. Overall, they represent up to 10% of the tumor volume [174]

Fig. 57 Low-grade mucoepidermoid carcinoma of the maxillary sinus. Nests of tumor cells with mucinous, clear, and squamoid morphology with partial cyst formation

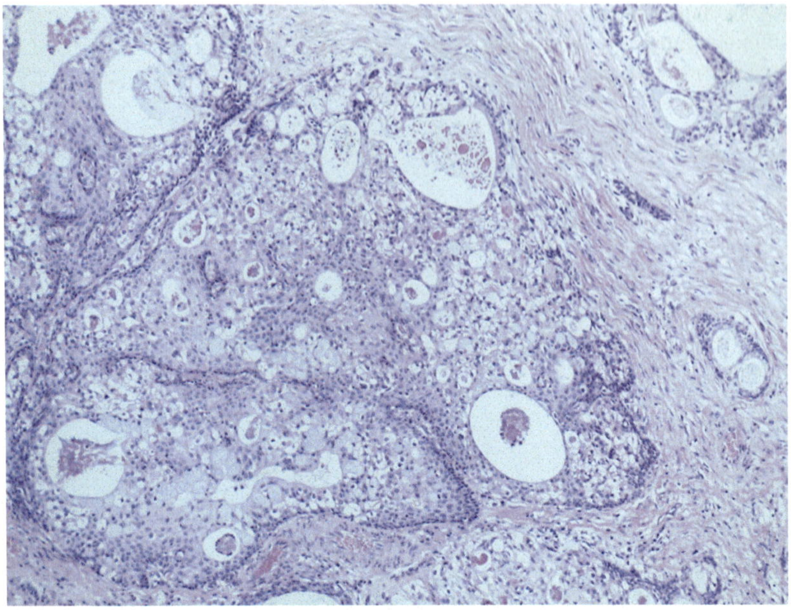

and can be interspersed between epidermoid and intermediate cells or may form solid proliferations or the lining of cystic spaces. A cystic component is frequently present, and it may consist of large spaces filled with mucinous material and lined by epithelium, small spaces with mucinous debris in the lumen, or dilated duct-like spaces containing mucinous and inflammatory debris [174]. MEC may arise from a preexisting sinonasal papilloma [28].

MECs can be separated in low, intermediate, and high grade based on the evaluation of the extent of the cystic component, neural invasion, necrosis, mitotic activity, and anaplasia. Most sinonasal tumors fall in the low- and intermediate-grade categories [174].

A few examples of sinonasal *epithelial-myoepithelial carcinoma* have been reported [178]. This tumor consists of tubular structures made of two distinct layers of cells, epithelial and myoepithelial, surrounded by a basement membrane of variable thickness. The inner epithelial layer is formed by cuboidal cells with scanty pale to eosinophilic cytoplasm and a round to oval nucleus. The outer myoepithelial layer consists of larger polygonal cells, often with clear cytoplasm.

Salivary duct carcinoma is exceedingly rare in the sinonasal tract [179]. Histologically, it resembles ductal carcinoma of the breast and consists of cribriform structures, solid nests, duct-like structures with papillary, "Roman bridge," and comedo patterns. Perineural and lympho-vascular invasion are frequently observed. Other salivary-type tumors reported in the sinonasal tract include *polymorphous adenocarcinoma* [180, 181], *basal cell adenocarcinoma* [182], and *myoepithelial carcinoma*, the latter with a round cell morphology that requires differential diagnosis with other sinonasal poorly differentiated carcinomas [183].

Finally, two examples of *secretory carcinoma* (synonym: mammary analogue secretory carcinoma) arising in the sinonasal tract have been recently reported [184]. This case is a rare salivary gland-type carcinoma characterized by a t(12;15)(p13;q25) translocation, resulting in an *ETV6-NTRK3* gene fusion, that needs to be distinguished from a potential molecular mimicker, the *ETV6*-rearranged low-grade sinonasal adenocarcinoma [171]. The histologic features of these entities are distinctive enough to allow their separation, since secretory carcinoma presents abundant hyalinized septae and pronounced secretory features that are not present in low-grade non-ITAC that in turn are composed of glands arranged back-to-back with little intervening stroma and minimal to absent secretory features. Finally, ETV6-rearranged low-grade non-ITAC is positive for DOG-1, negative for mammaglobin, and negative or patchy positive for S100, with the opposite is true for secretory carcinoma.

Immunohistochemistry

ACC is positive for pancytokeratin and cytokeratin 5/6, with different intensity according to the tumor cell type. The myoepithelial and/or basal components are variably reactive with S100 protein, calponin, smooth muscle actin, and p63, while actins and glial fibrillary acidic protein are weakly and focally positive in a minority of cases. CD117 is expressed mainly in the epithelial cells. P16 is positive virtually in all cases, with a nuclear and cytoplasmic localization, but true sinonasal ACC is negative for high-risk HPV [176].

MEC is also positive for pancytokeratin and cytokeratin 5/6, the latter with reactivity distributed mainly in the basal and intermediate cell components. P63 shows diffuse nuclear staining in the epidermoid cells, while the goblet-type mucinous epithelium is positive for CEA. CD117 and S100 show partial staining in rare cases.

Molecular Features

ACC presents a specific chromosomal translocation t(6;9) with formation of the fusion gene *MYB-NFIB* and overexpression of the oncogene *MYB* [185] which is diagnostically helpful. In sinonasal ACC, this rearrangement has been detected in 63% of the cases [176]. MEC is specifically associated with a t(11;19) translocation that results in a *CRTC1-MAML2* fusion [186, 187]. Secretory carcinoma is characterized by a t(12;15)(p13;q25) translocation that results in a *ETV6-NTRK3* fusion transcript [184].

Differential Diagnosis

In the sinonasal region, the main differential diagnosis of ACC is with HPV-related multiphenotypic carcinoma. Indeed, this tumor had been initially designated as HPV-related carcinoma with adenoid cystic carcinoma-like features to emphasize its histologic similarities with true ACC, particularly with the solid variant. The distinctive features of this entity are the presence of dysplasia of the surface epithelium, presence of squamous differentiation of the surface epithelium and less frequently within the invasive component, association with high-risk HPV, and absence of the *MYB-NFIB* gene fusion.

MEC must be separated from adenosquamous carcinoma, from other sinonasal adenocarcinomas, and from necrotizing sialometaplasia. Adenosquamous carcinoma is a biphasic tumor with adenocarcinoma and squamous cell carcinoma components. The squamous differentiation is usually evident, with keratin pearl formation, dyskeratosis, or individual cell keratinization, all features absent in MEC. Mucinous ITAC is easily separated from MEC because it does not present an epidermoid component, and it is positive for cytokeratin 20 and CDX2. Finally, necrotizing sialometaplasia lacks cellular atypia and presents a characteristic lobular growth without signs of invasion.

Treatment and Prognosis

Most patients with sinonasal ACC and MEC have been treated with surgery alone or with surgery and radiotherapy. The majority of ACC presents in advanced local stage, while lymph node and distant metastases are infrequent [173, 176]. The overall 5-year survival rate is approximately 65%, and the 10-year survival rate is 35–40% [173, 176]. Presentation in the nasal cavity and M0 disease stage are associated with a better survival [173]. Neural, bone, and lymphovascular invasion as well as high tumor grade are associated with poor prognosis [176].

Patients with MEC present more often with low stage disease and develop local recurrence in 35–40%. The overall 5-year survival rate is approximately 45%, and the 10-year survival rate is 20% [174]. Factors associated with worst prognosis include tumor size >4 cm, involvement of multiple anatomic sites or of ethmoid sinus, high tumor grade, high mitotic count, presence of atypical mitotic figures, development of recurrence, and advanced tumor stage [174].

Teratocarcinosarcoma

Definition

Sinonasal teratocarcinosarcoma (SNTCS) is an aggressive sinonasal tumor with combined histologic features of teratoma and carcinosarcoma, lacking malignant germ cell components [188, 189]. It is currently considered to derive from somatic pluripotent stem cells of the neuroepithelium related to the olfactory membrane.

Clinical Features

SNTCS is a rare neoplasm with fewer than 100 reported cases. However, a number of cases have been reported in the literature as examples of malignant teratoma or other germ cell tumors. It arises primarily in the sinonasal region and anterior skull base, involving mainly the nasal cavities, the ethmoid, and maxillary sinuses. Patients most commonly present with nasal obstruction and epistaxis, but frontal headaches, visual changes, proptosis, anosmia or hyposmia, airway obstruction, and frontal lobe-related neurologic changes have been reported as well [190]. It presents in adults (average of 53 years) with a clear predilection for mole subjects (7:1) [190].

Pathologic Features

SNTCSs are usually large and destructive lesions, with extensive areas of necrosis. Histologically, SNTCS is composed of a mixture of epithelial, mesenchymal, and neuroepithelial elements. The epithelial components may show features of keratinizing and non-keratinizing squamous epithelium, including nests of immature squamous epithelium with clear cell features (so-called fetal appearing) (Fig. 58). Other common epithelial elements are glandular and duct-like structures and ciliated epithelium. The mesenchymal component presents usually fibroblastic and myofibroblastic features, but areas with smooth muscle, skeletal muscle (Fig. 59), adipocytic, cartilage, and osseous differentiation can be seen as well. The neuroepithelial component consists of immature round cells (Fig. 60), sometimes with rosette formation, that may be associated with a fibrillary background. Ganglion-like cells can also be present (Fig. 61).

Immunohistochemical Profile

Staining of the different elements depends on their differentiation. The epithelial components are positive for cytokeratins and EMA. Actin, desmin, and myogenin are positive in the smooth

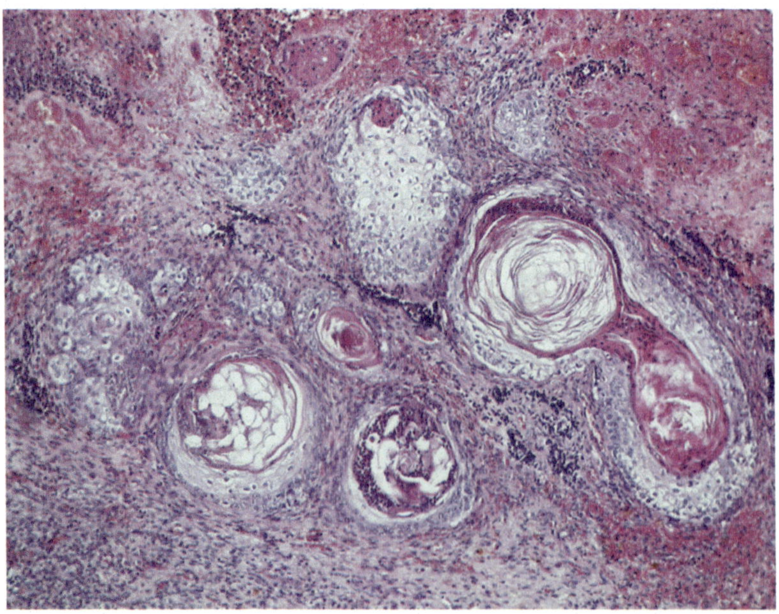

Fig. 58 Sinonasal teratocarcinosarcoma. Area showing islands of well-differentiated keratinizing epithelium

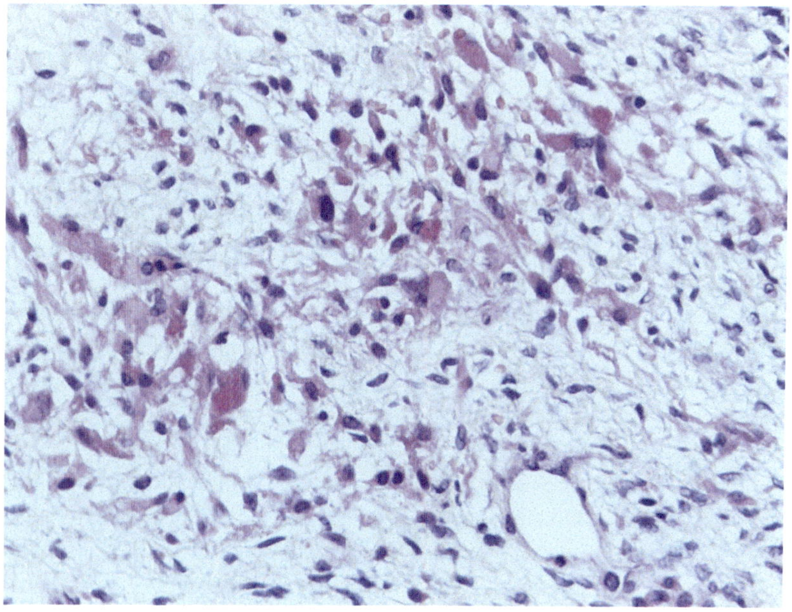

Fig. 59 Scattered rhabdomyoblasts with large eosinophilic cytoplasm are present in the mesenchymal component of this case

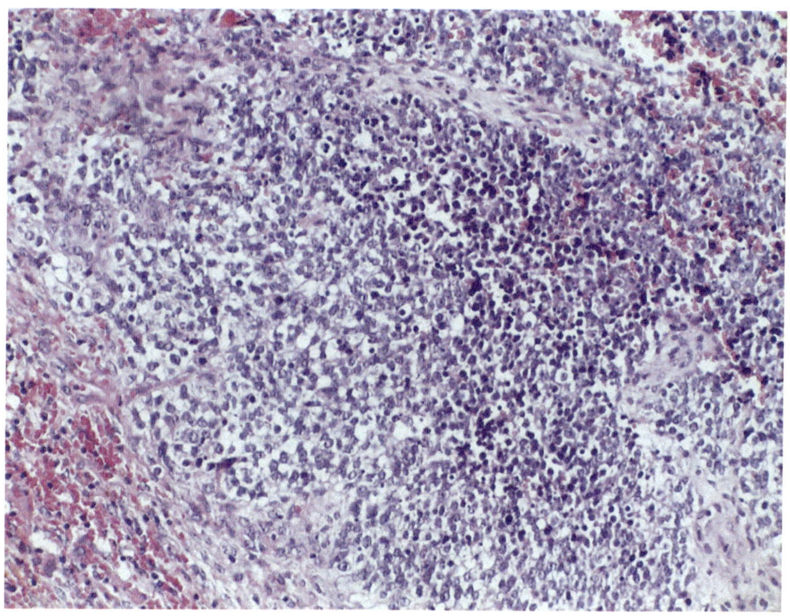

Fig. 60 Primitive round cell area in teratocarcinosarcoma

muscle and skeletal muscle components. The neuroectodermal components not only stain positively for neuroendocrine markers, such as synaptophysin and chromogranin A, but also for CD99. PLAP, alpha-fetoprotein, hCG, and CD30 are negative.

Molecular Features

SNTCS lacks the amplification of 12q which is usually present in germ cell tumors [191]. An activating p.S45F mutation in the β-catenin gene has been identified in one example of SNTCS [192]. Immunohistochemical nuclear staining for

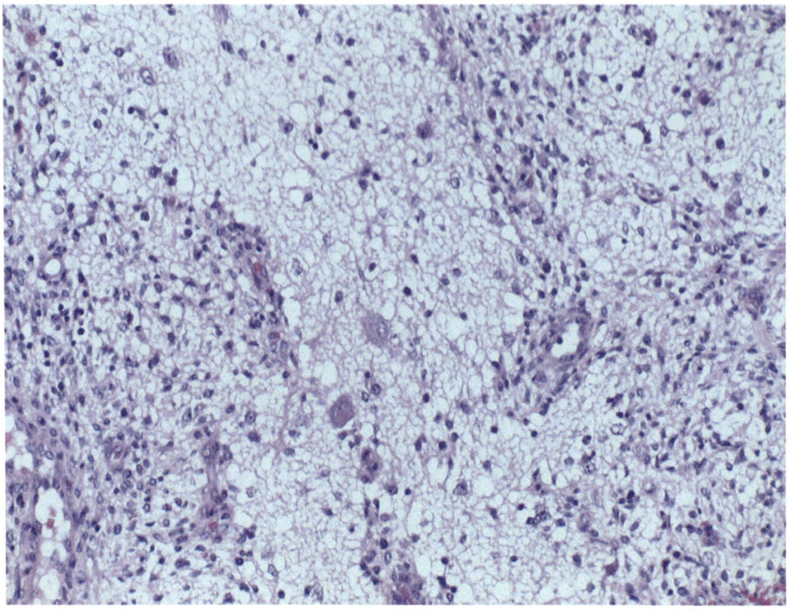

Fig. 61 Large ganglion-like cells in a fibrillary background

β-catenin was confirmed in the index case and in one further archival case [192].

Differential Diagnosis

The diagnosis of SNTCS can be challenging because of its rarity and phenotypic diversity, as it is indicated by an initial identification rate of 50% [190]. Extensive sampling is therefore recommended, in order to identify the different tumor components. Olfactory neuroblastoma, squamous cell carcinoma, adenocarcinoma, adenosquamous carcinoma, and various sarcoma types are the main differential diagnosis.

Treatment and Prognosis

SNTCS is an aggressive neoplasm, with destructive local growth and frequent lymph node and distant metastases [190, 193]. Radical surgical resection followed by radiation therapy is the most common treatment performed [190, 193].

References

1. Michaels L, Young M. Histogenesis of papillomas of the nose and paranasal sinuses. Arch Pathol Lab Med. 1995;119:821–6.
2. Bishop JA. OSPs and ESPs and ISPs, Oh My! An Update on Sinonasal (Schneiderian) Papillomas.
3. Barnes L. Schneiderian papillomas and nonsalivary glandular neoplasms of the head and neck. Mod Pathol. 2002;15:279–97.
4. Sarioglu S. Update on inverted epithelial lesions of the sinonasal and nasopharyngeal regions. Head Neck Pathol. 2007;1:44–9.
5. Outzen KE, Grøntveld A, Jørgensen K, Clausen PP, Ladefoged C. Inverted papilloma: incidence and late results of surgical treatment. Rhinology. 1996;34:114–8.
6. Buchwald C, Franzmann MB, Tos M. Sinonasal papillomas: a report of 82 cases in Copenhagen County, including a longitudinal epidemiological and clinical study. Laryngoscope. 1995;105:72–9.
7. Errico A, Zajacova J, Cacciatore A, et al. Occupational risk factors for sinonasal inverted papilloma: a case-control study. Occup Environ Med. 2013;70:703–8.
8. Sham CL, Lee DL, van Hasselt CA, Tong MC. A case-control study of the risk factors associated with sinonasal inverted papilloma. Am J Rhinol Allergy. 2010;24:e37–40.
9. Deitmer T, Wiener C. Is there an occupational etiology of inverted papilloma of the nose and sinuses? Acta Otolaryngol. 1996;116:762–5.
10. Moon IJ, Lee DY, Suh MW, et al. Cigarette smoking increases risk of recurrence for sinonasal inverted papilloma. Am J Rhinol Allergy. 2010;24:325–9.
11. Hong SL, Kim BH, Lee JH, Cho KS, Roh HJ. Smoking and malignancy in sinonasal inverted papilloma. Laryngoscope. 2013;123:1087–91.
12. Schwerer MJ, Kraft K, Baczako K, et al. Co-expression of cytokeratins typical for columnar and squamous differentiation in sinonasal inverted papillomas. Am J Pathol. 2001;115:747–54.

13. Udager AM, Rolland DCM, McHugh JB, et al. High-frequency targetable EGFR mutations in sinonasal squamous cell carcinomas arising from inverted sinonasal papilloma. Cancer Res. 2015;75:2600–6.
14. Udager AM, McHugh JB, Goudsmit CM, et al. Human papillomavirus (HPV) and somatic EGFR mutations are essential, mutually exclusive oncogenic mechanisms for inverted sinonasal papillomas and associated sinonasal squamous cell carcinomas. Ann Oncol. 2018;29:466–71.
15. Udager AM, McHugh JB, Betz BL, et al. Activating KRAS mutations are characteristic of oncocytic sinonasal papilloma and associated sinonasal squamous cell carcinoma. J Pathol. 2016;239:394–8.
16. Syrjänen K, Syrjänen S. Detection of human papillomavirus in sinonasal papillomas: systematic review and meta-analysis. Laryngoscope. 2013;123:181–92.
17. Stoddard DG Jr, Keeney MG, Gao G, et al. Transcriptional activity of HPV in inverted papilloma demonstrated by in situ hybridization for E6/E7 mRNA. Otolaryngol Head Neck Surg. 2015;152:752–8.
18. Rooper LM, Bishop JA, Westra WH. Transcriptionally active high-risk human papillomavirus is not a common etiologic agent in the malignant transformation of inverted Schneiderian papillomas. Head Neck Pathol. 2017;11:346–53.
19. Lawson W, Schlecht NF, Brandwein-Gensler M. The role of the human papillomavirus in the pathogenesis of Schneiderian inverted papillomas: an analytic overview of the evidence. Head Neck Pathol. 2008;2:49–59.
20. Lewis JS Jr, Chernock RD, Haynes W, El-Mofty SK. Low-grade papillary Schneiderian carcinoma, a unique and deceptively bland malignant neoplasm: report of a case. Am J Surg Pathol. 2015;39:714–21.
21. Jeong HJ, Roh J, Lee BJ, Cho KJ. Low-grade papillary Schneiderian carcinoma: a case report. Head Neck Pathol. 2018;12:131–5.
22. Reh DD, Lane AP. The role of endoscopic sinus surgery in the management of sinonasal inverted papilloma. Curr Opin Otolaryngol Head Neck Surg. 2009;17:6–10.
23. Busquets JM, Hwang PH. Endoscopic resection of sinonasal inverted papilloma: a meta-analysis. Otolaryngol Head Neck Surg. 2006;134:476–82.
24. Karkos PD, Fyrmpas G, Carrie SC, Swift AC. Endoscopic versus open surgical interventions for inverted nasal papilloma: a systematic review. Clin Otolaryngol. 2006;31:499–503.
25. Minovi A, Kollert M, Draf W, Bockmuhl U. Inverted papilloma: feasibility of endonasal surgery and long-term results of 87 cases. Rhinology. 2006;44:205–10.
26. Lombardi D, Tomenzoli D, Buttà L, et al. Limitations and complications of endoscopic surgery for treatment for sinonasal inverted papilloma: a reassessment after 212 cases. Head Neck. 2011;33:1154–61.
27. Anari S, Carrie S. Sinonasal inverted papilloma: narrative review. J Laryngol Otol. 2010;124:705–15.
28. Nudell J, Chiosea S, Thompson LD. Carcinoma ex-Schneiderian papilloma (malignant transformation): a clinicopathologic and immunophenotypic study of 20 cases combined with a comprehensive review of the literature. Head Neck Pathol. 2014;8:269–86.
29. Miyazaki T, Haku Y, Yoshizawa A, et al. Clinical features of nasal and sinonasal inverted papilloma associated with malignancy. Auris Nasus Larynx. 2018;45:1014–9.
30. Kaufman MR, Brandwein MS, Lawson W. Sinonasal papillomas: clinicopathologic review of 40 patients with inverted and oncocytic Schneiderian papillomas. Laryngoscope. 2002;112:1372–7.
31. Blumberg JM, Escobar-Stein J, Vining EM, Prasad ML. Low-grade, nonintestinal nonsalivary sinonasal adenocarcinoma associated with an exophytic Schneiderian papilloma: a case report. Int J Surg Pathol. 2015;23:662–6.
32. Kapadia SB, Barnes L, Pelzman K, Mirani N, Heffner DK, Bedetti C. Carcinoma ex oncocytic Schneiderian (cylindrical cell) papilloma. Am J Otolaryngol. 1993;14:332–8.
33. Katori H, Nozawa A, Tsukuda M. Histopathological parameters of recurrence and malignant transformation in sinonasal inverted papilloma. Acta Otolaryngol. 2006;126:214–8.
34. Batsakis JG, Suarez P. Schneiderian papillomas and carcinomas: a review. Adv Anat Pathol. 2001;8:53–64.
35. Vento SI, Numminen J, Kinnunen I, et al. Pleomorphic adenoma in the nasal cavity: a clinicopathological study of ten cases in Finland. Eur Arch Otorhinolaryngol. 2016;273:3741–5.
36. Kuan EC, Diaz MFP, Chiu AG, Bergsneider M, Wang MB, Suh JD. Sinonasal and skull base pleomorphic adenoma: a case series and literature review. Int Forum Allergy Rhinol. 2015;5:460–8.
37. Compagno J, Wong RT. Intranasal mixed tumors (pleomorphic adenomas): a clinicopathologic study of 40 cases. Am J Clin Pathol. 1977;68:213–8.
38. Hirai S, Matsumoto T, Suda K. Pleomorphic adenoma in nasal cavity: immunohistochemical study of three cases. Auris Nasus Larynx. 2002;29:291–5.
39. Lam PW, Chan JK, Sin VC. Nasal pleomorphic adenoma with skeletal muscle differentiation: potential misdiagnosis as rhabdomyosarcoma. Hum Pathol. 1997;28:1299–302.
40. Bégin LR, Rochon L, Frenkiel S. Spindle cell myoepithelioma of the nasal cavity. Am J Surg Pathol. 1991;15:184–90.
41. Hodzic Z, Rowan NR, Kashiwazaki R, Willson TJ, Wang EW, Lee SE. A systematic review of sinonasal oncocytomas and oncocytic carcinomas: diagnosis, management, and technical considerations. Int Forum Allergy Rhinol. 2017;7:514–24.
42. Nonomura N, Niijima H, Kimura O, Ikarashi F, Nakano Y, Kimura K. Immunohistochemical study of pleomorphic adenoma of the nasal septum. Auris Nasus Larynx. 1992;19:125–31.

43. Freeman SB, Kennedy KS, Parker GS, et al. Metastasing pleomorphic adenoma of the nasal septum. Arch Otolaryngol Head Neck Surg. 1990;116:1331–3.
44. Toluie S, Thompson LD. Sinonasal tract adenoid cystic carcinoma ex-pleomorphic adenoma: a clinicopathologic and immunophenotypic study of 9 cases combined with a comprehensive review of the literature. Head Neck Pathol. 2012;6:409–21.
45. Cimino-Mathews A, Lin BM, Chang SS, Boahene KD, Bishop JA. Carcinoma ex pleomorphic adenoma of the nasal cavity. Head Neck Pathol. 2011;5:405–9.
46. Cho KJ, El-Naggar AK, Mahanupab P, Luna MA, Batsakis JG. Carcinoma ex-pleomorphic adenoma of the nasal cavity: a report of two cases. J Laryngol Otol. 1995;109:677–9.
47. Schafer DR, Thompson LD, Smith BC, Wenig BM. Primary ameloblastoma of the sinonasal tract: a clinicopathologic study of 24 cases. Cancer. 1998;82:667–74.
48. Guilemany JM, Ballesteros F, Alós L, et al. Plexiform ameloblastoma presenting as a sinonasal tumor. Eur Arch Otorhinolaryngol. 2004;261:304–6.
49. Leong SC, Karkos PD, Krajacevic J, Islam R, Kent SE. Ameloblastoma of the sinonasal tract: a case report. Ear Nose Throat J. 2010;89:70–1.
50. Altini M, Coleman H, Doglioni C, Favia G, Maiorano E. Calretinin expression in ameloblastomas. Histopathology. 2000;37:27–32.
51. Verduin L, Bishop J, Mills SE. Gnathic and peripheral ameloblastomas lack human papillomavirus DNA. Ann Diagn Pathol. 2015;19:306–9.
52. Sanghvi S, Khan MN, Patel NR, Yeldandi S, Baredes S, Eloy JA. Epidemiology of sinonasal squamous cell carcinoma: a comprehensive analysis of 4994 patients. Laryngoscope. 2014;124:76–83.
53. Dubal PM, Bhojwani A, Patel TD, et al. Squamous cell carcinoma of the maxillary sinus: a population-based analysis. Laryngoscope. 2016;126:399–404.
54. Paleri V, Orvidas LJ, Wight RG, Bradley PJ. Verrucous carcinoma of the paranasal sinuses: case report and clinical update. Head Neck. 2004;26:184–9.
55. Strojan P, Soba E, Gale N, Auersperg M. Verrucous carcinoma of the temporal bone and maxillary antrum: two unusual presentations of a rare tumor. Onkologie. 2006;29:463–8.
56. Alos L, Moyano S, Nadal A, et al. Human papillomaviruses are identified in a subgroup of sinonasal squamous cell carcinomas with favorable outcome. Cancer. 2009;115:2701–9.
57. Laco J, Sieglová K, Vošmiková H, et al. The presence of high-risk human papillomavirus (HPV) E6/E7 mRNA transcripts in a subset of sinonasal carcinomas is evidence of involvement of HPV in its etiopathogenesis. Virchows Arch. 2015; 467:405–15.
58. Larque AB, Hakim S, Ordi J, et al. High-risk human papillomavirus is transcriptionally active in a subset of sinonasal squamous cell carcinomas. Mod Pathol. 2014;27:343–51.
59. Bishop JA, Guo TW, Smith DF, et al. Human papillomavirus related carcinomas of the sinonasal tract. Am J Surg Pathol. 2013;37:185–92.
60. El-Mofty SK, Lu DW. Prevalence of high-risk human papillomavirus DNA in nonkeratinizing (cylindrical cell) carcinoma of the sinonasal tract: a distinct clinicopathologic and molecular disease entity. Am J Surg Pathol. 2005;29:1367–72.
61. Lewis JS Jr. Sinonasal squamous cell carcinoma: a review with emphasis on emerging histologic subtypes and the role of human papillomavirus. Head Neck Pathol. 2016;10:60–7.
62. Kılıç S, Kılıç SS, Kim ES, Baredes S, Mahmoud O, Gray ST, Eloy JA. Significance of human papillomavirus positivity in sinonasal squamous cell carcinoma. Int Forum Allergy Rhinol. 2017;7:980–9.
63. Califano J, Koch W, Sidransky D, Westra WH. Inverted sinonasal papilloma: a molecular genetic appraisal of its putative status as a precursor to squamous cell carcinoma. Am J Pathol. 2000;156:333–7.
64. López F, Llorente JL, García-Inclán C, et al. Genomic profiling of sinonasal squamous cell carcinoma. Head Neck. 2011;33:145–53.
65. Chung CH, Guthrie VB, Masica DL, et al. Genomic alterations in head and neck squamous cell carcinoma determined by cancer gene-targeted sequencing. Ann Oncol. 2015;26:1216–23.
66. Kılıç S, Kılıç SS, Baredes S, et al. Comparison of endoscopic and open resection of sinonasal squamous cell carcinoma: a propensity score-matched analysis of 652 patients. Int Forum Allergy Rhinol. 2018;8:421–34.
67. Castelnuovo P, Turri-Zanoni M, Battaglia P, Antognoni P, Bossi P, Locatelli D. Sinonasal malignancies of anterior skull base: histology-driven treatment strategies. Otolaryngol Clin N Am. 2016;49:183–200.
68. Bossi P, Saba NF, Vermorken JB, et al. The role of systemic therapy in the management of sinonasal cancer: a critical review. Cancer Treat Rev. 2015;41:836–43.
69. Cantu G, Bimbi G, Miceli R, et al. Lymph node metastases in malignant tumors of the paranasal sinuses: prognostic value and treatment. Arch Otolaryngol Head Neck Surg. 2008;134:170–7.
70. Ansa B, Goodman M, Ward K, et al. Paranasal sinus squamous cell carcinoma incidence and survival based on Surveillance, Epidemiology, and End Results data, 1973 to 2009. Cancer. 2013;119:2602–10.
71. Gil Z, Carlson DL, Gupta A, et al. Patterns and incidence of neural invasion in patients with cancers of the paranasal sinuses. Arch Otolaryngol Head Neck Surg. 2009;135:173–9.
72. Vazquez A, Khan MN, Blake DM, Patel TD, Baredes S, Eloy JA. Sinonasal squamous cell carcinoma and the prognostic implications of its histologic variants:

a population-based study. Int Forum Allergy Rhinol. 2015;5:85–91.

73. Lin EM, Sparano A, Spalding A, et al. Sinonasal undifferentiated carcinoma: a 13-year experience at a single institution. Skull Base. 2010;20:61–7.
74. Frierson HF, Mills SE, Fechner RE, Taxy JB, Levine PA. Sinonasal undifferentiated carcinoma. An aggressive neoplasm derived from Schneiderian epithelium and distinct from olfactory neuroblastoma. Am J Surg Pathol. 1986;10:771–9.
75. Franchi A, Moroni M, Massi D, Paglierani M, Santucci M. Sinonasal undifferentiated carcinoma, nasopharyngeal-type undifferentiated carcinoma, and keratinizing and nonkeratinizing squamous cell carcinoma express different cytokeratin patterns. Am J Surg Pathol. 2002;26:1597–604.
76. Bourne TD, Bellizzi AM, Stelow EB, Loy AH, Levine PA, Wick MR, Mills SE. p63 expression in olfactory neuroblastoma and other small cell tumors of the sinonasal tract. Am J Clin Pathol. 2008;130:213–8.
77. Chapman-Fredricks J, Jorda M, Gomez-Fernandez C. A limited immunohistochemical panel helps differentiate small cell epithelial malignancies of the sinonasal cavity and nasopharynx. Appl Immunohistochem Mol Morphol. 2009;17:207–10.
78. Tilson MP, Bishop JA. Utility of p40 in the differential diagnosis of small round blue cell tumors of the sinonasal tract. Head Neck Pathol. 2014;8:141–5.
79. Cerilli LA, Holst VA, Brandwein MS, Stoler MH, Mills SE. Sinonasal undifferentiated carcinoma: immunohistochemical profile and lack of EBV association. Am J Surg Pathol. 2001;25:156–63.
80. Jeng YM, Sung MT, Fang CL, Huang HY, Mao TL, Cheng W, Hsiao CH. Sinonasal undifferentiated carcinoma and nasopharyngeal-type undifferentiated carcinoma: two clinically, biologically, and histopathologically distinct entities. Am J Surg Pathol. 2002;26:371–6.
81. Bishop JA, Guo TW, Smith DF, et al. Human papilloma virus related carcinomas of the sinonasal tract. Am J Surg Pathol. 2013;37:185–92.
82. Gray ST. Treatment outcomes and prognostic factors, including human papillomavirus, for sinonasal undifferentiated carcinoma: a retrospective review. Head Neck. 2015;37:366–74.
83. Jo VY, Chau NG, Hornick JL, Krane JF, Sholl LM. Recurrent IDH2 R172X mutations in sinonasal undifferentiated carcinoma. Mod Pathol. 2017;30:650–9.
84. Dogan S, Chute DJ, Xu B, et al. Frequent IDH2 R172 mutations in undifferentiated and poorly-differentiated sinonasal carcinomas. J Pathol. 2017;242:400–8.
85. Morand GB, Anderegg N, Vital D, et al. Outcome by treatment modality in sinonasal undifferentiated carcinoma (SNUC): a case-series, systematic review and meta-analysis. Oral Oncol. 2017;75:28–34.
86. Khan MN, Konuthula N, Parasher A, et al. Treatment modalities in sinonasal undifferentiated carcinoma: an analysis from the national cancer database. Int Forum Allergy Rhinol. 2017;7:205–10.
87. Bhasker S, Mallick S, Benson R, Bhanuprasad V, Sharma A, Thakar A. A multimodality approach to sinonasal undifferentiated carcinoma: a single institute experience. J Laryngol Otol. 2017;131:19–25.
88. Bishop JA, Westra JH. NUT midline carcinomas of the sinonasal tract. Am J Surg Pathol. 2012;36:1216–21.
89. Minato H, Kobayashi E, Nakada S, et al. Sinonasal NUT carcinoma: clinicopathological and cytogenetic analysis with autopsy findings. Hum Pathol. 2018;71:157–65.
90. Stelow EB. A review of NUT midline carcinoma. Head Neck Pathol. 2011;5:31–5.
91. Haack H, Johnson LA, Fry CJ, et al. Diagnosis of NUT midline carcinoma using a NUT-specific monoclonal antibody. Am J Surg Pathol. 2009;33:984–91.
92. French CA. Demystified molecular pathology of NUT midline carcinomas. J Clin Pathol. 2010;63:492–6.
93. French CA, Rahman S, Walsh EM, et al. NSD3-NUT fusion oncoprotein in NUT midline carcinoma: implications for a novel oncogenic mechanism. Cancer Discov. 2014;4:928–41.
94. French CA. Pathogenesis of NUT midline carcinoma. Ann Rev Pathol Mech Dis. 2012;7:247–65.
95. French CA, Ramirez CL, Kolmakova J, et al. BRD-NUT oncoproteins: a family of closely related nuclear proteins that block epithelial differentiation and maintain the growth of carcinoma cells. Oncogene. 2008;27:2237–42.
96. Stelow EBBA, Bellizzi AM, Taneja K, et al. NUT rearrangement in undifferentiated carcinomas of the upper aerodigestive tract. Am J Surg Pathol. 2008;32:828–34.
97. Bauer DE, Mitchell CM, Strait KM, et al. Clinicopathologic features and long-term outcomes of NUT midline carcinoma. Clin Cancer Res. 2012;18:5773–9.
98. Chau NG, Hurwitz S, Mitchell CM, et al. Intensive treatment and survival outcomes in NUT midline carcinoma of the head and neck. Cancer. 2016;122:3632–40.
99. Stathis A, Zucca E, Bekradda M, et al. Clinical response of carcinomas harboring the BRD4-NUT oncoprotein to the targeted bromodomain inhibitor OTX015/MK-8628. Cancer Discov. 2016;6:492–500.
100. Agaimy A, Koch M, Lell M, Semrau S, Dudek W, Wachter DL, Knöll A, Iro H, Haller F, Hartmann A. SMARCB1(INI1)-deficient sinonasal basaloid carcinoma: a novel member of the expanding family of SMARCB1-deficient neoplasms. Am J Surg Pathol. 2014;38:1274–81.
101. Bishop JA, Antonescu CR, Westra WH. SMARCB1 (INI-1)-deficient carcinomas of the sinonasal tract. Am J Surg Pathol. 2014;38:1282–9.
102. Bell D, Hanna EY, Agaimy A, Weissferdt A. Reappraisal of sinonasal undifferentiated

carcinoma: SMARCB1 (INI1)-deficient sinonasal carcinoma: a single-institution experience. Virchows Arch. 2015;467:649–56.
103. Agaimy A, Hartmann A, Antonescu CR, et al. SMARCB1 (INI-1)-deficient sinonasal carcinoma: a series of 39 cases expanding the morphologic and clinicopathologic spectrum of a recently described entity. Am J Surg Pathol. 2017;41:458–71.
104. Wasserman JK, Dickson BC, Perez-Ordonez B, de Almeida JR, Irish JC, Weinreb I. INI1 (SMARCB1)-deficient sinonasal carcinoma: a clinicopathologic report of 2 cases. Head Neck Pathol. 2017;11:256–61.
105. Chan JY, Wong EW, Ng SK, Vlantis AC. Non-nasopharyngeal head and neck lymphoepithelioma-like carcinoma in the United States: a population-based study. Head Neck. 2016;38(Suppl 1):E1294–300.
106. Rytkönen AE, Hirvikoski PP, Salo TA. Lymphoepithelial carcinoma: two case reports and a systematic review of oral and sinonasal cases. Head Neck Pathol. 2011;5:327–34.
107. Wenig BM. Lymphoepithelial-like carcinomas of the head and neck. Semin Diagn Pathol. 2015;32:74–86.
108. Zong Y, Liu K, Zhong B, et al. Epstein-Barr virus infection of sinonasal lymphoepithelial carcinoma in Guangzhou. Chin Med J (Engl). 2001;114:132–6.
109. Pointer KB, Ko HC, Brower JV, et al. Small cell carcinoma of the head and neck: an analysis of the National Cancer Database. Oral Oncol. 2017;69:92–8.
110. Likhacheva A, Rosenthal DI, Hanna E, et al. Sinonasal neuroendocrine carcinoma: impact of differentiation status on response and outcome. Head Neck Oncol. 2011;3:32.
111. Chu MW, Karakla DW, Silverberg M, et al. Primary carcinoid tumor of the frontal sinus: a case report. Ear Nose Throat J. 2010;89:E13–6.
112. Furuta A, Kudo M, Kanai K, et al. Typical carcinoid tumor arising in the nose and paranasal sinuses—case report. Auris Nasus Larynx. 2010;37:381–5.
113. Galm T, Turner N. Primary carcinoid tumour of nasal septum. J Laryngol Otol. 2009;123:789–92.
114. Patel TD, Vazquez A, Dubal PM, Baredes S, Liu JK, Eloy JA. Sinonasal neuroendocrine carcinoma: a population-based analysis of incidence and survival. Int Forum Allergy Rhinol. 2015;5:448–53.
115. Rivero A, Liang J. Sinonasal small cell neuroendocrine carcinoma: a systematic review of 80 patients. Int Forum Allergy Rhinol. 2016;6:744–51.
116. Pierce ST, Cibull ML, Metcalfe MS, Sloan D. Bone marrow metastases from small cell cancer of the head and neck. Head Neck. 1994;16:266–71.
117. Ma AT, Lei KI. Small cell neuroendocrine carcinoma of the ethmoid sinuses presenting with generalized seizure and syndrome of inappropriate antidiuretic hormone secretion: a case report and review of literature. Am J Otolaryngol. 2009;30:54–7.
118. Mineta H, Miura K, Takebayashi S, et al. Immunohistochemical analysis of small cell carcinoma of the head and neck: a report of four patients and a review of sixteen patients in the literature with ectopic hormone production. Ann Otol Rhinol Laryngol. 2001;110:76–82.
119. Wang CP, Hsieh CY, Chang YL, et al. Postirradiated neuroendocrine carcinoma of the sinonasal tract. Laryngoscope. 2008;118:804–9.
120. Bishop JA, Guo TW, Smith DF, Wang H, Ogawa T, Pai SI, Westra WH. Human papillomavirus-related carcinomas of the sinonasal tract. Am J Surg Pathol. 2013;37:185–92.
121. Thompson ED, Stelow EB, Mills SE, Westra WH, Bishop JA. Large cell neuroendocrine carcinoma of the head and neck: a clinicopathologic series of 10 cases with an emphasis on HPV status. Am J Surg Pathol. 2016;40:471–8.
122. Siwersson U, Kindblom LG. Oncocytic carcinoid of the nasal cavity and carcinoid of the lung in a child. Pathol Res Pract. 1984;178:562–9.
123. Kao HL, Chang WC, Li WY, et al. Head and neck large cell neuroendocrine carcinoma should be separated from atypical carcinoid on the basis of different clinical features, overall survival, and pathogenesis. Am J Surg Pathol. 2012;36:185–92.
124. Turri-Zanoni M, Maragliano R, Battaglia P, et al. The clinicopathological spectrum of olfactory neuroblastoma and sinonasal neuroendocrine neoplasms: refinements in diagnostic criteria and impact of multimodal treatments on survival. Oral Oncol. 2017;74:21–9.
125. Franchi A, Rocchetta D, Palomba A, Degli Innocenti DR, Castiglione F, Spinelli G. Primary combined neuroendocrine and squamous cell carcinoma of the maxillary sinus: report of a case with immunohistochemical and molecular characterization. Head Neck Pathol. 2015;9:107–13.
126. Kayakabe M, Takahashi K, Okamiya T, Segawa A, Oyama T, Chikamatsu K. Combined small cell carcinoma of the sinonasal tract associated with syndrome of inappropriate secretion of antidiuretic hormone: a case report. Oncol Lett. 2014;7:1253–6.
127. Serrano MF, El-Mofty SK, Gnepp DR, et al. Utility of high molecular weight cytokeratins, but not p63, in the differential diagnosis of neuroendocrine and basaloid carcinomas of the head and neck. Hum Pathol. 2008;39:591–8.
128. Alos L, Hakim S, Larque AB, et al. p16 overexpression in high-grade neuroendocrine carcinomas of the head and neck: potential diagnostic pitfall with HPV-related carcinomas. Virchows Arch. 2016;469:277–84.
129. Bishop JA, Ogawa T, Stelow EB, et al. Human papillomavirus-related carcinoma with adenoid cystic-like features: a peculiar variant of head and neck cancer restricted to the sinonasal tract. Am J Surg Pathol. 2013;37:836–44.
130. Bishop JA, Andreasen S, Hang JF, et al. HPV-related multiphenotypic sinonasal carcinoma: an expanded series of 49 cases of the tumor formerly known as HPV-related carcinoma with adenoid

cystic carcinoma-like features. Am J Surg Pathol. 2017;41:1690–701.
131. Andreasen S, Bishop JA, Hansen TV, et al. Human papillomavirus-related carcinoma with adenoid cystic-like features of the sinonasal tract: clinical and morphological characterization of six new cases. Histopathology. 2017;70:880–8.
132. Hang JF, Hsieh MS, Li WY, et al. Human papillomavirus-related carcinoma with adenoid cystic-like features: a series of five cases expanding the pathological spectrum. Histopathology. 2017;71:887–96.
133. Cantu G, Solero CL, Mariani L, et al. Intestinal type adenocarcinoma of the ethmoid sinus in wood and leather workers: a retrospective study of 153 cases. Head Neck. 2011;33:535–42.
134. Choussy O, Ferron C, Védrine PO, et al. Adenocarcinoma of Ethmoid: a GETTEC retrospective multicenter study of 418 cases. Laryngoscope. 2008;118:437–43.
135. Jankowski R, Georgel T, Vignaud JM, et al. Endoscopic surgery reveals that woodworkers' adenocarcinomas originate in the olfactory cleft. Rhinology. 2007;45:308–14.
136. Barnes L. Intestinal-type adenocarcinoma of the nasal cavity and paranasal sinuses. Am J Surg Pathol. 1986;10:192–202.
137. Franquemont DW, Fechner RE, Mills SE. Histologic classification of sinonasal intestinal-type adenocarcinoma. Am J Surg Pathol. 1991;15:368–75.
138. Vivanco B, Llorente JL, Perez-Escuredo J, Alvarez Marcos C, Fresno MF, Hermsen MA. Benign lesions in mucosa adjacent to intestinal-type sinonasal adenocarcinoma. Pathol Res Int. 2011;2011:230147.
139. Franchi A, Palomba A, Miligi L, et al. Intestinal metaplasia of the sinonasal mucosa adjacent to intestinal-type adenocarcinoma. A morphologic, immunohistochemical, and molecular study. Virchows Arch. 2015;466:161–8.
140. Kleinsasser O, Schroeder H-G. Adenocarcinoma of the inner nose after exposure to wood dust. Morphological findings and relationships between histopathology and clinical behavior in 79 cases. Arch Otolaryngol. 1988;245:1–15.
141. Franchi A, Gallo O, Santucci M. Clinical relevance of the histological classification of sinonasal intestinal-type adenocarcinomas. Hum Pathol. 1999;30:1140–5.
142. La Rosa S, Furlan D, Franzi F, et al. Mixed exocrine-neuroendocrine carcinoma of the nasal cavity: clinico-pathologic and molecular study of a case and review of the literature. Head Neck Pathol. 2013;7:76–84.
143. Jain R, Gramigna V, Sanchez-Marull R, Perez-Ordoñez B. Composite intestinal-type adenocarcinoma and small cell carcinoma of sinonasal tract. J Clin Pathol. 2009;62:634–7.
144. Franchi A, Massi D, Palomba A, Biancalani M, Santucci M. CDX-2, cytokeratin 7 and cytokeratin 20 immunohistochemical expression in the differential diagnosis of primary adenocarcinomas of the sinonasal tract. Virchows Arch. 2004;445:63–7.
145. Kennedy MT, Jordan RC, Berean KW, Perez-Ordoñez B. Expression pattern of CK7, CK20, CDX-2, and villin in intestinal-type sinonasal adenocarcinoma. J Clin Pathol. 2004;57:932–7.
146. Skalova A, Sar A, Laco J, et al. The role of SATB2 as a diagnostic marker of sinonasal intestinal-type adenocarcinoma. Appl Immunohistochem Mol Morphol. 2018;26:140–6.
147. Tilson MP, Gallia GL, Bishop JA. Among sinonasal tumors, CDX-2 immunoexpression is not restricted to intestinal-type adenocarcinomas. Head Neck Pathol. 2014;8:59–65.
148. Frattini M, Perrone F, Suardi S, et al. Phenotype-genotype correlation: challenge of intestinal-type adenocarcinoma of the nasal cavity and paranasal sinuses. Head Neck. 2006;28:909–15.
149. López-Hernández A, Pérez-Escuredo J, et al. Genomic profiling of intestinal-type sinonasal adenocarcinoma reveals subgroups of patients with distinct clinical outcomes. Head Neck. 2018;40:259–73.
150. Perrone F, Oggionni M, Birindelli S, et al. TP53, p14ARF, p16INK4a and H-ras gene molecular analysis in intestinal-type adenocarcinoma of the nasal cavity and paranasal sinuses. Int J Cancer. 2003;105:196–203.
151. Yom SS, Rashid A, Rosenthal DI, et al. Genetic analysis of sinonasal adenocarcinoma phenotypes: distinct alterations of histogenetic significance. Mod Pathol. 2005;18:315–9.
152. Franchi A, Palomba A, Fondi C, Miligi L, Paglierani M, Pepi M, Santucci M. Immunohistochemical investigation of tumorigenic pathways in sinonasal intestinal-type adenocarcinoma. A tissue microarray analysis of 62 cases. Histopathology. 2011;59:98–105.
153. Franchi A, Fondi C, Paglierani M, Pepi M, Gallo O, Santucci M. Epidermal growth factor receptor expression and gene copy number in sinonasal intestinal type adenocarcinoma. Oral Oncol. 2009;45:835–8.
154. García-Inclán C, López F, Pérez-Escuredo J, et al. EGFR status and KRAS/BRAF mutations in intestinal-type sinonasal adenocarcinomas. Cell Oncol (Dordr). 2012;35:443–50.
155. Lopez F, Inclan CG, Perez-Escuredo J, et al. KRAS and BRAF mutations in sinonasal cancer. Oral Oncol. 2012;48:692–7.
156. Projetti F, Durand K, Chaunavel A, et al. Epidermal growth factor receptor expression and KRAS and BRAF mutations: study of 39 sinonasal intestinal-type adenocarcinomas. Hum Pathol. 2013;44:2116–25.
157. Franchi A, Innocenti DRD, Palomba A, et al. Low prevalence of K-RAS, EGF-R and BRAF mutations in sinonasal adenocarcinomas. Implications for anti-EGFR treatments. Pathol Oncol Res. 2014;20:571–9.
158. Meccariello G, Deganello A, Choussy O, et al. Endoscopic nasal versus open approach for the

management of sinonasal adenocarcinoma: a pooled analysis of 1826 patients. Head Neck. 2016;38(Suppl 1):E2267–74.
159. Nicolai P, Schreiber A, Bolzoni Villaret A, et al. Intestinal type adenocarcinoma of the ethmoid: outcomes of a treatment regimen based on endoscopic surgery with or without radiotherapy. Head Neck. 2016;38(Suppl 1):E996–E1003.
160. Camp S, Van Gerven L, Poorten VV, et al. Long-term follow-up of 123 patients with adenocarcinoma of the sinonasal tract treated with endoscopic resection and postoperative radiation therapy. Head Neck. 2016;38:294–300.
161. Licitra L, Suardi S, Bossi P, et al. Prediction of TP53 status for primary cisplatin, fluorouracil, and leucovorin chemotherapy in ethmoid sinus intestinal-type adenocarcinoma. J Clin Oncol. 2004;22:4901–6.
162. Bossi P, Perrone F, Miceli R, et al. TP53 status as guide for the management of ethmoid sinus intestinal-type adenocarcinoma. Oral Oncol. 2013;49:413–9.
163. Fiaux-Camous D, Chevret S, Oker N, et al. Prognostic value of the seventh AJCC/UICC TNM classification of intestinal-type ethmoid adenocarcinoma: systematic review and risk prediction model. Head Neck. 2017;39:668–78.
164. Stelow EB, Jo VY, Mills SE, Carlson DL. A histologic and immunohistochemical study describing the diversity of tumors classified as sinonasal high-grade non intestinal adenocarcinomas. Am J Surg Pathol. 2011;35:971–80.
165. Purgina B, Bastaki JM, Duvvuri U, Seethala RR. A subset of sinonasal non-intestinal type adenocarcinomas are truly seromucinous adenocarcinomas: a morphologic and immunophenotypic assessment and description of a novel pitfall. Head Neck Pathol. 2015;9:436–46.
166. Jo VY, Mills SE, Cathro HP, Carlson DL, Stelow EB. Low-grade sinonasal adenocarcinomas: the association with and distinction from respiratory epithelial adenomatoid hamartomas and other glandular lesions. Am J Surg Pathol. 2009;33:401–8.
167. Zur KB, Brandwein M, Wang B, Som P, Gordon R, Urken ML. Primary description of a new entity, renal cell-like carcinoma of the nasal cavity: van Meegeren in the house of Vermeer. Arch Otolaryngol Head Neck Surg. 2002;128:441–7.
168. Storck K, Hadi UM, Simpson R, Ramer M, Brandwein-Gensler M. Sinonasal renal cell-like adenocarcinoma: a report on four patients. Head Neck Pathol. 2008;2:75–80.
169. Shen T, Shi Q, Velosa C, et al. Sinonasal renal cell-like adenocarcinomas: robust carbonic anhydrase expression. Hum Pathol. 2015;46:1598–606.
170. Franchi A, Palomba A, Massi D, et al. Low-grade salivary type tubulo-papillary adenocarcinoma of the sinonasal tract. Histopathology. 2006;48:881–4.
171. Andreasen S, Skálová A, Agaimy A, et al. ETV6 gene rearrangements characterize a morphologically distinct subset of sinonasal low-grade non-intestinal-type adenocarcinoma: a novel translocation-associated carcinoma restricted to the sinonasal tract. Am J Surg Pathol. 2017;41:1552–60.
172. Eveson J. Salivary gland-type carcinomas. WHO histological classification of tumors of the nasal cavity and paranasal sinuses. In: Barnes L, Eveson JW, Reichardt P, Sidransky D, editors. Pathology & genetics, head and neck tumors. Lyon: IARC Press; 2005. p. 24–5.
173. Unsal AA, Chung SY, Zhou AH, Baredes S, Eloy JA. Sinonasal adenoid cystic carcinoma: a population-based analysis of 694 cases. Int Forum Allergy Rhinol. 2017;7:312–20.
174. Wolfish EB, Nelson BL, Thompson LD. Sinonasal tract mucoepidermoid carcinoma: a clinicopathologic and immunophenotypic study of 19 cases combined with a comprehensive review of the literature. Head Neck Pathol. 2012;6:191–207.
175. Lupinetti AD, Roberts DB, Williams MD, et al. Sinonasal adenoid cystic carcinoma: the M. D. Anderson Cancer Center experience. Cancer. 2007;110:2726–31.
176. Thompson LD, Penner C, Ho NJ, et al. Sinonasal tract and nasopharyngeal adenoid cystic carcinoma: a clinicopathologic and immunophenotypic study of 86 cases. Head Neck Pathol. 2014;8:88–109.
177. Nagao T, Gaffey TA, Serizawa H, Sugano I, Ishida Y, Yamazaki K, Tokashiki R, Yoshida T, Minato H, Kay PA, Lewis JE. Dedifferentiated adenoid cystic carcinoma: a clinicopathologic study of 6 cases. Mod Pathol. 2003;16:1265–72.
178. Yamanegi K, Uwa N, Hirokawa M, et al. Epithelial-myoepithelial carcinoma arising in the nasal cavity. Auris Nasus Larynx. 2008;35:408–13.
179. Müller S, Mantsopoulos K, Iro H, Agaimy A. Salivary duct carcinoma of the sinonasal cavity: a case report and review of the literature. Head Neck. 2016;38:E2464–6.
180. Charous DD, Cunnane MF, Rosen MR, Keane WM. Recurrent polymorphous low-grade adenocarcinoma manifesting as a sinonasal mass: a case report. Ear Nose Throat J. 2005;84(354):356–7.
181. Lloreta J, Serrano S, Corominas JM, Ferrés-Padró E. Polymorphous low-grade adenocarcinoma arising in the nasal cavities with an associated undifferentiated carcinoma. Ultrastruct Pathol. 1995;19:365–70.
182. Fonseca I, Soares J. Basal cell adenocarcinoma of minor salivary and seromucous glands of the head and neck region. Semin Diagn Pathol. 1996;13:128–37.
183. Petersson F, Chao SS, Ng SB. Anaplastic myoepithelial carcinoma of the sinonasal tract: an underrecognized salivary-type tumor among the sinonasal small round blue cell malignancies?

Report of one case and a review of the literature. Head Neck Pathol. 2011;5:144–53.

184. Baneckova M, Agaimy A, Andreasen S, et al. Mammary analog secretory carcinoma of the nasal cavity: characterization of 2 cases and their distinction from other low-grade sinonasal adenocarcinomas. Am J Surg Pathol. 2018;42:735–43.
185. Brill LB 2nd, Kanner WA, Fehr A, et al. Analysis of MYB expression and MYB-NFIB gene fusions in adenoid cystic carcinoma and other salivary neoplasms. Mod Pathol. 2011;24:1169–76.
186. Tonon G, Modi S, Wu L, Kubo A, Coxon AB, Komiya T, O'Neil K, Stover K, El-Naggar A, Griffin JD, Kirsch IR, Kaye FJ. t(11;19)(q21;p13) translocation in mucoepidermoid carcinoma creates a novel fusion product that disrupts a Notch signaling pathway. Nat Genet. 2003;33:208–13.
187. Seethala RR, Dacic S, Cieply K, Kelly LM, Nikiforova MN. A reappraisal of the MECT1/MAML2 translocation in salivary mucoepidermoid carcinomas. Am J Surg Pathol. 2010;34:1106–21.
188. Franchi A, Wenig BM. Teratocarcinosarcoma. In: El-Naggar AK, Chan JKC, Grandis JR, Takata T, Slootweg PJ, editors. WHO classification of head and neck tumors. 4th ed. IARC: Lyon; 2017.
189. Heffner DK, Hyams VJ. Teratocarcinosarcoma (malignant teratoma?) of the nasal cavity and paranasal sinuses: a clinicopathologic study of 20 cases. Cancer. 1984;53:2140–54.
190. Misra P, Husain Q, Svider PF, Sanghvi S, Liu JK, Eloy JA. Management of sinonasal teratocarcinosarcoma: a systematic review. Am J Otolaryngol. 2014;35:5–11.
191. Salem F, Rosenblum MK, Jhanwar SC, Kancherla P, Ghossein RA, Carlson DL. Teratocarcinosarcoma of the nasal cavity and paranasal sinuses: report of 3 cases with assessment for chromosome 12p status. Hum Pathol. 2008;39:605–9.
192. Birkeland AC, Burgin SJ, Yanik M, et al. Pathogenetic analysis of sinonasal teratocarcinosarcomas reveal actionable β-catenin overexpression and a β-catenin mutation. J Neurol Surg B Skull Base. 2017;78:346–52.
193. Wei S, Carroll W, Lazenby A, Bell W, Lopez R, Said-Al-Naief N. Sinonasal teratocarcinosarcoma: report of a case with review of literature and treatment outcome. Ann Diagn Pathol. 2008;12:415–25.

Mesenchymal Tumors

Alessandro Franchi

Benign Mesenchymal Tumors

Hemangioma and Other Benign Vascular Lesions

Definition

Sinonasal hemangioma represents a group of benign proliferations of blood vessels arising in the sinonasal mucosa. Lobular capillary hemangioma (LCH; synonym: pyogenic granuloma) is the most frequent subtype observed at this anatomic site, followed by cavernous hemangioma (CH). Rare examples of epithelioid hemangioma and of epithelioid angiomatous nodule have also been reported [1–3].

Clinical Features

Hemangiomas of the sinonasal mucosa represent 10–15% of all hemangiomas of the head and neck. The most common presenting symptom is unilateral epistaxis, followed by nasal obstruction. Sinonasal hemangiomas occur over a wide age range (mean 40 years) [4], including cases arising in pediatric patients, without significant gender predilection. The most frequently involved subsites are the nasal septum (40%), followed by the inferior turbinate (30%), the vestibule (15%), the maxillary sinus (8%), and the uncinate process (7%) [5, 6].

CT scans and MR imaging are useful to define the extent of the tumor and bone involvement [7]. Although the etiology of sinonasal hemangiomas is unknown, a number of cases have been reported in pregnancy and in patients on oral contraceptive treatment, suggesting a possible hormonal involvement. There are also reports of development of hemangioma following local trauma (nasal packing, previous surgeries, insect sting).

Pathologic Features

Grossly, these lesions appear as red, exophytic masses that usually measure less than 1 cm [4]. LCH consists of a well-circumscribed proliferation of blood vessels lined by flat or plump endothelial cells without significant atypia, with a characteristic lobular architecture. At the center of the lobule, there is a larger dilated vessels, which is surrounded by small capillaries, often with a slit-like lumen or without any lumen (Figs. 1 and 2). These vessels are surrounded by pericytes, which are better appreciated with immunostains for actins. Mitotic activity is quite variable, ranging from 0 to 5 per high power field, but atypical forms are absent. The surface epithelium frequently shows erosion or ulceration, and an inflammatory infiltrate is present in most cases. The proliferating vascular lobules are

A. Franchi (✉)
Department of Translational Research and of New Technologies in Medicine and Surgery, University of Pisa, Pisa, Italy
e-mail: alessandro.franchi@unipi.it

A. Franchi (ed.), *Pathology of Sinonasal Tumors and Tumor-Like Lesions*,
https://doi.org/10.1007/978-3-030-29848-7_7

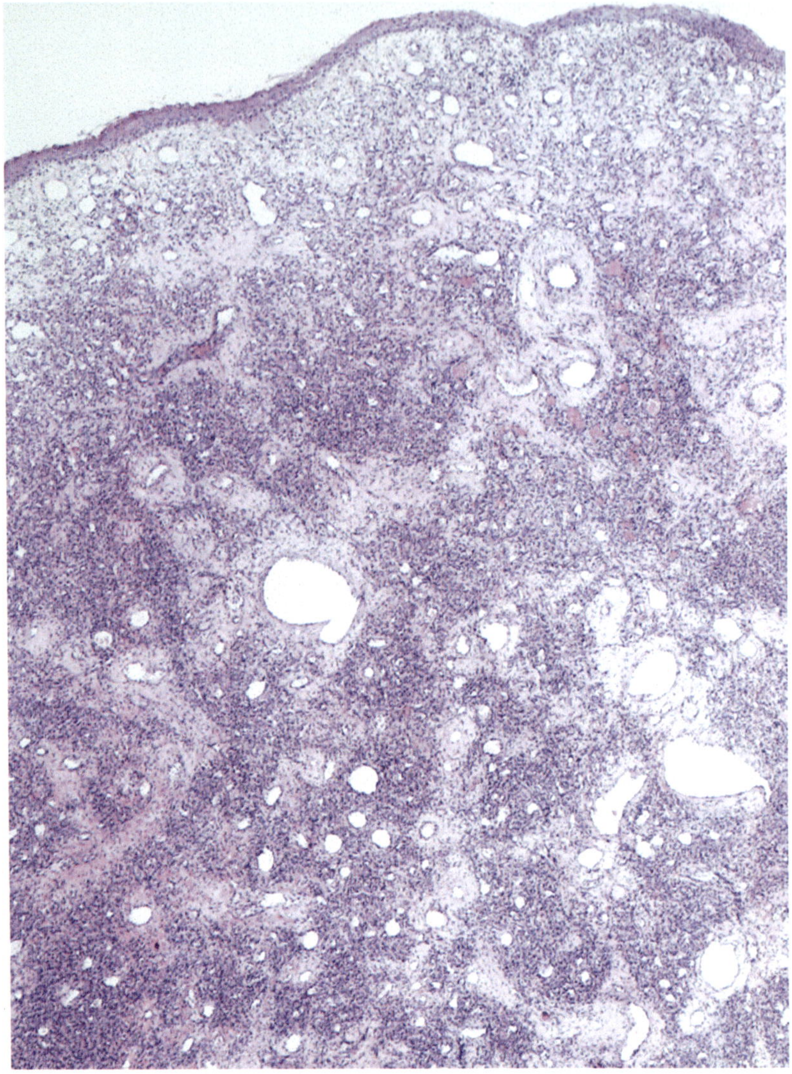

Fig. 1 Lobular capillary hemangioma of the nasal cavity. At the center of the lobule, there is a larger dilated vessels, which is surrounded by small capillaries

often arranged in a background of myxoid matrix. A subset of sinonasal hemangiomas presents extensive stromal myxoid change and hyalinization, which tends to obscure the lobular capillary arrangement, thus causing confusion with potentially more aggressive lesions [8].

CH consists of a proliferation of dilated thin-walled, blood-filled vascular spaces lined by flattened endothelial cells and separated by scant stromal tissue.

In epithelioid hemangioma, neoplastic vessels are lined by endothelial cells with an abundant eosinophil cytoplasm that protrudes in the lumen, and there is usually a dense inflammatory infiltrate with numerous eosinophils.

Epithelioid angiomatous nodule consists of a solid circumscribed proliferation of plump endothelial cells with abundant eosinophilic cytoplasm, focally organized to form vascular channels or showing cytoplasmic vacuoles [2, 3].

Immunohistochemical Profile

Endothelial cells are typically positive for CD31, CD34, ERG, and FLI1. Pericytes surrounding proliferating capillaries are positive for actins and desmin.

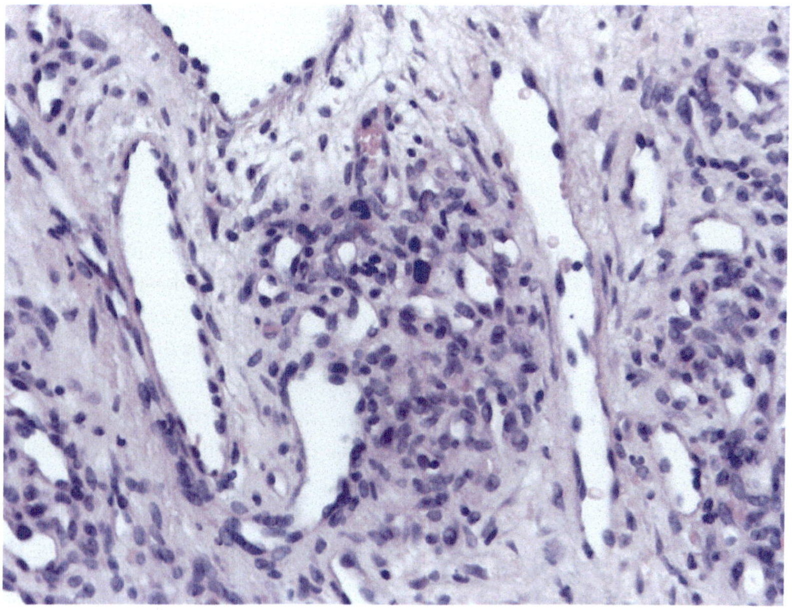

Fig. 2 Capillaries are lined by endothelial cells devoid of significant atypia

Molecular Features

A clonal deletion (q21.2q22.12) has been detected in one case of sinonasal LCH, supporting its neoplastic rather than reactive nature [9].

Differential Diagnosis

Sinonasal hemangiomas can be distinguished from juvenile angiofibroma because the latter does not show a hyalinized or myxoid stroma, and the proliferating vessels are of a thicker caliber and do not show a lobular arrangement. Angiomatous sinonasal polyps present areas of thrombosis and reorganization and lack the lobular growth pattern of true hemangiomas. Other mesenchymal tumors with prominent capillary vasculature, such as glomangiopericytoma and solitary fibrous tumor (SFT), can be easily distinguished from sinonasal hemangioma for the presence of a spindle cell neoplastic population with distinctive histologic and immunohistochemical features. Epithelioid hemangioma and angiomatous nodule must be distinguished from epithelioid hemangioendothelioma, a low-grade malignant neoplasm composed of strands or nests of tumor cells with frequent intracellular vacuoles within a myxoid or hyaline background.

Sinonasal angiosarcoma shows an infiltrative growth into surrounding soft tissues, formation of anastomosing vascular channels, endothelial cell multilayering, and nuclear atypia, all features lacking in sinonasal hemangiomas. Notably, angiosarcoma shows a solid growth pattern and lacks the lobular architecture of hemangioma.

Treatment and Prognosis

Sinonasal hemangiomas are removed surgically with an endoscopic excision with electrodessication of the tumor base. Preoperative embolization helps to reduce bleeding, and it is usually performed in large lesions and in pregnant women. Local recurrence after treatment occurs in 10–40% of cases [4, 10], and the second treatment is usually curative. Regression occurs in pregnancy-associated tumors after delivery.

Leiomyoma

Definition

Leiomyoma is a benign mesenchymal tumor with smooth muscle differentiation. In the sinonasal region, the majority of these lesions are associated with vessels, and therefore they belong to the group of angioleiomyoma (or vascular leiomyoma) [11, 12].

Clinical Features

They are rare tumors that occur in adult patients, with a slight predilection for female subjects. Presenting symptoms include intermittent nasal obstruction, chronic sinusitis-like symptoms, and recurrent epistaxis [12].

Pathologic Features

Grossly the lesions are tan-white, firm to rubbery in consistency, with a whorled cut surface, and measure in average 1 cm [12]. Microscopically, they are composed of well-differentiated, non-atypical smooth muscle cells with elongated fibrillary eosinophilic cytoplasm and blunt-ended cigar-shaped nucleus with inconspicuous nucleoli. The cells are arranged in intersecting fascicles with solid architecture or merging with the musculature of the vessel walls in angioleiomyoma (Fig. 3). Stromal changes, with myxoid and hyalinized areas, can be present. Mitotic figures are absent.

A mature adipocytic component consisting of scattered single adipocytes or of small aggregates and lobules within the lesions can be appreciated in some cases. The fatty component may represent up to 20% of the lesion [12].

Sinonasal smooth muscle tumors with low cellularity, mild to moderate pleomorphism, and presence of 1–4 mitotic figures have been designated as "smooth muscle tumors with unknown malignant potential" (SMTUMP) in analogy with those occurring at other anatomic sites [11]. These lesions may show local infiltrative growth with bone invasion, which is not observed in leiomyomas.

Immunohistochemical Features

Tumors are positive for alpha smooth muscle actin, h-Caldesmon, muscle-specific actin, and desmin. S100, CD34, and HMB45 are negative. The proliferation fraction (Ki-67) is <2% [12].

Differential Diagnosis

Juvenile angiofibroma may resemble angioleiomyoma for the polypoid appearance and rich vasculature. However, angiofibromas arise in male adolescents and histologically are less cellular, being formed by bland stellate to spindle cells set in a loose stroma with variably sized vessels devoid of an elastic lamina. The distinction from neurinoma is usually straightforward

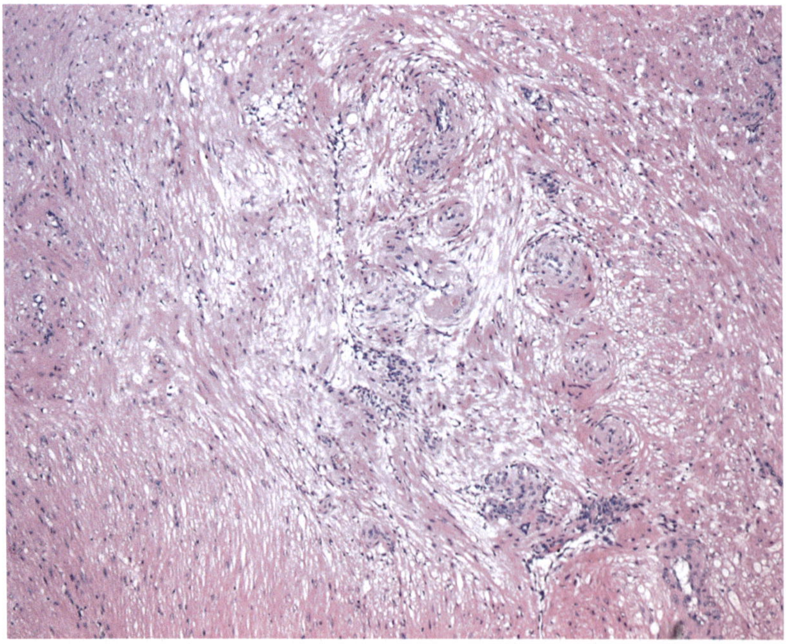

Fig. 3 Angioleiomyoma of the nasal cavity. Smooth muscle cells with elongated fibrillary eosinophilic cytoplasm are arranged in intersecting fascicles with solid architecture and merged with the musculature of the vessel walls

with the use of S100, actin, and desmin immunostains. Angioleiomyoma may be difficult to separate from sinonasal glomangiopericytoma. However, glomangiopericytoma is composed of short fascicles of ovoid to round cells that lack cytoplasmic eosinophilia, associated with a characteristic hemangiopericytomatous vascular pattern. Perivascular hyalinization is also present. Moreover, sinonasal glomangiopericytoma is usually negative for desmin and positive for β-catenin at the nuclear level. Finally, PECOMA may show some histologic overlap with angioleiomyoma, but characteristically there is co-expression of myogenic and melanocytic markers (HMB45).

Treatment and Prognosis

Sinonasal leiomyoma is a benign lesion that is cured after surgical excision.

Nodular Fasciitis

Definition

Nodular fasciitis (NF) is a benign neoplastic lesion composed of fibroblasts and myofibroblasts that predominantly affects children and young adults. It is characterized by a recurrent genetic alteration that results in a *MYH9-USP6* fusion [13, 14].

Clinical Features

NF most commonly arises in the extremities or trunk, but the soft tissues and the mucosal sites of the head and neck may also be involved. Sinonasal NF is extremely rare, with only few cases reported [15–18]. It arises mainly in children and young adults, and the clinical history is usually short (2–3-weeks), with a rapidly enlarging swelling, nasal obstruction, and discharge.

Pathologic Features

Nasal NF appears as a semitranslucent polypoid lesion, with a gelatinous appearance [15], which may displace the nasal bones and the septum, but without evidence of invasion. Cellularity is variable, ranging from highly cellular areas to hypocellular ones, which are rich in collagen. The extracellular matrix is at least focally myxoid in all cases, and cystic spaces are present in myxoid areas (Fig. 4). Cells are spindle or stellate in shape and are arranged in short fascicles, often with a storiform pattern (Fig. 5). Osteoclast-like giant cells and ganglion-like cells, as well as an infiltrate of mature lymphocytes are present in the majority of cases.

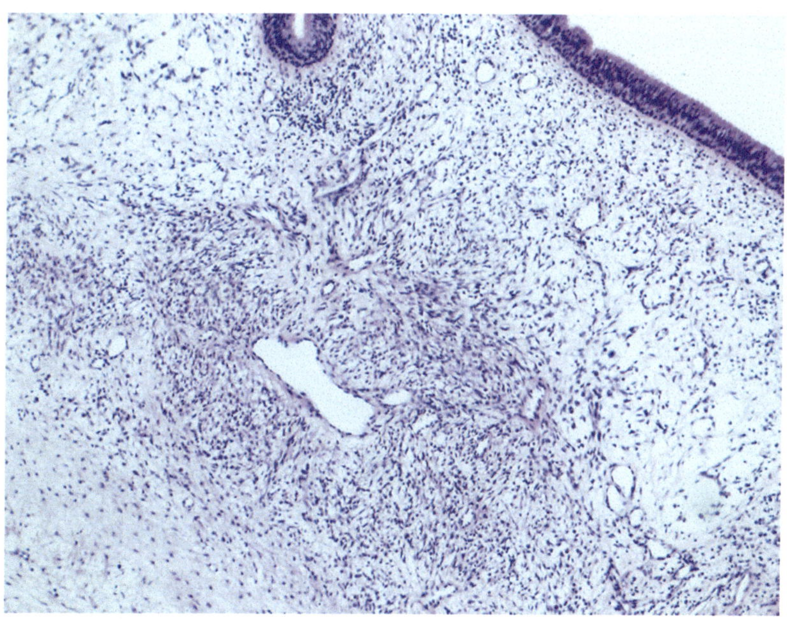

Fig. 4 Nodular fasciitis of the nasal cavity. A proliferation of bland spindle cells is present below the respiratory epithelium. They are separate by a moderate amount of myxoid matrix

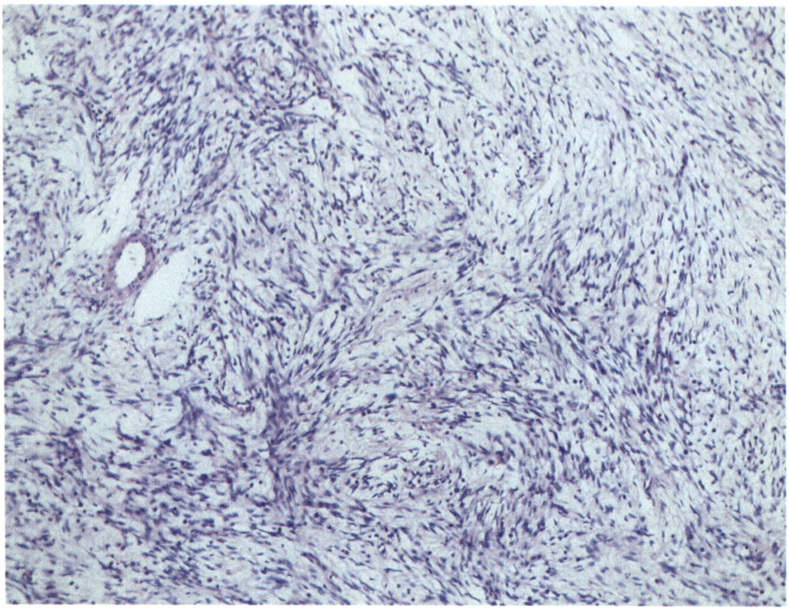

Fig. 5 Cells are spindle or stellate in shape and are arranged in short fascicles. Scattered lymphocytes are also present

Mitotic figures are easily identified, but no abnormal/atypical mitoses are present.

Immunohistochemical Profile

NF is variably positive for muscle markers, including actin and desmin, while myogenin, S-100, CD34, CD68, and factor XIIIa are negative.

Molecular Features

NF has a recurrent *USP6* gene rearrangement, whose identification is helpful in supporting the diagnosis, especially in lesions arising at unusual sites, like the sinonasal mucosa.

Differential Diagnosis

The differential diagnosis of NF is illustrated in Table 1. In children, a rapidly growing sinonasal mass and the macroscopic gelatinous appearance may cause concern for a malignant tumor, mainly embryonal rhabdomyosarcoma. The distinction is based on the positivity for myogenin and MYOD1 in rhabdomyosarcoma. Other malignancies to be considered in the differential diagnosis are fibrosarcoma, leiomyosarcoma (LMS), spindle cell carcinoma, and spindle cell melanoma, but they always show a degree of atypia which is not observed in NF. Desmoid-type fibromatosis occurs in the nasal cavity in pediatric patients and can be separated from NF based on a combination of morphologic features (elongated fascicles of uniform spindle cells with collagen production are distinctive features for desmoid fibromatosis) and positivity for β-catenin. Neurofibroma and Schwannoma can be easily ruled out with appropriate immunohistochemical markers.

Treatment and Prognosis

NF is a benign condition which is cured after surgical excision. If a lesion previously diagnosed as NF recurs, then the initial diagnosis should be critically reconsidered.

Fibroma

Definition

Nasal fibroma (NF) is a benign polypoid proliferation of fibroblasts set within abundant collagenous matrix (synonym: fibrous polyp). Sinonasal lesions classified as "fibroma" may originate as some other type of benign inflammatory, reactive, or neoplastic lesion (such as a nasal polyp), eventually being replaced with time by mature fibrous

Table 1 Summary of the diagnostic features of sinonasal spindle cell neoplasms

	Microscopic features	CK	EMA	CD34	CD31	SMA	DES	MYF4	S100	SOX10	STAT6	Beta catenin	Molecular changes
Nodular fasciitis	Plump spindle-shaped fibroblasts devoid of atypia, set in myxoid matrix often with discohesive areas; hypercellular areas with numerous nonatypical mitoses	–	–	–	–	–/+	–	–	–	–	–	–	*MYH9-USP6* fusion
Neurinoma	Unencapsulated proliferation of spindle cells, sometimes hypercellular; Antoni type A and B areas, Verocay bodies,	–	–	–	–	–	–	–	+	+	–	–	NA
Neurofibroma	Unencapsulated proliferation composed of irregular interlacing fascicles and bundles of spindled cells separated by collagen bundles or myxoid matrix	–	–	+	–	–	–	–	+	–	–	–	NA
Solitary fibrous tumor	Patternless proliferation of bland spindle cells, with alternating hypocellular and hypercellular areas, stromal hyalinization, and thin-walled branching vessels	–	–	+	–	–	–	–	–	–	+	–	*NAB2-STAT6* fusion
Glomangiopericytoma	Bland-looking ovoid to spindled cells with pale eosinophilic cytoplasm arranged in short fascicles; numerous capillary-sized vessels with frequent perithelial hyalinization	–	–	–	–	+	+	–	–	–	–	+	CTNNB1 mutations

(continued)

Table 1 (continued)

	Microscopic features	CK	EMA	CD34	CD31	SMA	DES	MYF4	S100	SOX10	STAT6	Beta catenin	Molecular changes
Desmoid-type fibromatosis	Poorly circumscribed proliferation of uniform, bland spindle cells arranged in elongated fascicles, with abundant collagen production	–	–	–	–	+	–	–	–	–		+	CTNNB1 mutations
Leiomyoma	Intersecting fascicles of elongated cells, with bright eosinophilic cytoplasm and ovoid cigar-shaped nucleus; no significant atypia; no mitosis	–	–	–	–	+	+	–	–	–	–	–	NA
Inflammatory myofibroblastic tumor	Proliferation of bland myofibroblasts accompanied by mixed inflammatory infiltrate	–	–	–	–	+	+	–	–	–	–	–	ALK gene rearrangements
Biphenotypic sinonasal sarcoma	Poorly circumscribed hypercellular proliferation of elongated uniform cells arranged in intersecting fascicles. “Staghorn” vessels are common.	–	–	–	–	+	+	–	+	–	–	–	*PAX3-MAML3* fusion
Spindle cell (sarcomatoid) carcinoma	Atypical spindle cells, often associated with areas showing epithelioid morphology; dysplastic surface epithelium	+	+	–	–	+	–	–	–	–	–		
Monophasic synovial sarcoma	Monomorphic spindle cells, with scant cytoplasm and ovoid nucleus, arranged in dense cellular sheets or in fascicles	+	+	–	–	–	–	–	–	–	–	–	*SS18-SSX* fusion
Fibrosarcoma	Proliferation of spindle cells arranged in fascicles with herringbone pattern	–	–	–	–	–	–	–	–	–	–	–	NA
Leiomyosarcoma	Interlacing bundles of spindle cells with variable degree of cellular atypia; mitotic figures	–	–	–	–	+	+	–	–	–	–	–	NA
Malignant peripheral nerve sheath tumor	Fascicular growth of spindle cells, with alternating hypo- and hypercellular areas	–	–	–	–	–	–	–	+ focal	+ focal	–	–	NA

Spindle cell rhabdomyosarcoma	Infiltrative fasciculated proliferation of spindle cells with ovoid nuclei and pale eosinophilic cytoplasm; cross-striation is sometimes seen	– (rare cases+)	–	–	–	–	+	+	– (rare cases +)	–	–	–	Rearrangements at 8q13 locus (*NCOA2*), *MYOD1* mutations
Spindle cell melanoma	Infiltrative fascicular proliferation of spindle cells with round nucleus with central nucleolus, granular cytoplasm; melanin pigment in some cases	– (+ in rare cases)	–	–	–	–	–	–	+	+	–	–	*KIT, NRAS* or *BRAF* mutations in a minority of cases
Kaposi sarcoma	Fascicular proliferation, intercellular erythrocytes, hyaline globules	–	–	+	+	–	–	–	–	–	–	–	HHV8 + by immunohistochemistry
Angiosarcoma	Anastomosing irregular vascular channels, lined by atypical spindle or epithelioid cells dissecting the stroma, cleft-like spaces, intracellular lumina	–	– (+ in rare cases)	+	+	–	–	–	–	–	–	–	

tissue [19]. Thus, NF probably represents a reparative/reactive process, rather than a true neoplasm.

Clinical Features

NF is usually an incidental finding and appears as a small (<1 cm), circumscribed, smooth surfaced nodule, most often arising from the nasal septum. Patients are adults (30–60 years).

Pathologic Features

The polypoid, sparsely cellular lesion consists of spindle and stellate fibroblasts and abundant collagenous matrix (Fig. 6).

Immunohistochemistry

NF is positive for vimentin, while actins, desmin, S100, and β-catenin are negative.

Differential Diagnosis

Distinction from benign and locally aggressive fibroblastic/myofibroblastic neoplasms is usually straightforward, being significantly less cellular lesions with no atypia and no expression of diagnostic immunohistochemical markers.

Treatment and Prognosis

Surgical removal of the lesion is curative.

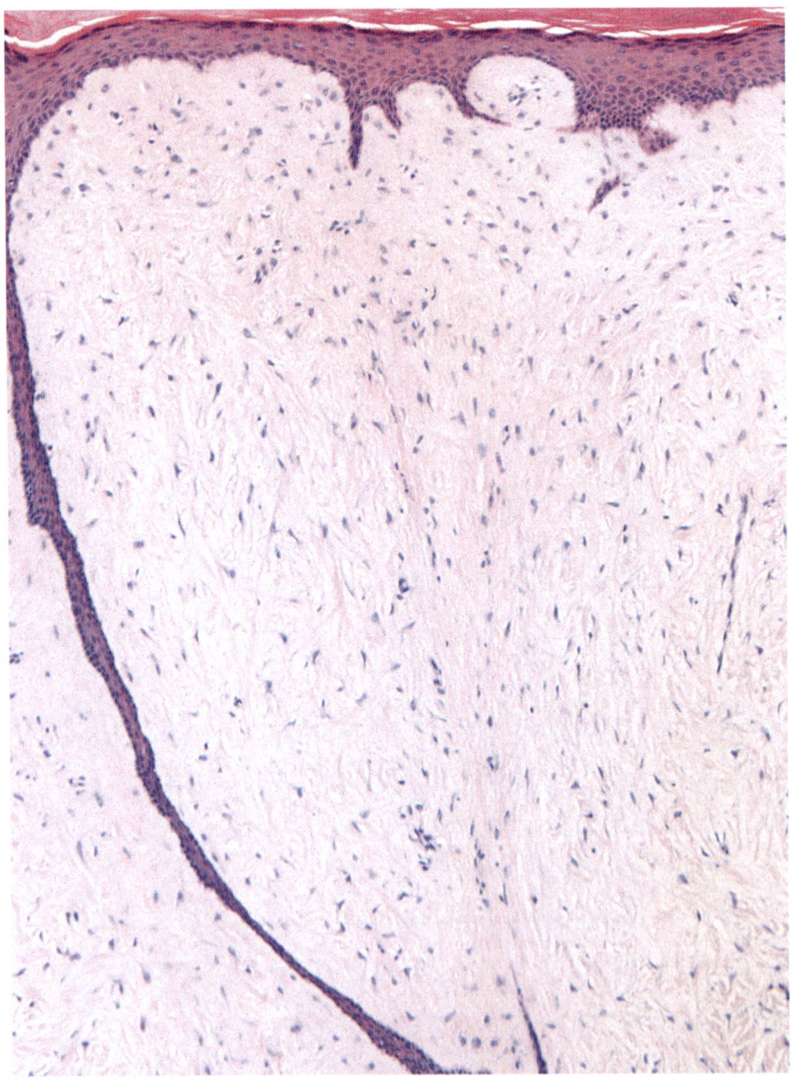

Fig. 6 Fibroma of the nasal septum. The lesion is covered by squamous epithelium and consists of spindle cells separated by abundant collagenous matrix

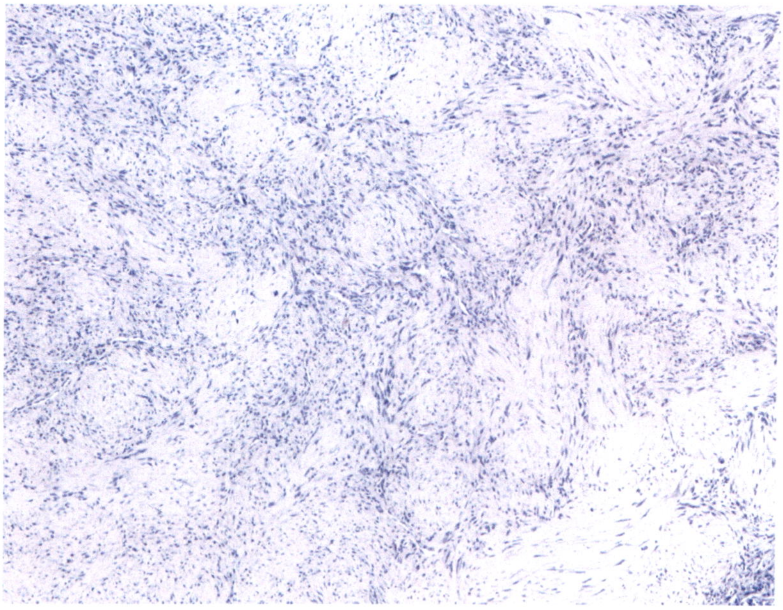

Fig. 7 Myofibroma presents a multinodular architecture with a characteristic biphasic pattern due to alternating hypo- and hypercellular areas

Myofibroma

Definition

Myofibroma (MF; synonym: infantile myofibroma) is a benign neoplasm composed of contractile myoid cells arranged around thin-walled blood vessels. It is one of the most common mesenchymal proliferations of the pediatric age, and it may present as a solitary lesion, as multicentric lesions without visceral involvement and multicentric lesions with visceral involvement. A subset of solitary and multiple non-visceral myofibromas are familial. Myopericytoma is a tumor of perivascular contractile cells that forms a morphologic continuum with myofibroma [20].

Clinical Features

Solitary myofibroma involves quite frequently the head and neck region, but there are only few cases reported with involvement of the nasal cavities [21–23]. Most cases are detected before 12 years of age, and boys appear to be more affected than girls for solitary lesions [24]. The primary symptoms are nasal obstruction and epistaxis [23].

Pathologic Features

MF presents a nodular or multinodular architecture with a characteristic biphasic pattern due to alternating hypo- and hypercellular areas (Fig. 7). In most cases, the central portion of the nodule is paucicellular and rich in hyaline collagen, while the periphery and the internodular areas are composed of plump spindle-shaped cells organized in fascicles or in solid sheets. The vascular component shows an "hemangiopericytoma-like" pattern, which is usually more prominent in the central region of the tumor. This is the reason why most myofibromas have been classified in the "hemangiopericytoma" category in the past.

Immunohistochemical Findings

Neoplastic cells are variably positive for actins, desmin, and h-Caldesmon. S100, cytokeratins, and β-catenin are negative.

Molecular Features

Somatic gain-of-function *PDGFRB* mutations occur at a high frequency in sporadic adult and infantile MF [25, 26]. These mutations are different from those occurring in the familial cases.

Differential Diagnosis

Desmoid fibromatosis has to be differentiated from MF because of its significantly more aggressive and destructive behavior. Infiltration of the adjacent tissues, absence of a biphasic pattern, and nuclear immunoreactivity for β-catenin are features supporting the diagnosis of desmoid fibromatosis. MF may sometimes be confused with spindle cell sarcomas, mainly low-grade myofibrosarcoma and leiomyosarcoma, for the presence of hypercellular areas and overlap of the immunoprofile. However, these sarcomas lack the typical biphasic pattern of MF and show at least focal cellular atypia.

Treatment and Prognosis

MF has a benign behavior, except for cases with multicentric visceral involvement, and conservative surgery is usually curative. Spontaneous regression has also been described.

Sinonasal PEComa

Definition

Perivascular epithelioid cell neoplasms (PEComas) are mesenchymal tumors composed of cells with features of both smooth muscle and melanocytic differentiation, associated with the wall of blood vessels. This family of tumors includes angiomyolipoma, clear cell sugar tumor of the lung, lymphangiomatosis, clear cell myomelanocytic tumor of the falciform ligament/ligamentum teres, and other unusual clear cell tumors arising at a variety of visceral or soft tissue sites.

Clinical Features

Only a few examples of true PEComa have been reported in the sinonasal region [27–33]. They occurred in the nasal cavities of adult patients and presented with nasal obstruction and/or bleeding. PEComas may develop in patients affected by tuberous sclerosis, an autosomal-dominant disease characterized by mutations or losses of *TSC1* or *TSC2* genes. However, none of the sinonasal PEComas reported so far was diagnosed in patients affected by tuberous sclerosis.

Pathologic Features

The lesion has a polypoid fleshy appearance and may be macroscopically pigmented. It consists of a nested proliferation of epithelioid and spindle cells with clear or granular cytoplasm and round nucleus with small but prominent eosinophilic nucleolus, arranged around thin-walled blood vessels (Fig. 8). The tumor cells may contain melanin pigment [33].

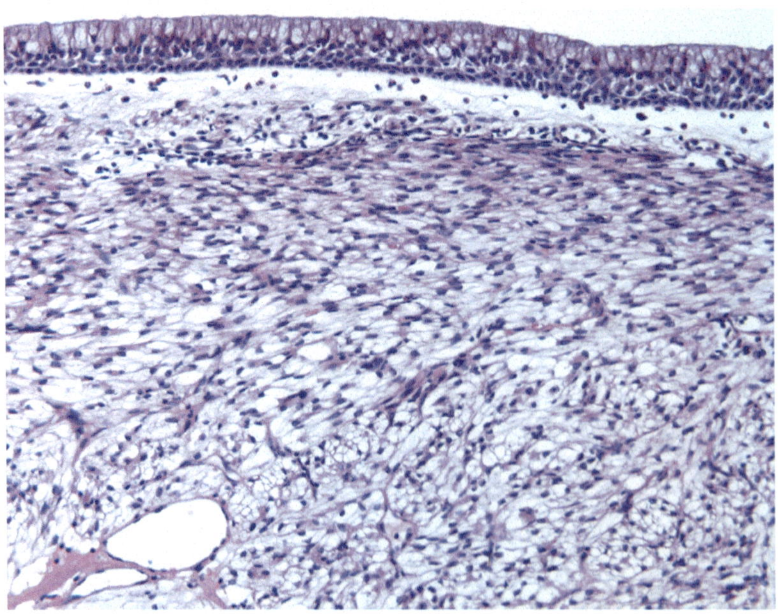

Fig. 8 Sinonasal PEComa. The tumor is formed by spindle-shaped tumor cells with clear cytoplasm

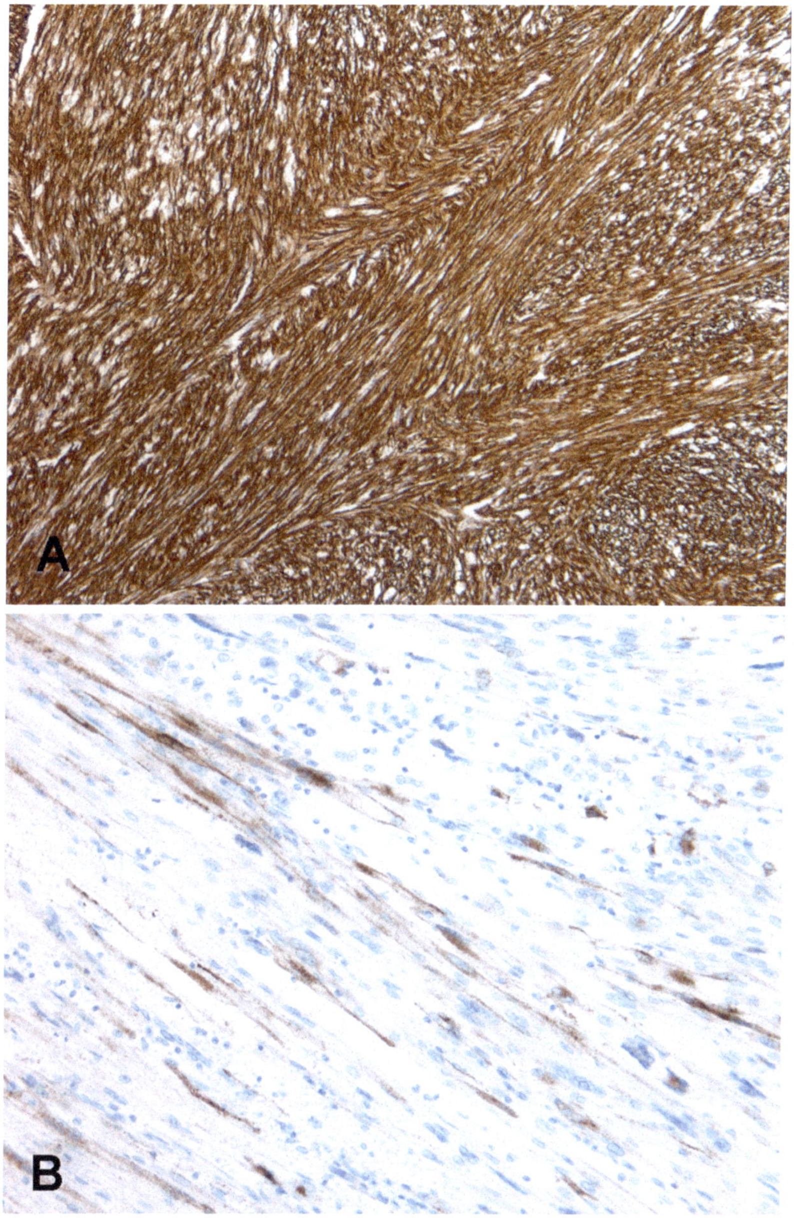

Fig. 9 Tumor cells are positive for smooth muscle actin (**a**) and HMB45 (**b**)

Immunohistochemical Findings

PEComas co-express muscle markers (smooth muscle actin and common muscle actin and less frequently h-Caldesmon and desmin) and melanocytic markers (HMB45, Melan-A, and less frequently MiTF) (Fig. 9). Nuclear expression of TFE3 is also frequently detected.

Molecular Features

A subset of PEComas presents a rearrangement of the *TFE3* gene [33, 34]. *TFE3* fusion-negative PEComas have been shown to harbor mainly *TSC2* mutations [34].

Differential Diagnosis

The main differential diagnosis in the nasal cavity is with melanoma. A diffuse and strong S100 expression and lack of smooth muscle actin immunoreactivity supports the diagnosis of melanoma. In addition, MUM1 is expressed in the majority of melanomas, while it is negative in PEComa [35]. Alveolar soft part sarcoma has been reported in the nasal cavity and shares with PEComa the nested growth pattern, the presence of epithelioid cells, and positivity for TFE3. However, alveolar soft part sarcoma does not show expression of actin and melanocytic markers.

Sinonasal leiomyoma can be separated based on the absence of expression of melanocytic markers.

Treatment and Prognosis

The cases described so far have been treated with surgery, and no recurrence has been reported [31].

Benign Peripheral Nerve Sheath Tumors

Definition

Schwannoma (synonyms: neurinoma, neurilemoma) is a benign peripheral nerve sheath tumor (BPNST) entirely composed of Schwann cells, while neurofibroma is a BPNST composed of Schwann cells, perineurial cells, and fibroblasts and contains residual myelinated and unmyelinated axons within the extracellular stroma.

Clinical Features

BPNSTs are relatively common in the head and neck region, but they rarely involve the sinonasal tract. They occur in adult subjects and headache, and nasal obstruction and epistaxis are the most common presenting symptoms [36, 37]. The majority of the lesions originate in the nasal cavities, and less frequently in a paranasal sinus. The nasal vestibule is the most common subsite for neurofibroma, while Schwannomas arise in the lateral wall and the vault of the nasal cavities. Extension in the skull base, in the anterior cranial fossa, and in the orbit may also occur through erosion of the bone [36]. Sinonasal neurofibromas may be seen in patients with neurofibromatosis type 1, while Schwannomas occur in patients affected by neurofibromatosis type 2.

Pathologic Features

Macroscopically, they appear as polypoid firm lesions usually yellow or white, often with areas of hemorrhage.

As for other anatomic sites, sinonasal Schwannomas are composed of Antoni type A and type B areas. Type A areas are formed by spindle cells with scant eosinophilic cytoplasm and elongated nucleus (Fig. 10), arranged in fascicles with nuclear palisading (Verocay bodies). In type B areas, neoplastic cells are loosely arranged in abundant matrix and accompanied by collections of lipid-laden macrophages. Numerous vessels, often with hyalinized walls, are present in

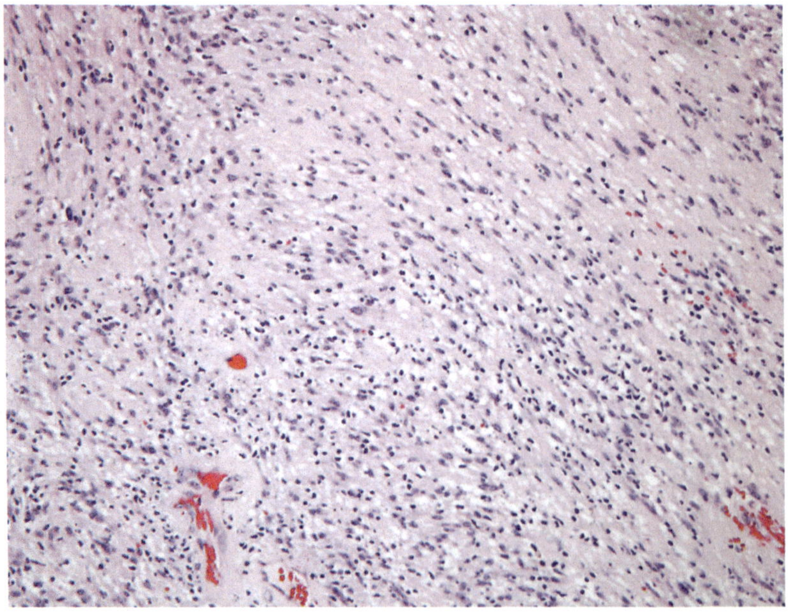

Fig. 10 Neurinoma of the ethmoid sinus. The tumor consists of spindle cells in a fibrillary background. Blood vessels with hyalinized wall are also present

the background (Fig. 10). Degenerative nuclear atypia and areas of hyalinization are present in the so-called ancient lesions. Some of the reported sinonasal Schwannomas had features of the *cellular* variant, being formed by Antoni type A areas, with fascicular pattern and lack of Verocay bodies. Sinonasal Schwannomas distinctively lack encapsulation and may show signs of invasion of bone and adjacent structures [38]. However, it is likely that at least part of the previously reported "invasive" Schwannomas represent indeed examples of biphenotypic sinonasal sarcoma (BSS).

Neurofibroma consists of a subepithelial unencapsulated proliferation of spindle cells with scant cytoplasms and undulating nuclei. They are arranged in short intersecting fascicles, forming small whorls or sometimes forming structures resembling Pacinian corpuscles. The background stroma is mainly myxoid with variable proportions of collagen bundles and contains a variable number of mast cells. Nerve twigs can be identified within the tumor, primarily at the periphery of the lesion. Scattered elements with enlarged hyperchromatic nucleus can be present, but hypercellularity, necrosis, and mitotic figures >4 × 10 high-power fields are not identified [37].

Finally, there are BPNSTs that consist of an admixture of different tumor types, including areas of Schwannoma, neurofibroma, and perineurioma (the so-called hybrid PNSTs). Exceptional examples of these tumor types have been documented in the sinonasal region [39, 40].

Immunohistochemical Profile

Schwannomas are diffusely and intensely positive for S100 protein, while in neurofibroma this marker is positive in 40–50% of cells. In addition, neurofibromas may contain a minor population of cells positive for CD34, claudin, EMA, and GLUT1. Residual axons can be highlighted with neurofilament markers. BPNSTs are also positive for SOX10 [41]. The Ki67 labeling index is usually low (1–5%) [42].

Differential Diagnosis

The main differential diagnosis of sinonasal BPNST is with biphenotypic sinonasal sarcoma (Table 1). Immunohistochemistry helps in the distinction, because both tumor types are positive for S100, but biphenotypic sinonasal sarcoma shows at least focal positive areas for a muscle marker (mainly actin or calponin, less frequently desmin). In addition, SOX10 is positive in BPNST but not in biphenotypic sinonasal sarcoma.

Treatment and Prognosis

Treatment is surgical with gross total resection via endoscopic endonasal approach, rhinotomy, or other sinonasal approaches [36]. Only three recurrences were documented in a series of 94 Schwannomas of the sinonasal tract and skull base [36, 43–45].

Meningioma

Definition

Meningioma is a tumor that arises from the meningothelial arachnoid cells.

Clinical Features

In rare instances, meningiomas occur as extracranial tumors, most often involving the head and neck region. Sinonasal and nasopharyngeal meningiomas represented approximately 25% of all head and neck extracranial meningiomas in a large series [46]. They develop either as a direct extension of an intracranial meningioma (secondary sinonasal meningiomas), or they originate from arachnoid cells that may be present in cranial nerve sheaths or vessels, or finally they develop without any apparent connection with cranial primaries, vessels, or nerves (primary, ectopic, or extra calvarial meningiomas) [46]. Thus, the diagnosis of primary sinonasal meningioma requires the exclusion of an intracranial mass or "dural enhancement" by imaging [47].

They occur over a wide age range, with a peak in the fifth decade and approximately equal gender distribution. The presenting symptoms are nonspecific (mass lesion, epistaxis, sinusitis, pain, nasal obstruction) and are present for a long duration (mean 4 years) [46, 48]. Most tumors involve the nasal cavity alone [48].

Pathologic Features

The surface epithelium is usually intact, and the tumor is polypoid and expands into the bone. Calcifications are frequently present.

Histologically, the majority of sinonasal meningiomas are of the meningothelial type, being composed of nests of tumor cells with indistinct borders that tend to produce whorls. They have uniform round to oval nuclei with fine chromatin pattern and one or two small nucleoli [48]. Psammoma bodies are present. In the transitional form, the nests of tumor cells tend to be larger, the whorls are more conspicuous with the presence of spindle cells, and psammoma bodies are more numerous. A minority of cases presents features of atypical meningioma, with loss of architectural pattern, hypercellularity, increased mitotic activity, necrosis, and nuclear pleomorphism with prominent nucleoli.

Immunohistochemical Features

Meningiomas are typically positive for epithelial membrane antigen (often weakly and focally), cytokeratin 18, and vimentin. Occasional cases may be positive for pancytokeratin or other keratins, CD34, and S100 protein. GFAP, smooth muscle actin, and STAT6 are usually negative. Ki67-positive proliferative fraction is generally low.

Molecular Features

Although there are no specific studies conducted on the genetic alterations of sinonasal meningiomas, the intracranial counterparts have been extensively studied. Monosomy 22, in association or not with mutation of the NF2 gene, is the most frequent genetic alteration in meningiomas. Other recurrent chromosomal alterations include chromosome 1p deletions, gains at 1q25.1 and 1q25.3 in atypical meningiomas, losses involving the long arm of chromosome 6, monosomy 14/del(14q), chromosome 17 gains in malignant meningiomas, and losses at chromosome 18q [49].

Differential Diagnosis

The differential diagnosis of sinonasal meningioma includes several benign and malignant lesions, but their histologic features and immunohistochemical profile can usually separate among these tumors. Carcinomas are usually more atypical and pleomorphic and show a greater degree of cytokeratin expression or demonstrate squamous differentiation. Melanoma, paraganglioma, and olfactory neuroblastoma may resemble the growth pattern of meningioma, but their cytologic features and immunohistochemical profiles are consistently different from those of meningioma. The aggressive psammomatoid ossifying fibroma may be confused with meningioma for the presence of several psammoma bodies, but it shows a more compact growth pattern with the presence of osteoclasts and osteoblasts. Solitary fibrous tumor can be separated from fibroblastic meningioma because it shows STAT6 nuclear immunoreactivity. Sinonasal glomangiopericytoma shows a syncytial growth pattern that may resemble that of meningioma, but it is positive for smooth muscle actin and β-catenin.

Treatment and Prognosis

In general, sinonasal meningioma has a slow and indolent growth, and surgical removal is the treatment of choice. The 5-year disease-free survival rate is around 80%, and local recurrences are likely due to incomplete surgery [47].

Borderline Mesenchymal Tumors

Glomangiopericytoma

Definition

Sinonasal glomangiopericytoma (synonym: sinonasal hemangiopericytoma) is a site-specific tumor with perivascular myoid phenotype, which is closely related to glomus tumor and myopericytoma of the soft tissues [50–52].

Clinical Features

It is an uncommon tumor (<0.5% of all sinonasal neoplasms), which affects mainly adult subjects of either sex, with a peak in the sixth and seventh decades of life [51]. It presents with nasal obstruction and epistaxis and at clinical examination has a polypoid appearance [53]. Most lesions originate in the nasal cavity although the paranasal sinuses can also be affected. An association with oncogenic osteomalacia has been reported in rare cases [54–57].

Pathologic Features

It appears as a soft polypoid lesion, tan to reddish, with hemorrhagic areas on the cut surface, measuring in average 3 cm. Histologically, it consists of an unencapsulated growth of closely packed uniform spindle cells, without intervening matrix. Neoplastic cells are organized in short fascicles, often around vascular channels of varying sizes (Fig. 11). Perivascular hyalinization is commonly observed, as it is the presence of extravasated erythrocytes. Lipomatous change and presence of extra medullary hematopoiesis have been recorded in isolated cases [51]. The nucleus is oval and hyperchromatic, and the cytoplasm is eosinophilic (Fig. 12). Mitotic activity is low (1–2 × 10 high power fields) [51].

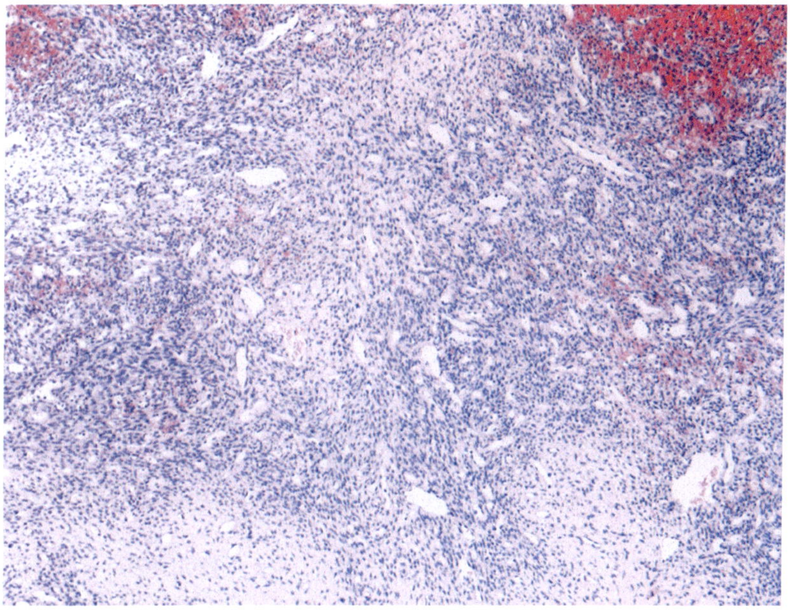

Fig. 11 Sinonasal glomangiopericytoma. Neoplastic cells are organized in short fascicles around vascular channels of varying sizes

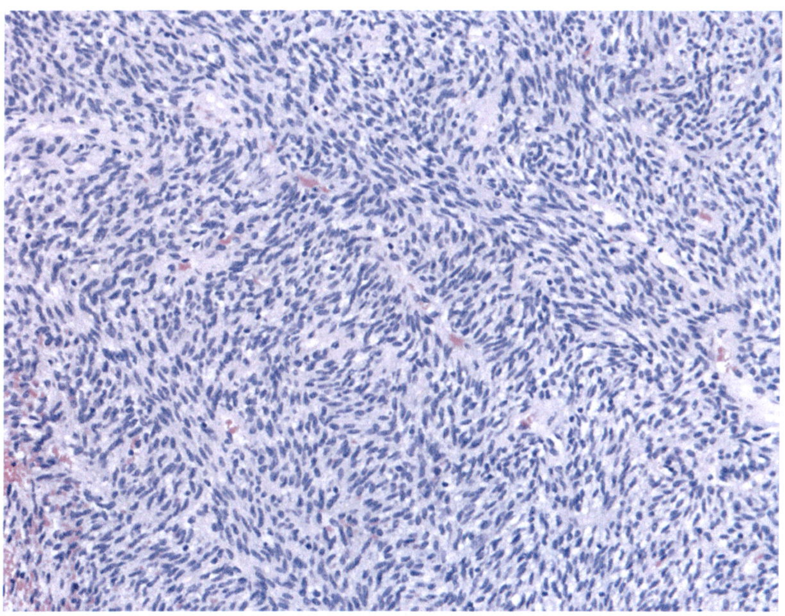

Fig. 12 At higher power, the nucleus of neoplastic cells is oval and hyperchromatic and the cytoplasm is eosinophilic

Degenerative atypia, including the presence of multinucleate elements, can occasionally be found. Increased mitotic activity, pleomorphism, and presence of necrosis are indicative of aggressive clinical behavior [51].

Immunohistochemical Profile

Sinonasal glomangiopericytoma is positive for vimentin and actins as well as for β-catenin [58]. Occasional cases may show focal immunoreactivity for CD34, S-100 protein, glial fibrillary acidic protein, and CD68 [51]. CD31, STAT6, cytokeratins, EMA, desmin, and CD117 are negative in neoplastic cells.

Molecular Features

Missense mutations within the amino-terminal region of the *CTNNB1* gene which encodes for β-catenin have been identified as the likely initiating molecular event driving sinonasal glomangiopericytoma tumorigenesis [59, 60]. These mutations prevent β-catenin phosphorylation and degradation and promote its nuclear accumulation, hence the intense and diffuse immunohistochemical positivity for β-catenin in these tumors [59, 60]. Nuclear overexpression of cyclin D1 is observed as well [60].

Differential Diagnosis

Solitary fibrous tumor may be confused with glomangiopericytoma because of the presence of prominent thin-walled dilated vessels. However, in solitary fibrous tumor neoplastic cells are more elongated and associated with variable degrees of collagen formation, including the presence of "ropey" collagen fibers that are usually not seen in glomangiopericytoma. By immunohistochemical analysis, solitary fibrous tumor shows diffuse positivity for CD34 and STAT6, which is not a feature of glomangiopericytoma [61] (Table 1). Nuclear positivity for β-catenin is not discriminant, because it is observed in both tumor types [58–60].

Biphenotypic sinonasal sarcoma is a spindle cell tumor which may show a hemangiopericytomatous vascular pattern, as well as immunoreactivity for actins and β-catenin, thus closely mimicking the histologic and immunohistochemical features of glomangiopericytoma [62]. However, biphenotypic sinonasal sarcoma shows at least focal positivity for S100 and presents a *PAX3* rearrangement that are not detected in glomangiopericytoma. Finally, sinonasal smooth muscle tumors share the positivity for actins with glomangiopericytoma, but they lack the prominent vascular network and the positivity for β-catenin.

Treatment and Prognosis

Surgery is the treatment of choice for sinonasal glomangiopericytoma varying from simple polypectomy without extended resection to wide excision with tumor-free margins [63]. Overall, it is a low-grade indolent tumor with a 5-year-survival rate >90%; local recurrence develops in 20–40% of cases, even several years after diagnosis. Aggressive behavior is rare, and it is associated with larger tumor dimensions (>5 cm), bone invasion, nuclear pleomorphism, brisk mitotic activity, and necrosis.

Desmoid Fibromatosis

Definition

Desmoid fibromatosis (synonym: aggressive fibromatosis) is a locally aggressive, non-metastasizing, fibroblastic/myofibroblastic tumor.

Clinical Features

In the head and neck region, the involvement of the sinonasal tract is infrequent. Patients are most frequently in first three decades of life, and there is a slight male predominance [64, 65]. The maxillary sinus is the most frequently involved site, followed by the nasal cavity, and the most common presenting symptoms are swelling and pain or tenderness [64].

Pathologic Features

Desmoid fibromatosis appears as a firm, white, poorly circumscribed, infiltrating lesion, with a whorled, fascicular appearance on the cut surface. Microscopically, there is a proliferation of bland looking spindle cells arranged in long fascicles, separated by abundant collagen (Fig. 13). The

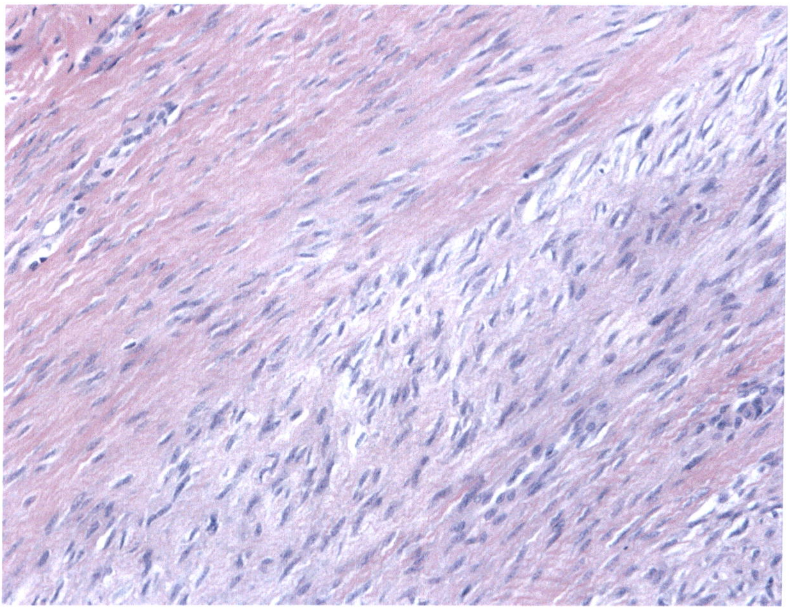

Fig. 13 Desmoid fibromatosis presents as a proliferation of uniform bland-looking spindle cells arranged in long fascicles, separated by abundant collagen

stroma may also show myxoid areas or keloidal collagen fibers. Mitotic figures are absent or rare, and necrosis is not present. Destructive infiltration of bone is commonly seen [64].

Immunohistochemical Findings

Tumor cells are variably positive for actins and desmin. Nuclear positivity for β-catenin is detected in 75–80% of cases, and it is useful to support the diagnosis [66, 67]. However, it should be remembered that β-catenin nuclear immunoreactivity is found also in other spindle cell sinonasal neoplasms that may be entered in the differential diagnosis with desmoid fibromatosis, including glomangiopericytoma and biphenotypic sinonasal sarcoma [58].

Molecular Features

Activating mutations of *CTNNB1*, the β-catenin encoding gene are detected in approximately 85% of sporadic cases [68], while tumors associated with Gardner-type FAP syndrome show germline mutations of the APC gene. However, APC mutations are sometimes detected also in sporadic cases [69].

Differential Diagnosis

Desmoid fibromatosis needs to be distinguished from several benign and malignant conditions (Table 1). Reactive fibrosis lacks the fascicular pattern of fibromatosis and the nuclear immunoreactivity for β-catenin. Nasal fibroma is a small polypoid lesion that originates from the vestibule or the septum and does not show an infiltrative and fasciculated growth pattern. Similarly, nodular fasciitis lacks the long fascicles of desmoid fibromatosis, is more cellular, presents extravasated erythrocytes, and is not immunoreactive for β-catenin. In sinonasal glomangiopericytoma, neoplastic cells are closely packed, without collagen production, and in addition there is a well-developed vascular network, often with perivascular hyalinosis. Among malignancies, low-grade myofibroblastic sarcoma is very similar to desmoid fibromatosis, but it is more cellular and presents focal atypia and mitoses. Fibrosarcoma and leiomyosarcoma are significantly more cellular and atypical than desmoid fibromatosis and lack positivity for β-catenin.

Treatment and Prognosis

Desmoid fibromatosis shows a high propensity to recur after initial treatment although in the sinonasal region the rate is lower than other sites [64]. Surgery remains the mainstay of treatment, although currently an aggressive approach aiming at negative margins is debated and a wait-and-see policy as initial strategy is being adopted.

Solitary Fibrous Tumor

Definition

Solitary fibrous tumor (SFT) is a fibroblastic neoplasm associated with a specific *NAB2-STAT6* gene fusion. In the past, most cases were included in the diagnostic category of hemangiopericytoma.

Clinical Features

Head and neck sites are rarely involved (except for the meninges). SFT arising in the sinonasal tract represent 20–30% of all the head and neck SFTs [70, 71]. Patients are adults, with no gender predilection [70–72], who present with nasal obstruction and epistaxis.

Pathologic Features

They appear as polypoid, firm, white lesion. Histologically, they are identical to the pleural counterpart and consist of a proliferation of bland looking, uniform spindle cells, with no specific architectural arrangement, embedded within collagen matrix (Fig. 14). The tumor involves the nasal mucosa and is nonencapsulated, sometimes invading the bone structures. Cellularity is variable, with hypercellular sparsely collagenized areas adjacent to densely collagenized hypocellular regions. A prominent vascular component, with interlaced thin-walled dilated capillary vessels, is usually present (Fig. 15). Giant-cell angiofibroma-like histology with multinucleated cells surrounding pseudoangiomatous spaces has been observed in rare sinonasal cases [70]. In typical cases, mitotic activity is low, and necrosis is not present.

Immunohistochemical Findings

Immunohistochemically, neoplastic cells are positive for STAT6 (nuclear) (Fig. 16), CD34, and bcl-2, while actins, S100 protein, cytokeratins, and EMA are negative. Nuclear immunoreactivity for β-catenin has been reported [58].

Molecular Features

SFT presents a specific translocation *NAB2-STAT6* which may be useful for purposes of differential diagnosis, especially in atypical forms.

Differential Diagnosis

The main differential diagnoses are sinonasal glomangiopericytoma and nasopharyngeal angiofibroma (Table 1). Neoplastic cells in glomangiopericytoma are plumper, closely packed with no collagen matrix deposition, and show positivity for actins and negativity for CD34 and STAT6.

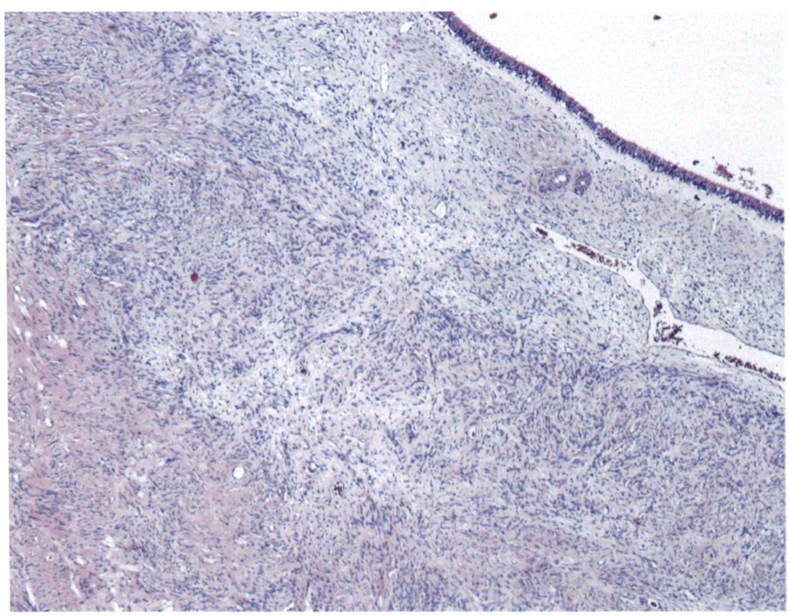

Fig. 14 Sinonasal solitary fibrous tumor presenting as a variably cellular proliferation, with alternating collagen-rich areas and cellular areas

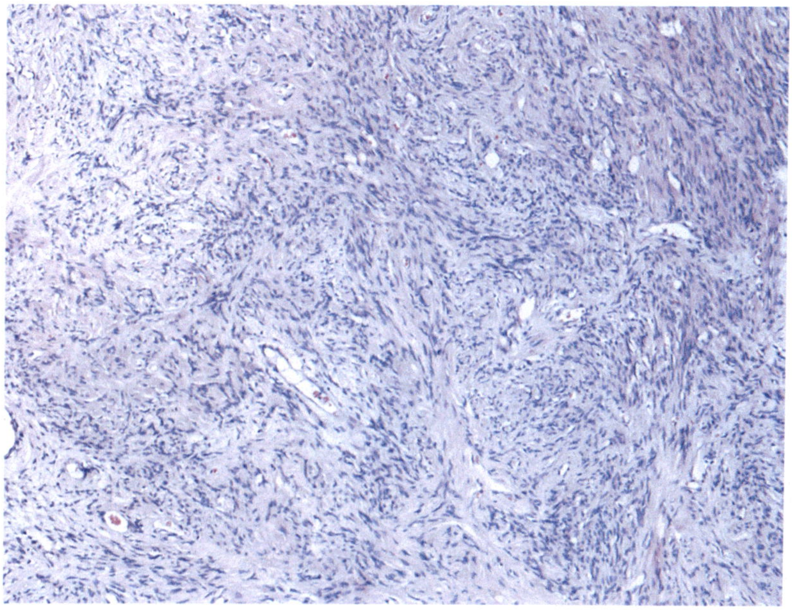

Fig. 15 Neoplastic cells are bland and arranged around vessels without a specific pattern

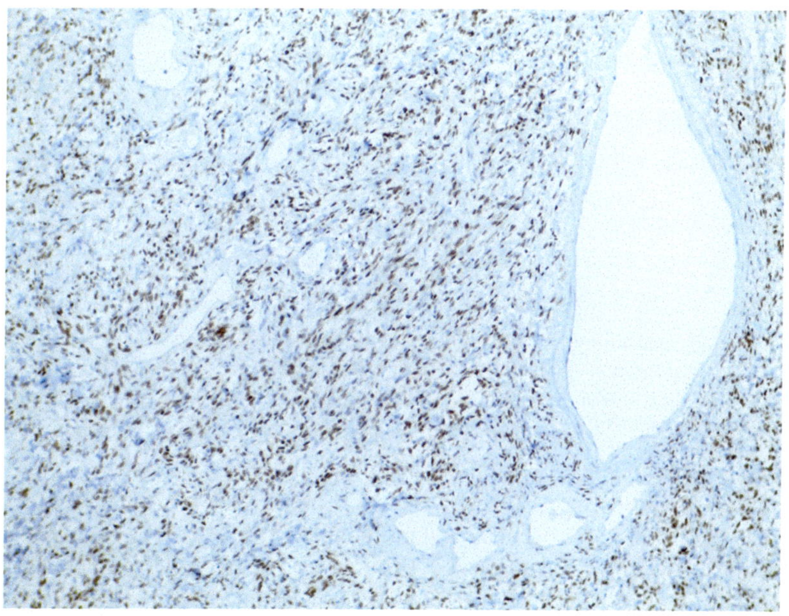

Fig. 16 Neoplastic cells present nuclear staining for STAT6

Nasopharyngeal angiofibroma is a rare benign neoplasm which affects almost exclusively boys and adolescent to young men. Histologically, it may resemble SFT, being formed of a network of dilated capillary vessels set in a fibrous stroma containing stellate fibroblasts, which, however, are negative for CD34 and STAT6.

Treatment and Prognosis

Nasal solitary fibrous tumor has a locally aggressive behavior, with recurrences occurring in up to 40% of the cases [71]. Infiltrative growth, with extension in the paranasal sinuses, as well as in the nasopharynx or to the anterior cranial fossa is frequently observed [73, 74]. Distant metastases have been documented in a minority of cases [71]. Size and mitotic rate ≥4 per 10 high power fields are associated with worst prognosis. Complete surgical removal is the treatment of choice.

Phosphaturic Mesenchymal Tumor

Definition

Phosphaturic mesenchymal tumor (PMT) is an intermediate rarely metastasizing tumor of uncertain histogenesis that induces osteomalacia in most patients (*tumor induced* or *oncogenic* osteomalacia), through the production of fibroblast growth factor 23 (FGF23) by neoplastic cells. This hormone inhibits sodium-phosphate co-transport in the proximal tubular cells of the kidney, determining phosphaturia and bone demineralization.

Clinical Features

Approximately 5% of all PMTs are located in the head and neck, and half of these cases occur in the nasal cavity [75, 76]. Patients are affected over a wide age range (3–73 years) without gender predilection. Local symptoms include episodes of epistaxis, anosmia, and nasal obstruction. The presence of paraneoplastic oncogenic osteomalacia is indicated by bone pain, progressive muscle weakness, and fractures. This paraneoplastic syndrome may not be apparent in all cases at the time of diagnosis. A minority of cases with PMT histologic features is not associated with oncogenic osteomalacia. Preoperative laboratory values show hypophosphatemia, normocalcemia or borderline hypocalcemia, increased alkaline phosphatase, a low serum 25-hydroxyvitamin D level and phosphaturia. Serum FGF-23 levels are elevated in most but not all cases.

Pathologic Features

The tumor is small and well circumscribed in most cases, gray-white or tan, with myxoid areas and foci of calcifications. It consists of a population of bland-looking spindle or ovoid cells that produce variable, usually small, amount of extracellular matrix with a peculiar appearance, ranging from myxoid to hyalinized or "smudgy" appearing or sometimes resembling cartilage or osteoid (Fig. 17). However, sinonasal tumors tend to be more cellular and to produce less extracellular matrix [77]. The matrix presents foci of calcification often showing a characteristic "grungy" or flocculent pattern. Scattered

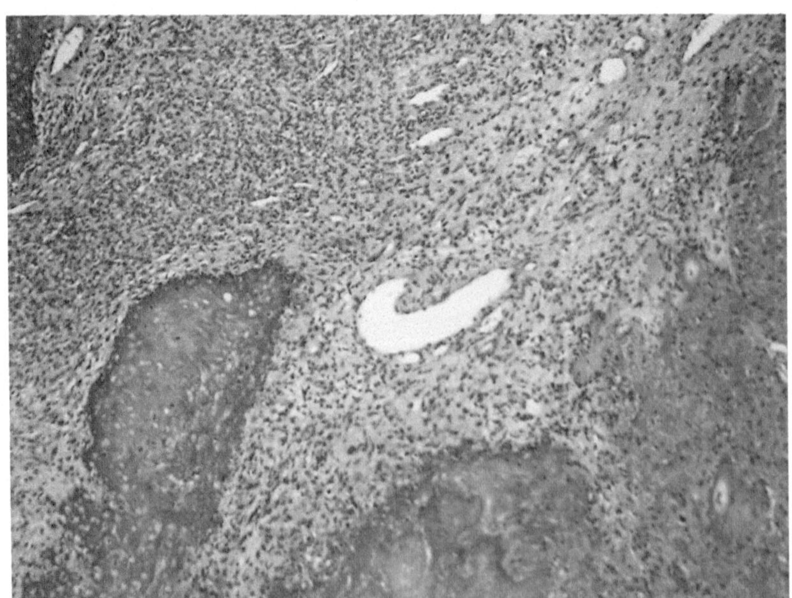

Fig. 17 Phosphaturic mesenchymal tumor. The tumor consists of a uniform population of bland ovoid cells that produce calcified extracellular matrix. Dilated vessels are present in the background

osteoclast-like giant cells can be present, as well as areas of hemorrhage. A prominent vascular component is detected in most cases, particularly in those arising in the sinonasal region, often consisting in dilated capillary vessels with a hemangiopericytoma-like pattern. Areas of mature adipocytes can be present as well. Mitotic activity is low or absent.

Immunohistochemical Findings

Positivity for FGF23 can be detected by immunohistochemistry in 80–90% of cases, but it does not correlate with the serum levels of the growth factor, and it is not specific for PMT, being expressed also in other mesenchymal tumors. Other consistently expressed markers include CD56, ERG, SATB2, and somatostatin receptor 2A, while DOG1, β-catenin, S100, and STAT6 are negative [77].

Molecular Features

PMT shows mutually exclusive gene translocations involving the *FN1-FGFR1* and *FN1-FGF1* genes with a frequency of 40–45% and 5%, respectively [77–79].

Differential Diagnosis

The differential diagnosis of sinonasal PMT is broad due to the variable histologic appearance and includes vascular tumors, glomangiopericytoma, solitary fibrous tumor, as well as matrix forming tumors of cartilage and osteoblastic lineage. The distinction from glomangiopericytoma and solitary fibrous tumor is facilitated by the differences in the immunoprofile, since PMT is positive for SATB2 and negative for β-catenin and STAT6.

Treatment and Prognosis

PMT behaves as a benign tumor, with high rate of local recurrence if incompletely excised. Rare examples showed a malignant clinical course and presented increased cellularity, high nuclear grade, and brisk mitotic activity. Surgical removal of the tumor is followed by resolution of osteomalacia.

Myxoma

Definition

Sinonasal myxoma (SM) is a benign/locally aggressive tumor of uncertain histogenesis, characterized by bland spindle to stellate cells embedded in abundant hypovascular myxoid to fibromyxoid stroma. In the head and neck, myxomas develop more frequently in gnatic sites than in extragnatic sites, and mandibular myxomas are more common than maxillary/sinonasal myxomas [80]. Tumors arising in non-tooth bearing areas and lacking odontogenic epithelium at the histologic level should be kept distinguished from "odontogenic myxomas" [80].

Clinical Features

SM is a rare tumor which occurs over a wide age range, developing both in pediatric and adult patients [80–84]. They present as slowly growing swellings of the involved region, causing sinonasal or ocular symptoms. Tumors primarily involving the sinonasal tract most often arise in the maxillary antrum and tend to extend into nasal cavity. In addition, SM may destroy the bone and extend in the orbit, skull base, and cranial cavity.

Pathologic Features

Grossly, myxomas are well circumscribed but nonencapsulated and appear as a gelatinous mass. Histologically, they consist of stellate and spindled-shaped cells embedded in abundant myxoid matrix (Fig. 18). Neoplastic cells are bland, present oval, and hyperchromatic nuclei, and the cytoplasm is slightly basophilic and sometimes vacuolated. A delicate capillary network is present in the background. Mitotic activity is absent or low, and necrosis is not observed. Odontogenic epithelium should not be seen. Lesions showing a greater degree of collagenous matrix production may be designated as fibromyxomas.

Immunohistochemical Profile

Neoplastic cells are positive for vimentin and negative for S100, SOX10, smooth muscle actin, desmin, myogenin, CD34, STAT6, and MUC4.

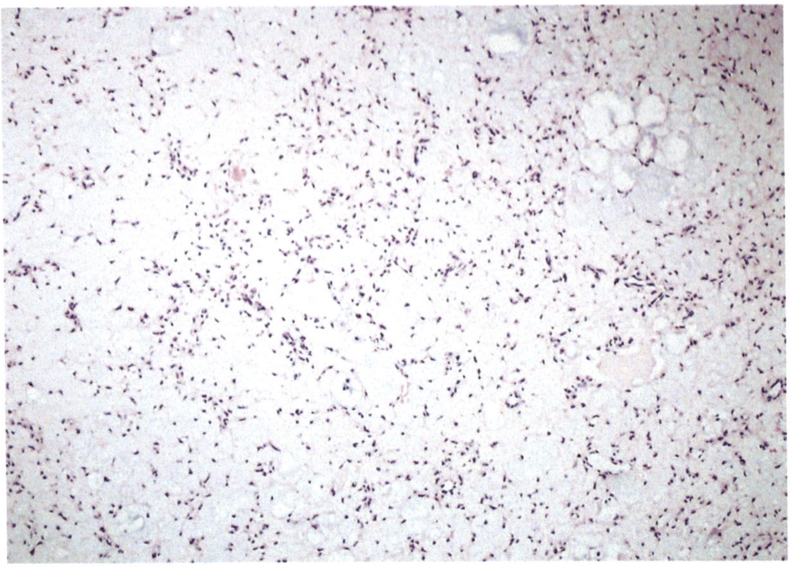

Fig. 18 Sinonasal myxoma consists of stellate and spindled shaped cells embedded in abundant myxoid matrix

Differential Diagnosis

SM may be confused with several benign and malignant lesions. Inflammatory polyp can be separated because it presents abundant mixed inflammatory infiltrate and edematous rather than mucinous stromal changes. Angiofibroma occurs almost exclusively in male adolescents and presents a more collagenized stromal background with prominent vasculature. Neurofibroma may closely resemble the appearance of myxoma, but neoplastic cells show a wavy nucleus and are positive for S100 protein. More importantly, SM should be distinguished from sarcomas with prominent myxoid matrix component. Embryonal rhabdomyosarcoma (RMS) is the main diagnostic differential concern in infants and can be distinguished because it presents increased cellularity and atypia and for the different immunohistochemical profile that includes positivity for desmin and myogenin.

Treatment and Prognosis

Treatment consists of wide local resection with clear margins. Incomplete surgery results in a high risk of local recurrence [80]. Metastases have not been reported.

Malignant Mesenchymal Tumors

Fibrosarcoma

Definition

Fibrosarcoma (FS; synonym: adult-type fibrosarcoma) is a malignant spindle cell tumor that lacks any form of differentiation other than fibroblastic.

Clinical Features

It is a rare tumor that affects adult patients, with a mean age at diagnosis of 50 years and no significant gender predilection [85]. It most commonly arises in the maxillary sinus, and the nasal cavity is the second most frequent involved site [85]. Presenting symptoms include nasal obstruction, recurrent epistaxis, and rhinorrhea, as well as hyposmia and frequent sinusal cephalalgias [86]. Examples of radiation-induced sinonasal FS have been reported [87].

Pathologic Features

The tumor occupies the nasal cavities and the sinuses, often invading the bone. Histologically, FS is a variably cellular proliferation of spindle cells arranged in intersecting fascicles, often with

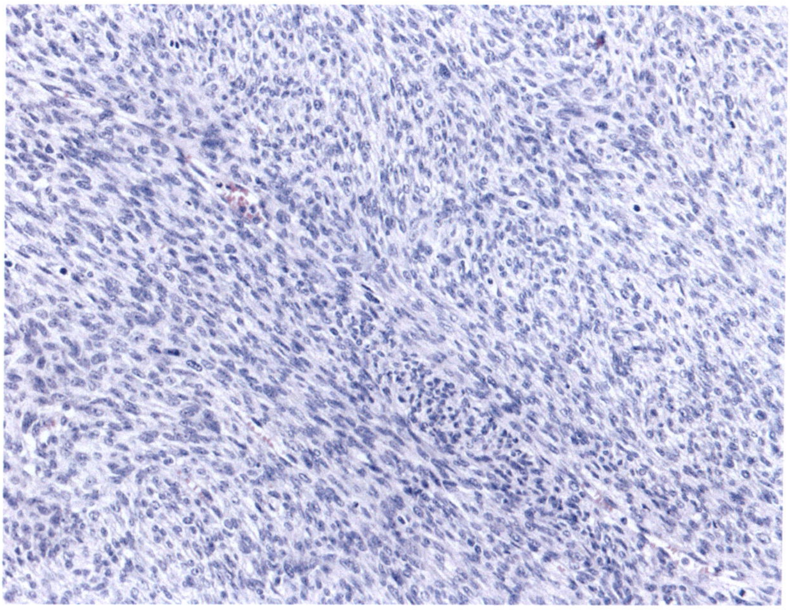

Fig. 19 Fibrosarcoma presents intersecting fascicles of spindle cells

a "herringbone" pattern, and with variable amount of collagen production (Fig. 19). Areas of myxoid matrix production can also be present. Cellular atypia is slight to moderate, whereas cellular pleomorphism is not observed.

Immunohistochemical Profile

Neoplastic cells are positive for vimentin and focally for actin. Epithelial markers, S100 protein, desmin, and myogenin are negative.

Differential Diagnosis

The histologic appearance of the tumor is not specific; thus, the diagnosis requires the exclusion of other entities with similar morphology, mainly sarcomatoid carcinoma, synovial sarcoma, leiomyosarcoma, spindle cell rhabdomyosarcoma, and spindle cell melanoma (Table 1). An appropriate immunohistochemical panel including epithelial, melanoma, and muscle markers helps to rule out these malignancies. The distinction from monophasic synovial sarcoma may require the analysis of SYT rearrangement. Negative nuclear staining for β-catenin supports the diagnosis of FS versus desmoid-type fibromatosis. Electron microscopy can demonstrate the fibroblastic differentiation of the tumor.

Treatment and Prognosis

The 5-year survival rate is around 75%, and high histologic grade is associated with poorer prognosis. Patients treated with surgery, with or without adjuvant radiotherapy, have an improved survival in comparison with for those treated with radiotherapy alone [85].

Undifferentiated Pleomorphic Sarcoma

Definition

Undifferentiated pleomorphic sarcoma (UPS; synonym: malignant fibrous histiocytoma) is a high-grade mesenchymal neoplasm that lacks a specific line of differentiation.

Clinical Features

UPS only rarely arises in the sinonasal region, where it is the second most common sarcoma after rhabdomyosarcoma. It occurs over a wide age range, with a median of 50 years [88, 89]. Sinonasal UPS may arise at the site of previous irradiation for nasopharyngeal carcinoma [88, 90]. Symptoms include pain in the facial region, swelling of the cheek, and nasal bleeding [91].

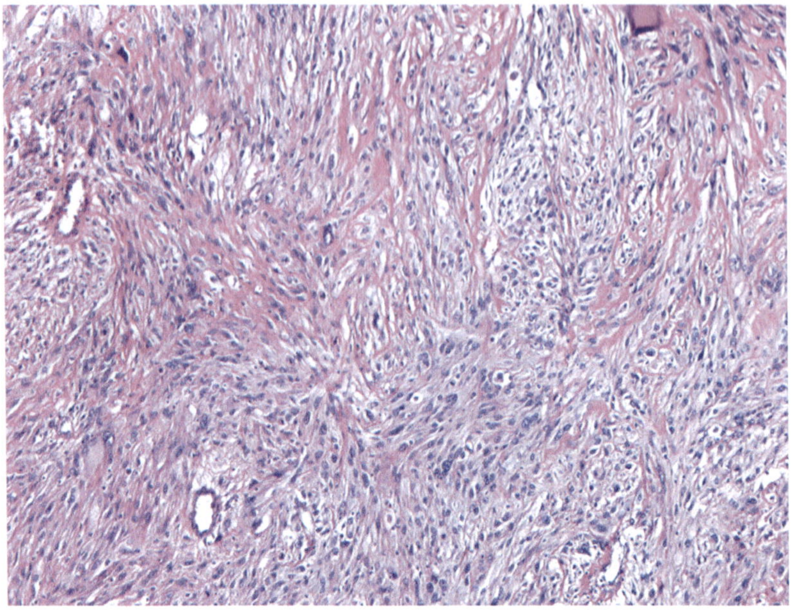

Fig. 20 Undifferentiated pleomorphic sarcoma. The tumor consists of polymorphic spindle cells with no specific line of differentiation

The main site of origin is the maxillary sinus, followed by the nasal cavities.

Pathologic Features

It consists of a proliferation of atypical spindle cells and large, often multinucleated pleomorphic cells, with patternless arrangement or with fascicular and storiform architecture (Fig. 20).

Immunohistochemical Profile

Neoplastic cells may show limited reactivity for actin, whereas desmin, myogenin, S100 protein, and epithelial markers are negative.

Differential Diagnosis

Sinonasal UPS is a diagnosis of exclusion, and other high-grade pleomorphic malignancies must be ruled out, including sarcomatoid carcinoma, melanoma, lymphomas, and other sarcomas, mainly rhabdomyosarcoma, leiomyosarcoma, and malignant peripheral nerve sheath tumor (MPNST).

Treatment and Prognosis

Surgery with or without radiotherapy is the mainstay for treatment. The 5-year survival rate ranges between 60 and 75%. Deaths are mainly due to local recurrence with invasion of the cranial cavity while distant metastases are infrequent. Sinonasal post radiation UPS has a worst prognosis than primary UPS (Wang CP).

Leiomyosarcoma

Definition

Leiomyosarcoma (LMS) is a sarcoma with smooth muscle differentiation. An origin from a vessel wall can be observed in the majority of cases [11].

Clinical Features

LMS is very rare in the sinonasal tract, being the third histotype in frequency after rhabdomyosarcoma and undifferentiated sarcoma [92, 93]. Most cases affect adult patients, with a slight female predilection [11]. They present with nasal stuffiness and bleeding, and involvement of the nasal cavities is more frequent than that of a paranasal sinus alone or of both [11]. A history of retinoblastoma and of previous irradiation of the head and neck is reported in a significant number of patients [94].

Pathologic Features

The tumor is usually polypoid, firm in consistency, and white to gray. Bone invasion can be present. In the better differentiated areas, it consists of intersecting fascicles of spindle cells with elongated eosinophilic fibrillary cytoplasm and blunt-ended, cigar-shaped nucleus (Fig. 21). Atypical cells, with enlarged hyperchromatic nuclei, are variably present. In high-grade lesions, there are evident pleomorphism, atypical mitotic figures, and areas of necrosis.

Immunohistochemical Profile

Smooth muscle differentiation can be confirmed by the positivity for at least two markers among smooth muscle actin, common muscle actin, desmin, and h-Caldesmon. Other markers, like S100, HMB45, and EBER, are negative [94]. Loss of RB expression is a frequent finding [94].

Differential Diagnosis

The differential diagnosis includes spindle cell carcinoma, melanoma, fibrosarcoma, synovial sarcoma, malignant peripheral nerve sheath tumor among malignant tumors, leiomyoma, glomangiopericytoma, and desmoid fibromatosis among benign/borderline tumors. In general, these latter tumors lack significant atypia and have low or absent mitotic activity.

Examples of the so-called smooth muscle tumors with unknown malignant potential (SMTUMP) have been reported in nasal cavities [11]. They can be separated from leiomyomas and LMS mainly based on the presence of atypia and on the mitotic count (1–4 mitotic figures/10 high power field) [11].

Finally, metastatic leiomyosarcoma from another site should also be ruled out [94].

Treatment and Prognosis

In most cases, the initial treatment has been surgical excision, while the efficacy of radiotherapy and chemotherapy is not yet well established [95]. Local recurrence is more frequent in large lesions with bone invasion that are less amenable to radical surgery. Late metastatic disease has been reported, and therefore long-term follow-up is recommended [94, 96].

Rhabdomyosarcoma

Definition

Rhabdomyosarcoma (RMS) is malignant mesenchymal tumor with skeletal muscle differentiation.

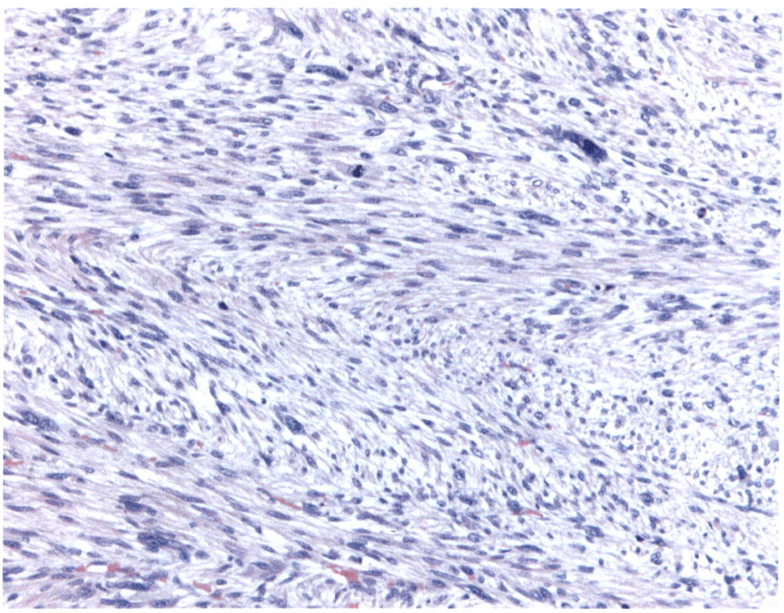

Fig. 21 Leiomyosarcoma consists of intersecting fascicles of spindle and pleomorphic cells with eosinophilic cytoplasm

In the nasal cavities and paranasal sinuses, the embryonal and alveolar subtypes are the most frequent, while pleomorphic and spindle cell variants are extremely rare.

Clinical Features

Sinonasal RMS account for approximately 15% of all RMSs arising in the head and neck [97]. It is the most common sinonasal malignancy in the pediatric age, and the majority of cases occur before the age of 12, with a slight male predominance [98]. However, RMS occurs also in adult patients, with the alveolar type being the most frequent in this age group [92, 97]. The presenting symptoms are nonspecific and often of relatively short duration, indicating a rapid clinical onset, and the tumor is in advanced stage at presentation, with involvement of more than one anatomic site [97, 99]. In rare cases, RMS is part of a genetic syndrome, including Li-Fraumeni, Beckwith–Wiedemann, neurofibromatosis type 1, Costello, Noonan, and Gorlin syndromes.

Pathologic Features

Embryonal RMS is the most common type and presents as a soft, fleshy, often polypoid mass. It is formed by rhabdomyoblasts in various stages of differentiation, appearing as undifferentiated round or spindle cells, with scant cytoplasm and small hyperchromatic nuclei, set in a myxoid background, and varying number of larger more differentiated cells with bright eosinophilic cytoplasm, sometimes showing cross striations (Fig. 22). Cellular and hypocellular areas with stromal hyalinization are present. Cellular pleomorphism may also be detected. The botryoid variant has a polypoid architecture and presents linear aggregates of neoplastic cells below the epithelial surface, resulting in a grading of cellularity.

The alveolar RMS is characterized by the presence of fibrovascular septa separating dyscohesive aggregates of monomorphic atypical round to oval neoplastic cells with eosinophilic cytoplasm (Fig. 23). Giant cells with multiple peripheral nuclei may be present. As the name implies, in the solid variant of alveolar RMS, fibrovascular septa are absent, and neoplastic cells form solid sheets.

In the spindle cell variant, neoplastic cells are arranged in fascicles and present elongated pale eosinophilic cytoplasm and oval nuclei (Fig. 24). In addition, small numbers of spindled or polygonal rhabdomyoblasts with hyperchromatic, eccentric nuclei and abundant brightly eosinophilic cytoplasm are scattered throughout the

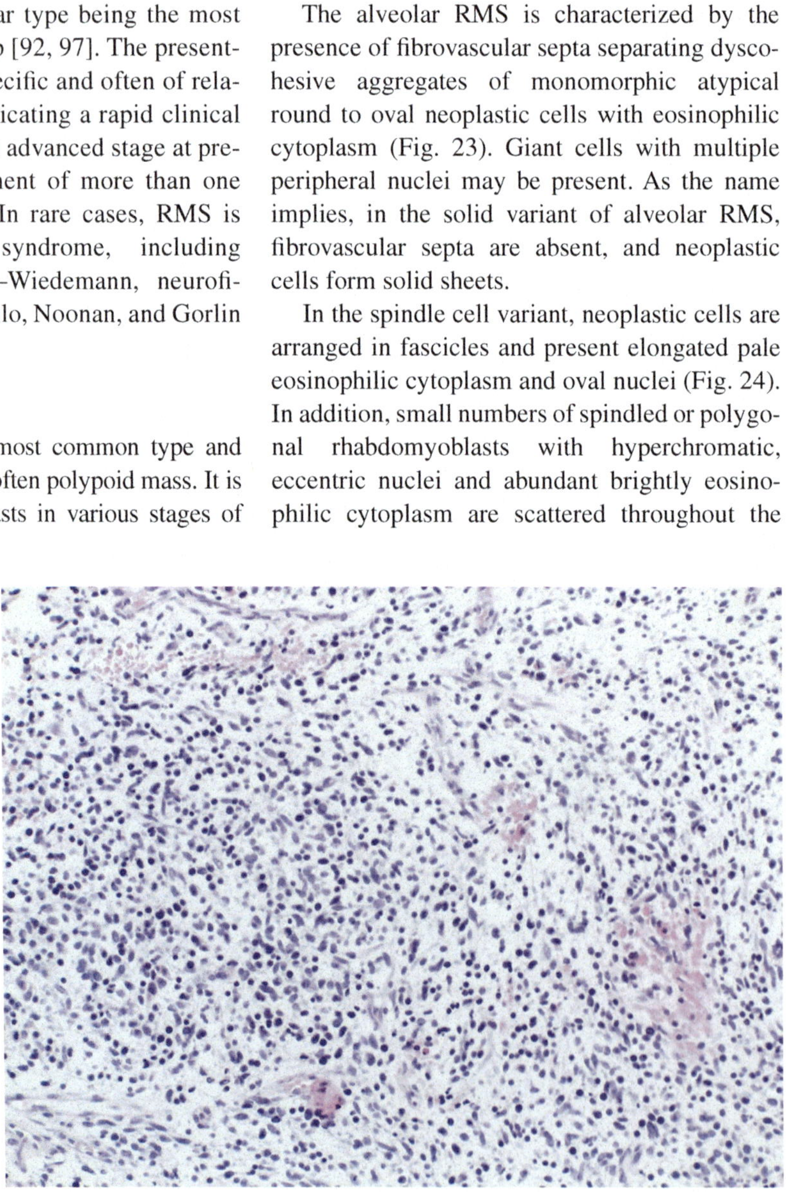

Fig. 22 Embryonal rhabdomyosarcoma. The tumor consists of a proliferation of undifferentiated round cells and larger cells with rhabdomyoblastic features

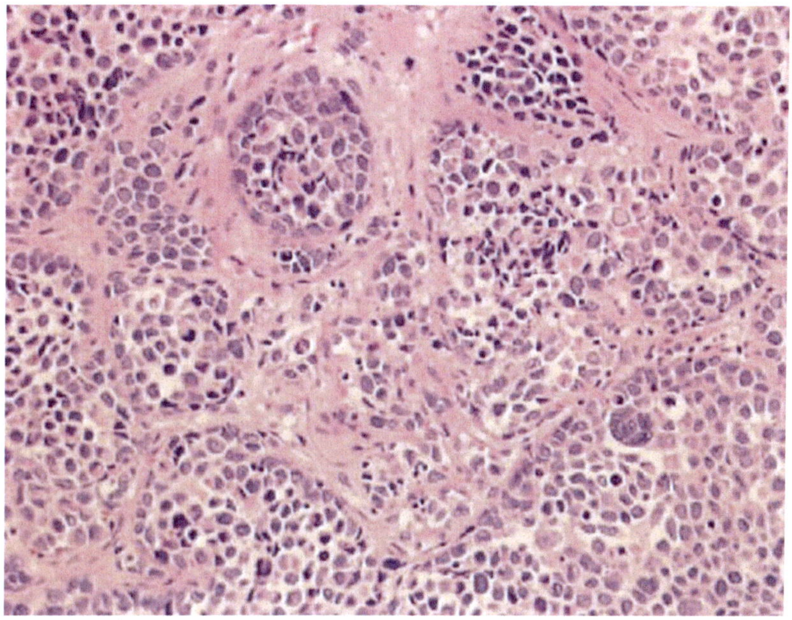

Fig. 23 Alveolar rhabdomyosarcoma. The tumor cells tend to aggregate in alveolar structures separated by fibrous septa

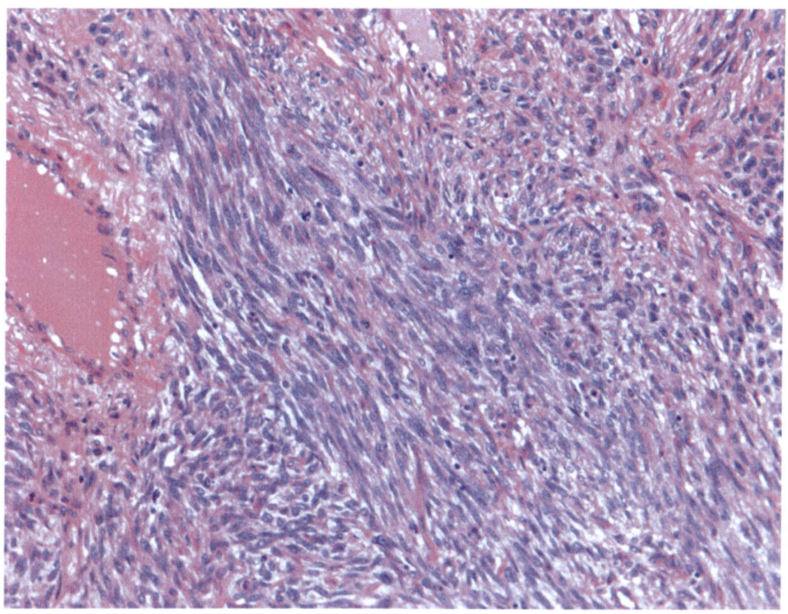

Fig. 24 Spindle cell rhabdomyosarcoma. Spindle cells with eosinophilic cytoplasm are arranged in intersecting fascicles

tumor. A minority of cases shows prominent stromal hyalinization.

In pleomorphic RMS, neoplastic cells show high variability in size and shape, and large rhabdomyoblasts with eosinophilic cytoplasm can be identified.

Immunohistochemical Profile

RMS is typically positive for desmin and myogenin (MYF4). Other positive markers include MYOD1, fast myosin, myoglobin, and common muscle actin, while smooth muscle actin is detected in a minority of cases. Some RMSs,

Table 2 Summary of the diagnostic features of sinonasal "round cell" sarcomas

	Histologic features	Immunohistochemical markers	Diagnostic gene fusion(s)
Rhabdomyosarcoma	Loose myxoid areas, subepithelial cellular areas, solid, alveolar	Myogenin, desmin, actin	*PAX3* or *PAX7-FOXO1* (alveolar rhabdomyosarcoma)
Ewing sarcoma	Solid, pseudorosettes	CD99, variable expression of neuroectodermal markers and cytokeratins	*EWSR1-FLI1* or other ETS family members
Desmoplastic small round cell tumor	Solid areas separated by desmoplastic stroma	Cytokeratins, desmin, WT1, neuron-specific enolase, CD99	*EWSR1-WT1*
Synovial sarcoma (poorly differentiated)	Solid, prominent vascular channels	Cytokeratins, EMA, TLE1	*SS18-SSX1* or *SSX2*
Mesenchymal chondrosarcoma	Biphasic, small cells, and islands of cartilage	SOX9	*HEY1-NCOA2*
Small cell osteosarcoma	Solid, osteoid deposition	SATB2	Not determined

especially of the alveolar subtype, may express non-myogenic markers, including cytokeratins of different classes (often with a dot-like paranuclear pattern), EMA, CD56, chromogranin, CD56, synaptophysin, S100, CD20, and CD99 [99].

Molecular Features

The genetic hallmarks of alveolar RMS are the t(2;13)(q35;q14) translocation, which results in the *PAX3-FOXO1* fusion and occurs in 70–80% of the cases or the t(1;13) (q36;q14), which results in the *PAX7-FOXO1* fusion and is less frequently identified. Spindle cell RMS presents recurrent *NCOA2* and *VGLL2* fusions in pediatric patients or *MYOD1* mutations in older children and adults [100–103]. Embryonal RMS and pleomorphic RMS have no recurrent chromosomal abnormality of diagnostic value.

Differential Diagnosis

Embryonal RMS often presents as a polypoid lesion and histologically shows a myxoid background; thus, it may be confused with the far more common sinonasal polyp. Presence of rhabdomyoblasts and positivity of neoplastic cells for desmin and myogenin (usually focal) help in the distinction. The differential diagnosis with alveolar RMS is based on the more uniform round cell cytologic appearance of the latter that is also more widely positive for myogenin. Detection of the *PAX* gene rearrangements is also helpful in the distinction.

The differential diagnosis of alveolar RMS includes a wide array of sinonasal round cell malignancies [104] (Table 2). The identification of rhabdomyoblasts with bright eosinophilic cytoplasm is a helpful diagnostic feature, but they are often absent, especially in small biopsies. Thus, immunohistochemistry and search for the *PAX* gene rearrangements are the most useful tools. Positivity for myogenin, MYOD1, and desmin support the diagnosis of alveolar RMS, and these markers should always be included in the evaluation of a sinonasal round cell malignancy. However, there are some important caveats in interpreting the results of the immunohistochemical studies in this tumor type because of the relatively frequent expression of non-myogenic markers that may be the source of confusion with undifferentiated tumors of other lineages. In particular, the expression of cytokeratins may lead to an erroneous diagnosis of poorly differentiated carcinoma, and the expression of neural markers (synaptophysin and CD56) raises the possibility of neuroendocrine tumors (neuroendocrine carcinoma, olfactory neuroblastoma).

Another possible pitfall is the presence of skeletal muscle differentiation in sinonasal tumors other than rhabdomyosarcoma, including malignant triton tumor, olfactory neuroblastoma, teratocarcinosarcoma, and melanoma [105]. However, a careful evaluation of the non-rhabdomyosarcomatous components will help prevent misdiagnosis in most instances.

The differential diagnosis of spindle cell RMS includes leiomyosarcoma, biphenotypic sinonasal sarcoma, and MPNST with rhabdomyoblastic differentiation (malignant triton tumor). Both leiomyosarcoma and biphenotypic sinonasal sarcoma are negative for myogenin and MYOD1. However, it should also be remembered that a subset of biphenotypic sinonasal sarcomas presents focal rhabdomyoblastic differentiation and *PAX3-NCOA1* fusions [106]. In MPNST, cells with rhabdomyoblastic differentiation are scattered and often present cross striations, while pleomorphic RMS can be separated from other high-grade pleomorphic malignancies of the nasal cavities based on the positivity for desmin and myogenin.

Treatment and Prognosis

Sinonasal RMS is treated with a multimodal approach that includes primary chemoradiation with or without surgery. Although the sinonasal region is an unfavorable site for RMS of the head and neck region, younger patients as well as embryonal and botryoid subtypes respond well to multimodality treatment [107]. Conversely, patients affected by alveolar RMS present more often with metastases, have a higher recurrence rate, and decreased survival [99, 107]. Higher TNM stage is also an indicator of poorer prognosis [107].

Kaposi Sarcoma

Definition

Kaposi sarcoma (KS) is a locally aggressive vascular tumor or tumor-like lesion, associated with infection by human herpesvirus 8 (HHV-8).

Clinical Features

Primary manifestation of the KS in the nasal mucosa is exceedingly rare, and there are only a few cases reported in the literature [108–114]. The majority were in patients with AIDS, one developed in an immunocompetent subject [110], and one in a patient under immunosuppressive treatment [109]. Chronic sinus congestion, nasal obstruction, and episodes of epistaxis were the presenting signs. All cases developed in the mucosa of the nasal cavity.

Pathologic Features

The nasal mucosa is occupied by a proliferation of mildly atypical plump spindle cells arranged in intersecting ill-defined fascicles and forming slit- and sieve-like vascular spaces containing erythrocytes (Fig. 25). Extravasated erythrocytes and lymphocytes are also identified. Hyaline globules are present inside and outside the spindle cells.

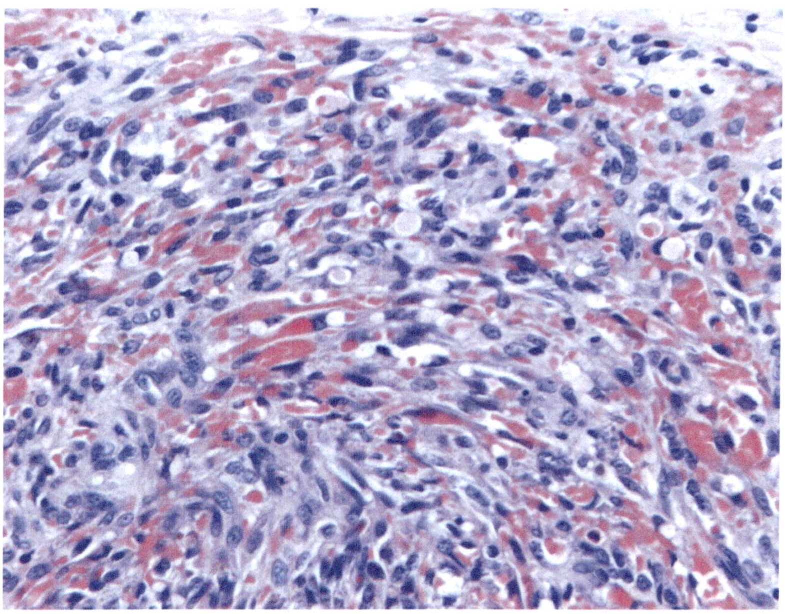

Fig. 25 Kaposi sarcoma. The tumor consists of mildly atypical plump spindle cells arranged in intersecting ill-defined fascicles forming slit-like vascular spaces containing erythrocytes. Hyaline globules are also present

Immunohistochemical Profile

Neoplastic cells are variably positive for the endothelial markers CD31, CD34, FLI1, ERG, and podoplanin (D2–40) and show nuclear positivity for HHV8.

Differential Diagnosis

In the sinonasal tract, lobular capillary hemangioma (pyogenic granuloma), glomangiopericytoma, and angiosarcoma are the main differential diagnostic considerations. Clinicopathological features, immunohistochemical studies (in particular HHV8), help to exclude these entities.

Treatment and Prognosis

The behavior and the treatment of KS depend on a several factors including the type of the disease, site and extent of the lesion, the immunocompetence, and the general medical condition of the patient. Surgical excision, radiotherapy, chemotherapy, and the adjustment of immunosuppressive medications can be considered. Antiretroviral therapy is also to be considered in AIDS patients. Local recurrence may occur, but survival is more dependent on the immunologic status of the patient.

Epithelioid Hemangioendothelioma

Definition

Epithelioid hemangioendothelioma (EHE) is a low-grade malignant vascular neoplasm, composed of epithelioid endothelial cells within a distinctive myxohyaline stroma.

Clinical Features

EHE rarely involves the head and neck region, and only a handful of cases have been reported in the nasal cavities [115–120]. It occurs over a wide age range with no significant gender predilection.

Pathologic Features

Histologically, it appears as a proliferation of epithelioid cells, either in solid sheets, cords, or short strands, embedded within a collagenous to fibromyxoid stroma (Fig. 26). These cells present intracytoplasmic lumina (vacuoles) often containing erythrocytes, which is the evidence of their endothelial differentiation. Mitotic figures are rarely detected.

Immunohistochemical Profile

Neoplastic cells are immunoreactive for endothelial markers including CD31, CD34, FLI1, and

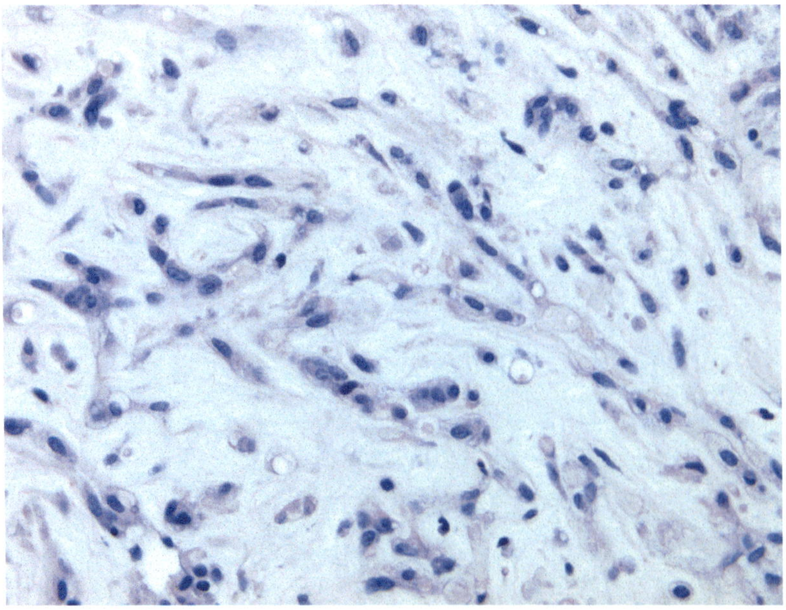

Fig. 26 Epithelioid hemangioendothelioma appears as a proliferation of epithelioid cells arranged in cords or short strands, embedded within a fibromyxoid stroma. Intracytoplasmic lumina containing erythrocytes are visible in this field

ERG. Cytokeratin expression is present in about 25–30% of cases.

Molecular Features

Most cases of EHE with classic morphology present a *WWTR1-CAMTA1* fusion [121]. A subset of EHE with distinct morphology (well-formed vascular channels and large neoplastic cells with eosinophilic cytoplasm) presents a *YAP1-TFE3* gene fusion and strong TFE3 expression by immunohistochemistry [122].

Differential Diagnosis

EHE may be difficult to distinguish from carcinomas and adenocarcinomas for the overlapping histologic features and for cytokeratin positivity, but expression of vascular endothelial markers helps to rule out this possibility. Epithelioid hemangioma lacks the myxohyaline stromal background and the cytologic atypia of EHE. In addition, capillary-sized vessels and the presence of a mixed inflammatory background are not features of EHE. In challenging cases, the lack of *CAMTA1*, *WWTR1*, and *TFE3* gene rearrangements in epithelioid hemangioma is helpful in the differential diagnosis. The distinction between EHE and epithelioid angiosarcoma is based on the presence of marked cytologic atypia and high mitotic rate in the latter tumor.

Treatment and Prognosis

The sinonasal cases reported so far behaved as locally aggressive lesions, with invasion of the skull base in one instance [116], and infrequent local relapse. Lymph node metastases may also rarely occur; thus, clinical monitoring should include lymph node evaluation [115].

Angiosarcoma

Definition

Angiosarcoma is a high-grade malignant neoplasm with vascular endothelial differentiation. In the head and neck region, it typically involves the skin and superficial soft tissues, particularly of the scalp, while cases primarily involving the sinonasal tract are exceedingly rare [123].

Clinical Features

In the small series reported so far, there was a slight male predominance, and the mean age was 47 years. The majority of the cases involved the nasal cavity, followed by the maxillary sinus, with a predominance of tumors involving only one anatomic site. The tumors appeared as polypoid lesions and were often ulcerated and hemorrhagic [123]. Rare cases have developed after radiation exposure or after exposure to vinyl chloride.

Pathologic Features

Histologically, angiosarcomas are highly infiltrative lesions, consisting mainly of anastomosing irregular cleft-like vascular channels dissecting the stroma or of rudimentary vessels and cavernous spaces (Fig. 27). These vascular spaces contain erythrocytes and are lined by atypical endothelial cells with spindle or epithelioid morphology, often forming multiple layers or papillae. Areas of solid growth, composed of sheets of epithelioid cells or fascicles of spindle cells, can be present, often associated with abundant extravasated erythrocytes. Single epithelioid cells may present an intracytoplasmic pseudolumen-containing erythrocytes. Mitotic activity is usually brisk, and atypical mitotic figures are easily identified.

Immunohistochemical Features

Neoplastic cells are immunoreactive for CD31, CD34, factor VIIRA, ERG, FLI1, and variably positive for podoplanin. Cytokeratins and EMA are frequently positive, especially in cases with epithelioid morphology.

Differential Diagnosis

Among benign vascular lesions, lobular capillary hemangioma (pyogenic granuloma) may be confused with angiosarcoma because it appears as a cellular lesion with brisk mitotic activity. However, lobular capillary hemangioma has a distinct lobular architecture, with larger vessels, often with a thick wall, in the center of the lesion and lobules composed of closely packed capillar-

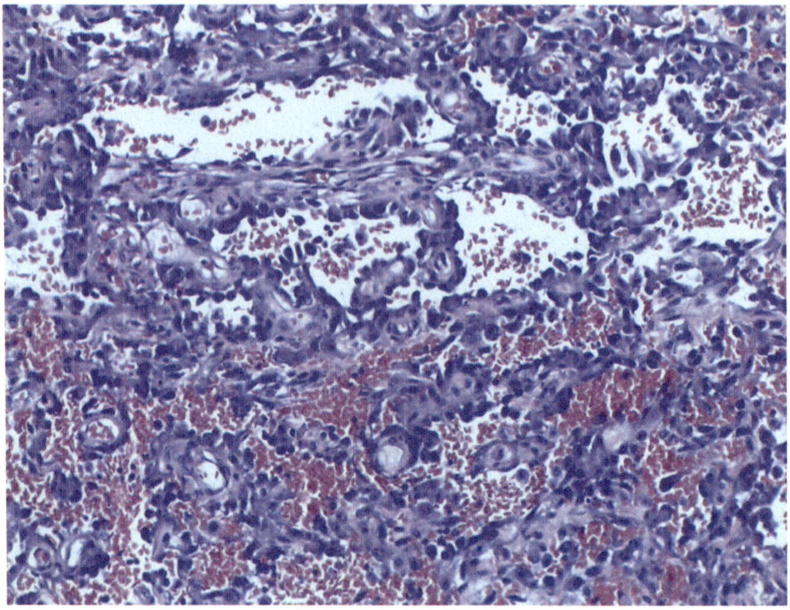

Fig. 27 Angiosarcoma presents as a proliferation of anastomosing irregular vascular channels, lined by atypical endothelial cells protruding in the lumen

ies with slit-like or indistinct lumina that seem to branch towards the periphery. In addition, the endothelial cells are not atypical. Intravascular papillary hyperplasia (Masson's hyperplasia) may resemble angiosarcoma for its complex architecture, but the endothelial cells are not atypical, and the lesion develops in the process of recanalization of a thrombosed vessel which is usually easy to identify. The epithelioid angiomatous nodule is an unencapsulated lesion composed of large polygonal epithelioid cells with vesicular nuclei but without the prominent nuclear atypia, brisk mitotic activity, and necrosis present in angiosarcoma [2].

Sinonasal Kaposi sarcoma is exceedingly rare, and HHV8 positivity helps in distinguishing the more cellular and atypical lesions from angiosarcoma.

Finally, positivity for cytokeratins and epithelioid morphology may elicit a diagnosis of carcinoma, but positivity for vascular endothelial markers helps to rule out this possibility.

Treatment and Prognosis

Patients have been treated with surgery alone or with surgery followed by radiotherapy and chemotherapy, without significant difference in the outcome [123]. Tumors larger than 4 cm, and tumors involving the maxillary sinuses tended to do worse [123].

Malignant Peripheral Nerve Sheath Tumor

Definition

Malignant peripheral nerve sheath tumor (MPNST; synonyms: malignant Schwannoma, neurofibrosarcoma) is a tumor showing variable differentiation towards one of the cellular components of the peripheral nerve sheath, including Schwann cells, fibroblasts, and perineurial cells. It originates from a nerve or from a pre-existing neurofibroma.

Clinical Features

Although MPNST is relatively frequent in the head and neck region, sinonasal involvement is rare, representing <5% of all sinonasal sarcomas in adult patients in a recent analysis [92]. About 25% of all MPNST are associated with neurofibromatosis type 1. They occur mainly in adult patients, although cases associated with NF1 tend to occur in younger patients [124, 125].

Pathologic Features

MPNST is typically a spindle cell tumor composed of elongated intersecting fascicles, with alternating cellular and myxoid areas (Fig. 28). Neoplastic cells have oval or wavy nuclei and scant amphophilic cytoplasm. Mitotic activity is usually brisk, and areas of necrosis can be identified. The presence of cells with rhabdomyoblastic differentiation characterizes the so-called triton tumor [126]. Other heterologous components that can be present include osteosarcoma, chondrosarcoma, angiosarcoma, and epithelial (usually glandular) elements. Rare cases of MPNST with epithelioid morphology have been described in the sinonasal mucosa [127].

Immunohistochemical Profile

MPNST is usually negative or only focally positive for S100 protein, with the exception of the epithelioid variant that is diffusely and intensely positive [128]. Nuclear positivity for SOX10 is identified in approximately 50% of the cases, usually in only a minor proportion of neoplastic cells. Loss of HK27me3 has been recently reported as a frequent event in MPNSTs, in particular NF1-associated tumors, but the specificity of this finding must be confirmed [128].

Differential Diagnosis

The main differential diagnosis of sinonasal MPNST is with biphenotypic sinonasal sarcoma, for the overlapping spindle cell morphology and S100 positivity. In addition, a minority of biphenotypic sinonasal sarcomas presents foci of rhabdomyoblastic differentiation, raising the differential diagnosis of a malignant Triton tumor. However, biphenotypic sinonasal sarcoma is usually less cellular and mitotically active; it is also positive for smooth muscle markers and lacks evidence of Schwann cell differentiation on electron microscopy. Moreover, it presents a *PAX3* gene rearrangement that is diagnostically useful.

Other entities to be considered in the differential diagnosis of MPNST are fibrosarcoma, synovial sarcoma, leiomyosarcoma, spindle cell carcinoma, and melanoma. These tumors usually can be excluded based on their histologic features and on appropriate immunostains.

Spindle cell melanoma may closely mimic the appearance of MPNST [129]. The diagnosis of melanoma is supported by the presence of larger nuclei, prominent eosinophilic nucleoli, amphophilic cytoplasm, immunoreactivity for

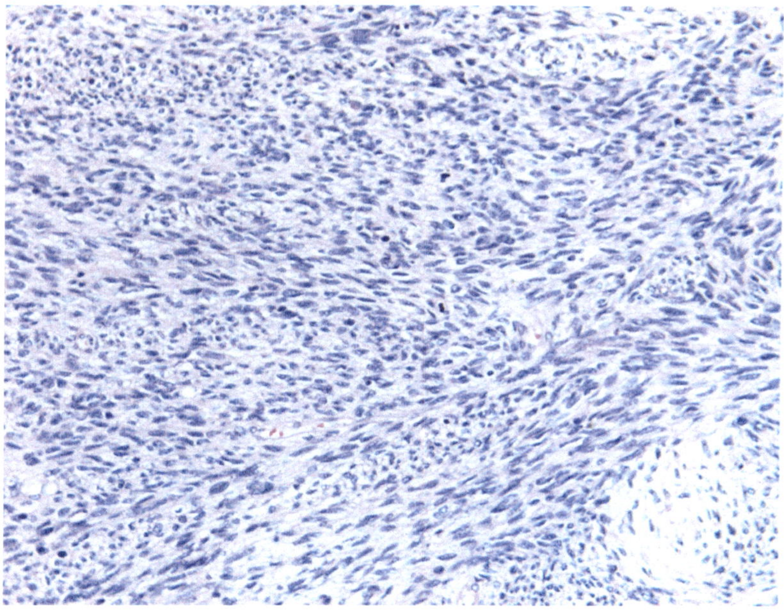

Fig. 28 Malignant peripheral nerve sheath tumor presents as a proliferation of atypical spindle cells organized in fascicles with brisk mitotic activity

S-100 protein and HMB-45, as well as the ultrastructural demonstration of melanosomes or premelanosomes [129].

Treatment and Prognosis

Larger tumors and tumors that prominently involved the maxillary sinus tended to have a worse prognosis [126].

Biphenotypic Sinonasal Sarcoma

Definition

Biphenotypic sinonasal sarcoma (BSS) (synonym: low-grade sinonasal sarcoma with neural and myogenic features) is a locally aggressive spindle cell neoplasm with distinctive histologic, immunohistochemical, and molecular features that so far has been reported only in the sinonasal tract [130].

Clinical Features

BSS affects more frequently female subjects (M:F = 2:1), with a wide age range at presentation (25–85 years, mean 50 years). Presenting symptoms are nonspecific and include nasal obstruction, facial pressure, and congestion [130]. Facial pain and mild epiphora have been occasionally reported. Most tumors involve multiple sites in the sinonasal region, with the nasal cavity and the ethmoid being the most commonly involved areas [130].

Pathologic Features

The lesion appears as a polyp, which is usually more firm than typical inflammatory nasal polyps [130]. Histologically, there is a mucosal proliferation of bland, spindle cells with elongated and slender nuclei, arranged in fascicles with a herringbone pattern (Fig. 29). Typically, there is infiltration of bone structures, while necrosis is not seen and mitotic activity is low (Fig. 30). In some cases, there is a prominent vascular component with hemangiopericytomatous features. Focal rhabdomyoblastic differentiation, consisting in the presence of large cells with eosinophilic cytoplasm and focal cross-striations, has been rarely observed [130].

In the majority of the cases, the spindle cell proliferation is accompanied by an epithelial proliferation, which consists of invaginated surface respiratory epithelium forming gland-like structures beneath the mucosal surface (Fig. 31). These epithelial elements are intimately associated with the neoplastic spindle cell component, imparting a biphasic pattern to the lesion.

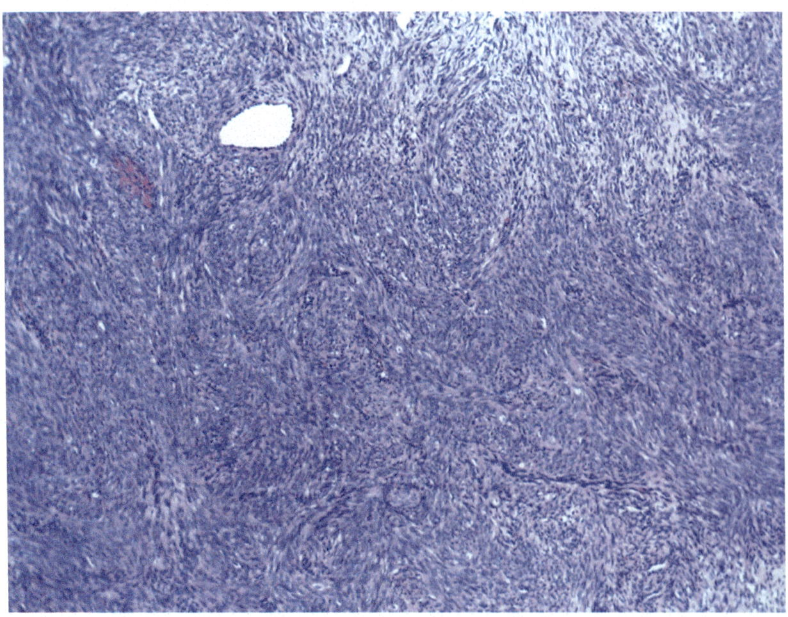

Fig. 29 Biphenotypic sinonasal sarcoma presents with a proliferation of bland, spindle cells with elongated and slender nuclei, arranged in fascicles with a herringbone pattern

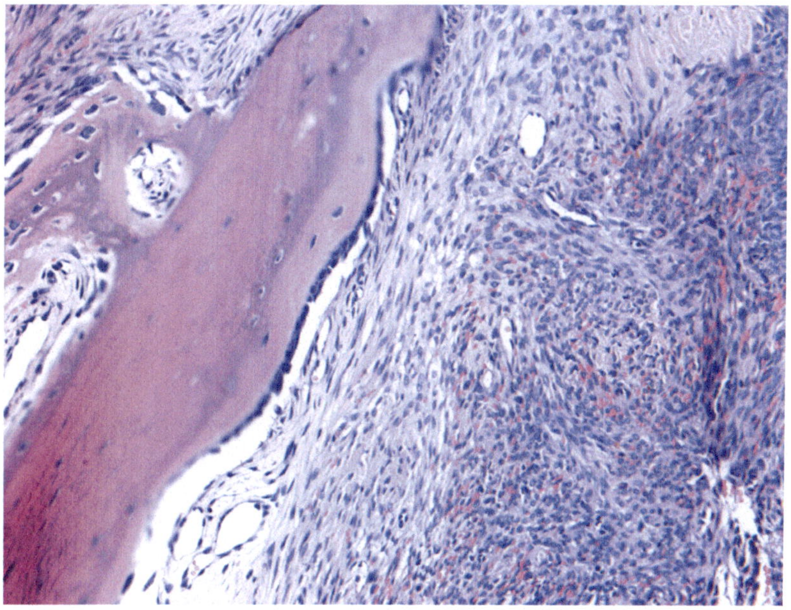

Fig. 30 The tumor infiltrates bone

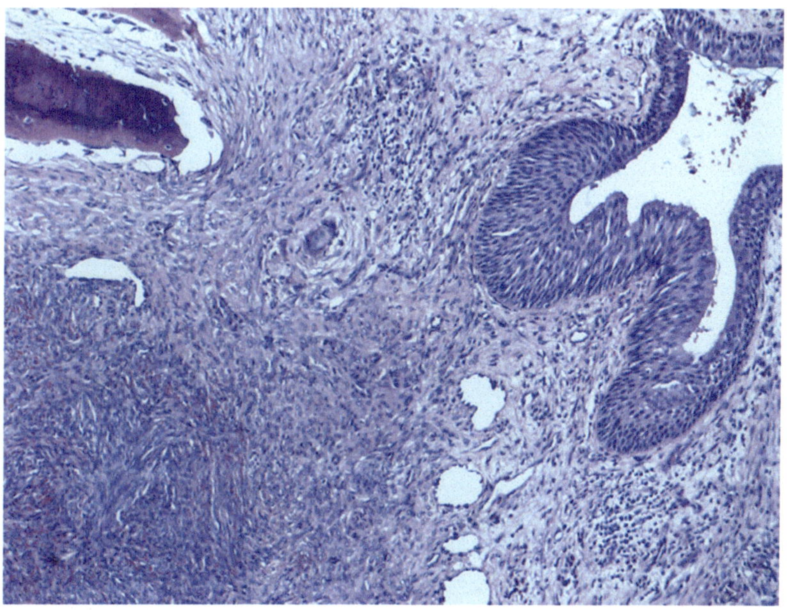

Fig. 31 The spindle cell proliferation is accompanied by an epithelial proliferation, which consists of invaginated surface respiratory epithelium forming gland-like structures

Immunohistochemical Profile

The neoplastic cells show a variable (focal to diffuse) immunoreactivity with S100 protein (nuclear and cytoplasmic) (Fig. 32a) and a muscle marker including smooth muscle actin, muscle-specific actin, or calponin (Fig. 32b), while immunoreactivity for desmin is only rarely seen [62, 130]. MYOD1 and myogenin are positive in cases showing areas of rhabdomyoblastic differentiation. Nuclear β-catenin staining can be detected in 90% of the cases, and positivity for factor XIIIa is also frequently observed [62]. Isolated keratin and EMA positive cells may also be seen. SOX10 has been consistently negative in

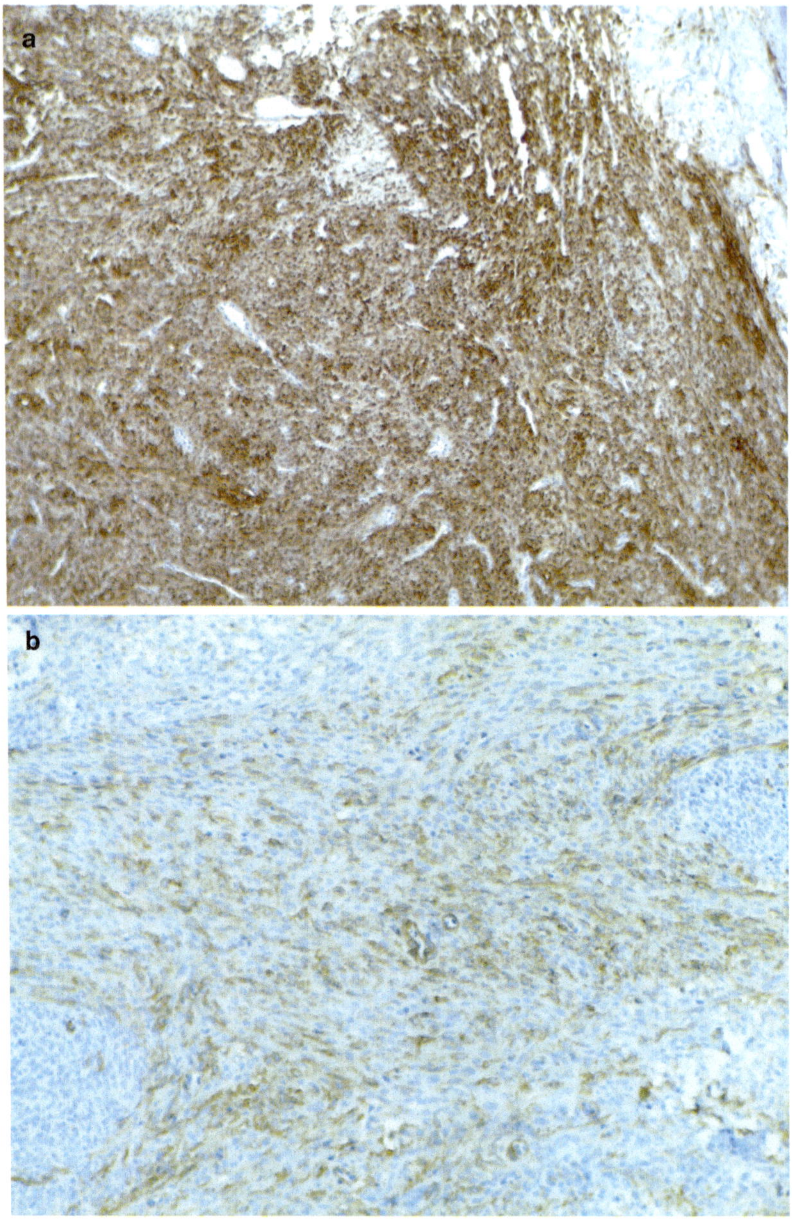

Fig. 32 The tumor is positive for S100 (**a**) and smooth muscle actin (**b**)

the tumors tested [62, 130]. In a recent study, immunohistochemical expression of PAX3 was highly sensitive and specific for the diagnosis of BSS [131].

Molecular Features Genetic Profile

The majority of BSS has a recurrent translocation t(2;4)(q35;q31.1) with a *PAX3–MAML3* fusion transcript that results in the activation of PAX3 response elements. Alternative fusions include *PAX3–FOXO1* and *PAX3–NCOA1*, the latter being associated with the presence of rhabdomyoblastic differentiation [132–135].

Differential Diagnosis

BSS must be distinguished from other spindle cell neoplasms of the nasal cavity (Table 1). Peripheral nerve sheath tumors are at the top of the list of differential diagnoses, for the overlap in morphology and immunohistochemical features (S100 positivity). However, most peripheral nerve sheath tumors are also positive for SOX10 (100% of Schwannomas and 50–60% of malignant peripheral nerve sheath tumors), which is negative in BSS. In addition, positive staining for smooth muscle markers is against the diagnosis of peripheral nerve sheath tumor. Malignant peripheral nerve sheath tumor is a high-grade tumor, with higher cellularity, presence of necrosis, and brisk mitotic activity, which are not features of BSS. In leiomyosarcoma neoplastic cells present oval, cigar-shaped nuclei and eosinophilic cytoplasm, and positivity for smooth muscle actin and desmin is more diffuse than in BSS. Synovial sarcoma (SS), both monophasic and biphasic, also shows a higher degree of cellularity and atypia. However, SS and BSS may show some overlap in their immunoprofile, with SS occasionally expressing S100 and muscle markers and BSS expressing EMA and cytokeratins, but their genetic profiles are mutually exclusive. Sinonasal glomangiopericytoma may resemble histologically BSS, mainly for the presence of prominent background vasculature, but neoplastic cells are more "myoid" in appearance, with ovoid nuclei and eosinophilic cytoplasm. There is some overlap in the immunoprofile, because of the positivity for smooth muscle actin and β-catenin, but glomangiopericytoma is negative for S100. Solitary fibrous tumor may mimic quite closely the histologic appearance of BSS, but it is positive for CD34 and STAT6, while smooth muscle actin and S100 are not detected.

Finally, sinonasal papilloma of the inverted type can also be considered in the differential diagnosis, because of the surface epithelial proliferation that accompanies the spindle cell neoplastic population. The latter may be not sampled in small biopsies or may be overlooked, leading to the erroneous diagnosis of sinonasal inverted papilloma.

Treatment and Prognosis

BSS is a low-grade sarcoma, with propensity for local invasion, and the natural history is characterized by repeated recurrences. So far, only one tumor-related death has been reported, which occurred after two local recurrences [62]. The treatment is surgical.

Synovial Sarcoma

Definition

Synovial sarcoma (SS) is a malignant mesenchymal neoplasm characterized by variable degrees of epithelial differentiation and by a specific chromosomal translocation t(X;18)(p11;q11).

Clinical Features

SS represents less than 10% of all head and neck sarcomas, where it most commonly arises in the parapharyngeal space [136]. It is extremely rare in the sinonasal tract. Most patients are young adults, and the paranasal sinuses are involved in the majority of cases [137].

Pathologic Features

Monophasic and biphasic forms are recognized. In the sinonasal tract, most SS are monophasic [137], being formed by a uniform population of spindle cells arranged in fascicles, with oval nucleus and scant cytoplasm (Fig. 33). Variable amounts of collagen are present between neoplastic cells, and myxoid change is observed in rare cases. A prominent background vasculature, with dilated branching vessels, is usually present. Areas of calcification and ossification can be found.

In the biphasic form, besides a spindle cell component identical to that of monophasic SS, there is an epithelial component consisting of well-formed gland-like structures lined by cuboidal to columnar cells with ovoid nucleus and abundant weakly eosinophilic cytoplasm (Fig. 34). Less frequently, epithelial cells are arranged in solid nests or cords.

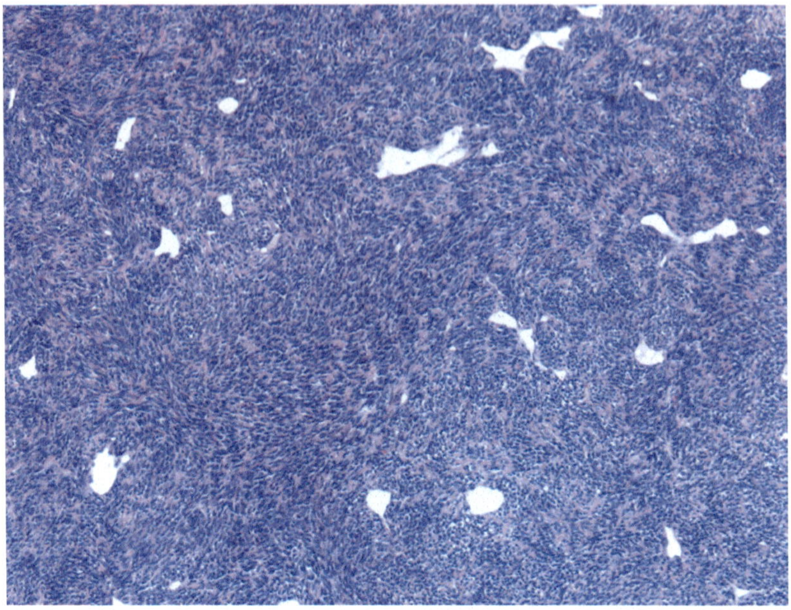

Fig. 33 Monophasic synovial sarcoma. Densely cellular area consisting of spindle cells arranged around dilated blood vessels

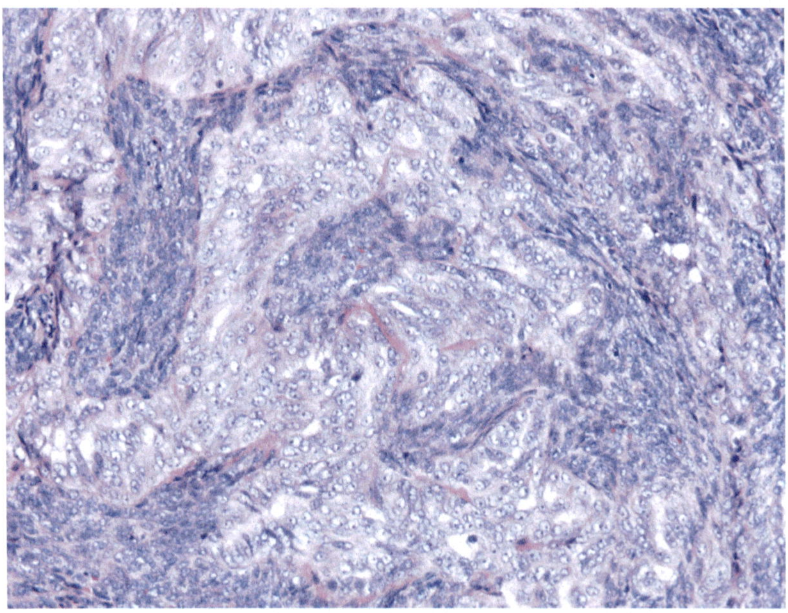

Fig. 34 Biphasic synovial sarcoma. A second population of epithelioid cells with abundant eosinophilic cytoplasm is present

Poorly differentiated round cell or spindle cell areas, with hypercellularity, nuclear atypia, brisk mitotic activity, and necrosis, can be associated with the classical monophasic and biphasic patterns or may exceptionally form the entire tumor [137].

Immunohistochemical Profile

SS is positive for epithelial markers, with EMA more expressed than cytokeratins. The immunoreactivity is more consistent in the epithelial component biphasic tumors, while in the monophasic and poorly differentiated forms, positivity is usually focal. SS is also positive for CD99 and bcl-2. Nuclear positivity for TLE2 is present in 80–90% of the cases, but this marker is not entirely specific, being expressed also in MPNST and solitary fibrous tumor [138]. Nuclear expression of β-catenin is frequently seen in SS, which may be the source of confusion with sinonasal glomangiopericytoma [58]. CD34 and S100 are negative or expressed in few cells in rare cases.

Molecular Features

SS presents a specific translocation t(X;18)(p11;q11) which is detected in >95% of the cases. This translocation results in *SS18-SSX1* or *SS18-SSX2* fusions and only rarely in the *SS18-SSX4* fusion. The identification of this rearrangement by FISH with SS18 break apart probes or by classic cytogenetics or RT-PCR-based techniques is important to confirm the diagnosis.

Differential Diagnosis

In the sinonasal tract, monophasic SS must be distinguished from spindle cell carcinoma, because of overlapping morphological and immunohistochemical features. Spindle cell carcinoma is associated with dysplasia/carcinoma in situ of the surface epithelium and may present areas of conventional squamous cell carcinoma. Malignant peripheral nerve sheath tumor is usually negative for epithelial markers and often associated with neurofibromatosis. Solitary fibrous tumor presents variable cellularity, and it is positive for CD34 and STAT6. For the differential diagnosis with biphenotypic sinonasal sarcoma, see previous section. Biphasic tumors require to be distinguished from adenocarcinomas, while for poorly differentiated round cell tumors, the main differential diagnosis is with Ewing sarcoma, small cell neuroendocrine carcinoma, and rhabdomyosarcoma. Search for the t(X;18) is an important diagnostic aid to distinguish SS from histologic mimickers.

Treatment and Prognosis

Surgery is the primary mode of treatment in sinonasal SS, but adjuvant chemo- and radiotherapy have been administered alone or in combination. The clinical course is characterized by frequent local recurrences and death for disease occurred in approximately half of the patients [137].

Mesenchymal Chondrosarcoma

Definition

Mesenchymal chondrosarcoma (MC) is a rare and aggressive subtype of chondrosarcoma, which is characterized by a biphasic pattern consisting of a round cell undifferentiated component combined with cartilaginous islands.

Clinical Features

Only few cases of sinonasal MC have been reported [139, 140]. There is a predominance of female patients, with a median age of 40 years. Presenting symptoms include nasal obstruction, epistaxis, mass effect, or a combination of these [139]. The maxillary sinus is the most common site of origin, followed by the ethmoid sinuses and the nasal cavity [139].

Pathologic Features

The undifferentiated round cells grow in solid sheets or in nests and are associated with prominent vascular structures, often showing a pattern resembling sinonasal glomangiopericytoma. The cartilage component is variably represented and consists in nodules merging with the round cell component, often showing areas of calcification (Fig. 35). Osteoid-like matrix may also be produced by neoplastic cells. Osteoclast-like multinucleated giant cells can be present.

Immunohistochemical Profile

Neoplastic cells are positive for SOX9 [141], but this marker is not entirely specific [142]. CD99 and desmin are also variably expressed.

Molecular Features

MC presents a recurrent *HEY1-NCOA2* fusion which is absent in other chondrosarcomas.

Differential Diagnosis

MC must be entered in the differential diagnosis with other round cell sinonasal neoplasms

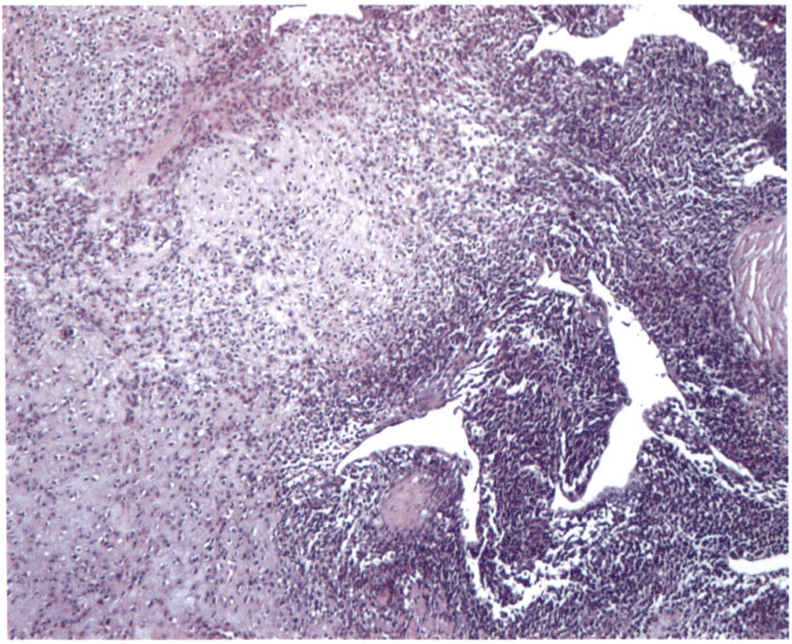

Fig. 35 Mesenchymal chondrosarcoma consists of undifferentiated round cells (right) and nodules of cartilage (left)

(Table 2). If the cartilaginous component can be recognized, the diagnosis is usually straightforward. If not, as it frequently occurs in small biopsy material, the differential diagnosis includes Ewing sarcoma, rhabdomyosarcoma, synovial sarcoma, small cell osteosarcoma, and undifferentiated carcinomas. The identification of the *HEY1-NCOA2* fusion by fluorescent in situ hybridization or other methods distinguishes MC from other round cell malignancies.

Treatment and Prognosis

Surgery has been the primary treatment modality, often combined with radiation therapy and chemotherapy [139]. In a small cohort of 13 patients, the disease-free 5-year and 10-year survival rates were 64% and 55%, respectively, with an overall mean survival of 12.1 years [139]. Local recurrence predicts a poor prognosis.

References

1. Kurihara K, Saiki T, Takeda T, Kobayashi J. Epithelioid hemangioma of the maxillary sinus: a case report. J Oral Maxillofac Surg. 1995;53:1221–3.
2. Leroy X, Mortuaire G, Chevalier D, Aubert S. Epithelioid angiomatous nodule of the nasal cavity. Pathol Res Pract. 2008;204:929–32.
3. Wong WK, Lim DH, Ong CW. Epithelioid angiomatous nodule of the nasal cavity: report of 2 cases. Auris Nasus Larynx. 2015;42:341–4.
4. Smith SC, Patel RM, Lucas DR, McHugh JB. Sinonasal lobular capillary hemangioma: a clinicopathologic study of 34 cases characterizing potential for local recurrence. Head Neck Pathol. 2013;7:129–34.
5. Kim JS, Kwon SH. Sinonasal hemangioma: diagnosis, treatment, and follow-up of 37 patients at a single center. J Oral Maxillofac Surg. 2017;75:1775–83.
6. Puxeddu R, Berlucchi M, Ledda GP, Parodo G, Farina D, Nicolai P. Lobular capillary hemangioma of the nasal cavity: a retrospective study on 40 patients. Am J Rhinol. 2006;20:480–4.
7. Iwata N, Hattori K, Nakagawa T, Tsujimura T. Hemangioma of the nasal cavity: a clinicopathologic study. Auris Nasus Larynx. 2002;29:335–9.
8. Guo R, Folpe AL. Extensively myxoid and hyalinized sinonasal capillary hemangiomas: a clinicopathologic study of 16 cases of a distinctive and potentially confusing hemangioma variant. Am J Surg Pathol. 2015;39:1584–90.
9. Truss L, Dobin SM, Donner LR. Deletion (21) (q21.2q22.12) as a sole clonal cytogenetic abnormality in a lobular capillary hemangioma of the nasal cavity. Cancer Genet Cytogenet. 2006;170:69–70.
10. Mills SE, Cooper PH, Fechner RE. Lobular capillary hemangioma: the underlying lesion of pyogenic granuloma. A study of 73 cases from the oral and nasal mucous membranes. Am J Surg Pathol. 1980;4:470–9.
11. Huang HY, Antonescu CR. Sinonasal smooth muscle cell tumors: a clinicopathologic and immunohis-

tochemical analysis of 12 cases with emphasis on the low-grade end of the spectrum. Arch Pathol Lab Med. 2003;127:297–304.
12. Agaimy A, Michal M, Thompson LD, Michal M. Angioleiomyoma of the sinonasal tract: analysis of 16 cases and review of the literature. Head Neck Pathol. 2015;9:463–73.
13. Amary MF, Ye H, Berisha F, Tirabosco R, Presneau N, Flanagan AM. Detection of USP6 gene rearrangement in nodular fasciitis: an important diagnostic tool. Virchows Arch. 2013;463:97–8.
14. Erickson-Johnson MR, Chou MM, Evers BR, et al. Nodular fasciitis: a novel model of transient neoplasia induced by MYH9-USP6 gene fusion. Lab Investig. 2011;91:1427–33.
15. Harrison HC, Motbey J, Kan AE, de Silva M. Nodular fasciitis of the nose in a child. Int J Pediatr Otorhinolaryngol. 1995;33:257–64.
16. Weinreb I, Shaw AJ, Perez-Ordoñez B, Goldblum JR, Rubin BP. Nodular fasciitis of the head and neck region: a clinicopathologic description in a series of 30 cases. J Cutan Pathol. 2009;36:1168–73.
17. Alsaied AS, Lotfy MA. Maxillary sinus nodular fasciitis. Saudi Med J. 2014;35:88–92.
18. Mullin D, Lindsay FW, Keefe MA. Nodular fasciitis of the nasal cavity: a case report. Ear Nose Throat J. 2007;86:748–51.
19. Fu YS, Perzin KH. Nonepithelial tumors of the nasal cavity, paranasal sinuses, and nasopharynx. A clinicopathologic study. VI. Fibrous tissue tumors (fibroma, fibromatosis, fibrosarcoma). Cancer. 1976;37:2912–28.
20. Wilson T, Hellquist HB, Ray S, Pickles J. Intranasal myopericytoma. A tumour with perivascular myoid differentiation: the changing nomenclature for haemangiopericytoma. J Laryngol Otol. 2007;121:786–9.
21. Beck JC, Devaney KO, Weatherly RA, Koopmann CF Jr, Lesperance MM. Pediatric myofibromatosis of the head and neck. Arch Otolaryngol Head Neck Surg. 1999;125:39–44.
22. Swaika S, Thomas B, Kapilamoorthy TR. Solitary infantile myofibroma of left ethmoid sinus with intracranial extension. Pediatr Neurol. 2016;57:107–8.
23. Josephson GD, Patel S, Duckworth L, Goldstein J. Infantile myofibroma of the nasal cavity; a case report and review of the literature. Int J Pediatr Otorhinolaryngol. 2010;74:1452–4.
24. Loundon N, Dedieuleveult T, Ayache D, Roger G, Josset P, Garabedian EN. Head and neck infantile myofibromatosis—a report of three cases. Int J Pediatr Otorhinolaryngol. 1999;51:181–6.
25. Arts FA, Sciot R, Brichard B, et al. PDGFRB gain-of-function mutations in sporadic infantile myofibromatosis. Hum Mol Genet. 2017;26(10):1801–10.
26. Agaimy A, Bieg M, Michal M, et al. Recurrent somatic PDGFRB mutations in sporadic infantile/solitary adult myofibromas but not in angioleiomyomas and myopericytomas. Am J Surg Pathol. 2017;41:195–203.
27. Banerjee SS, Eyden B, Trenholm PW, Sheikh MY, Wakamatsu K, Ancans J, Rosai J. Monotypic angiomyolipoma of the nasal cavity: a heretofore undescribed occurrence. Int J Surg Pathol. 2001;9:309–15.
28. Kuroda N, Goda M, Kazakov DV, Hes O, Michal M, Lee GH. Perivascular epithelioid cell tumor of the nasal cavity with TFE3 expression. Pathol Int. 2009;59:769–70.
29. Panelos J, Gallo O, Scala I, Franchi A. PEComa of the nasal septum. Otolaryngol Head Neck Surg. 2009;141:543–4.
30. Bocciolini C, Fornelli A, Casadei GP, Cattani MG, Dall'Olio D. PEComa of the nasal cavity with worrisome histologic features and benign behavior: a case report. Ann Otol Rhinol Laryngol. 2013;122:725–8.
31. Afrogheh A, Schneider J, Bezuidenhout AF, Hille J. PEComa of the nose: report of a case with immunohistochemical and ultrastructural studies and a review of the literature. Head Neck Pathol. 2014;8:122–6.
32. Bandhlish A, Barnes LE, Rabban JT, McHugh JB. Perivascular epithelioid cell tumors (PEComas) of the head and neck: report of three cases and review of the literature. Head Neck Pathol. 2011;5:233–40.
33. McGregor SM, Alikhan MB, John RA, Kotler H, Bridge JA, Mujacic I, Kadri S, Segal J, Krausz T. Melanotic PEComa of the sinonasal mucosa with NONO-TFE3 fusion: an elusive mimic of sinonasal melanoma. Am J Surg Pathol. 2017;41:717–22.
34. Thway K, Fisher C. PEComa: morphology and genetics of a complex tumor family. Ann Diagn Pathol. 2015;19:359–68.
35. Ferenczi K, Lastra RR, Farkas T, et al. MUM-1 expression differentiates tumors in the PEComa family from clear cell sarcoma and melanoma. Int J Surg Pathol. 2012;20:29–36.
36. Sunaryo PL, Svider PF, Husain Q, Choudhry OJ, Eloy JA, Liu JK. Schwannomas of the sinonasal tract and anterior skull base: a systematic review of 94 cases. Am J Rhinol Allergy. 2014;28:39–49.
37. Azani AB, Bishop JA, Thompson LD. Sinonasal tract neurofibroma: a clinicopathologic series of 12 cases with a review of the literature. Head Neck Pathol. 2015;9:323–33.
38. Hasegawa SL, Mentzel T, Fletcher CD. Schwannomas of the sinonasal tract and nasopharynx. Mod Pathol. 1997;10:777–84.
39. Yang X, Zeng Y, Wang J. Hybrid schwannoma/perineurioma: report of 10 Chinese cases supporting a distinctive entity. Int J Surg Pathol. 2013;21:22–8.
40. Kuroda N, Kazakov DV, Hes O, Michal M, Goda M, Miyazaki K, Hayashi Y, Okamoto S, Lee GH. Hybrid peripheral nerve sheath tumor of the nasal cavity showing schwannomatous, neurofibromatous, and perineuriomatous areas. Med Mol Morphol. 2010;43:82–5.
41. Miettinen M, McCue PA, Sarlomo-Rikala M, et al. Sox10—a marker for not only schwannian and melanocytic neoplasms but also myoepithelial cell

tumors of soft tissue: a systematic analysis of 5134 tumors. Am J Surg Pathol. 2015;39:826–35.
42. Buob D, Wacrenier A, Chevalier D, Aubert S, Quinchon JF, Gosselin B, Leroy X. Schwannoma of the sinonasal tract: a clinicopathologic and immunohistochemical study of 5 cases. Arch Pathol Lab Med. 2003;127:1196–9.
43. Butler RT, Patel RM, McHugh JB. Head and neck schwannomas: 20-year experience of a single institution excluding cutaneous and acoustic sites. Head Neck Pathol. 2016;10:286–91.
44. Suh JD, Ramakrishnan VR, Zhang PJ, Wu AW, Wang MB, Palmer JN, Chiu AG. Diagnosis and endoscopic management of sinonasal schwannomas. ORL J Otorhinolaryngol Relat Spec. 2011;73:308–12.
45. Mey KH, Buchwald C, Daugaard S, Prause JU. Sinonasal schwannoma—a clinicopathological analysis of five rare cases. Rhinology. 2006;44:46–52.
46. Rushing EJ, Bouffard JP, McCall S, et al. Primary extracranial meningiomas: an analysis of 146 cases. Head Neck Pathol. 2009;3:116–30.
47. Thompson LDR, Fanburg-Smith JC. Update on select benign mesenchymal and meningothelial sinonasal tract lesions. Head Neck Pathol. 2016;10:95–108.
48. Thompson LD, Gyure KA. Extracranial sinonasal tract meningiomas: a clinicopathologic study of 30 cases with a review of the literature. Am J Surg Pathol. 2000;24:640–50.
49. Domingues P, González-Tablas M, Otero Á, et al. Genetic/molecular alterations of meningiomas and the signaling pathways targeted. Oncotarget. 2015;6:10671–88.
50. Granter SR, Badizadegan K, Fletcher CD. Myofibromatosis in adults, glomangiopericytoma, and myopericytoma: a spectrum of tumors showing perivascular myoid differentiation. Am J Surg Pathol. 1998;22:513–25.
51. Thompson LDR, Miettinen M, Wenig BM. Sinonasal-type hemangiopericytoma. A clinicopathologic and immunophenotypic analysis of 104 cases showing perivascular myoid differentiation. Am J Surg Pathol. 2003;27:737–49.
52. Thompson LDR, Flucke U, Wenig BM. Sinonasal glomangiopericytoma. In: El-Naggar AK, JKC C, Grandis JR, Takata T, Slootweg PJ, editors. WHO classification of head and neck tumors. 4th ed. Lyon: IARC; 2017. p. 44–5.
53. Catalano PJ, Brandwein M, Shah DK, et al. Sinonasal hemangiopericytomas: a clinicopathologic and immunohistochemical study of seven cases. Head Neck. 1996;18:42–53.
54. Ray S, Chakraborty PP, Biswas K, Ghosh S, Mukhopadhyay S, Chowdhury S. A case of oncogenic osteomalacia due to occult nasal sinus tumor. Clin Cases Miner Bone Metab. 2015;12:65–8.
55. Kabtouri H, Karmali R, Spinato L, Khamaktchian M, Bisschop P. Oncogenic osteomalacia induced by a sinonasal tumour: case report and review. B-ENT. 2014;10:149–55.
56. Lee GG, Dhong HJ, Park YS, Ko YH. Sinonasal glomangiopericytoma causing oncogenic osteomalacia. Clin Exp Otorhinolaryngol. 2014;7:145–8.
57. Jamal SA, Dickson BC, Radziunas I. Tumour induced osteomalacia due to a sinonasal hemangiopericytoma: a case report. World J Clin Cases. 2013;1:59–63.
58. Jo VY, Fletcher CDM. Nuclear β-catenin expression is frequent in sinonasal hemangiopericytoma and its mimics. Head Neck Pathol. 2017;11:119–23.
59. Haller F, Bieg M, Moskalev EA, et al. Recurrent mutations within the amino-terminal region of β-catenin are probable key molecular driver events in sinonasal hemangiopericytoma. Am J Pathol. 2015;185:563–71.
60. Lasota J, Felisiak-Golabek A, Aly FZ, Wang ZF, Thompson LD, Miettinen M. Nuclear expression and gain-of-function β-catenin mutation in glomangiopericytoma (sinonasal-type hemangiopericytoma): insight into pathogenesis and a diagnostic marker. Mod Pathol. 2015;28:715–20.
61. Agaimy A, Barthelmess S, Geddert H, et al. Phenotypical and molecular distinctness of sinonasal haemangiopericytoma compared to solitary fibrous tumour of the sinonasal tract. Histopathology. 2014;65:667–73.
62. Rooper LM, Huang SC, Antonescu CR, Westra WH, Bishop JA. Biphenotypic sinonasal sarcoma: an expanded immunoprofile including consistent nuclear β-catenin positivity and absence of SOX10 expression. Hum Pathol. 2016;55:44–50.
63. Herve S, Abd AI, Beautru R, et al. Management of sinonasal hemangiopericytomas. Rhinology. 1999;37:153–8.
64. Gnepp DR, Henley J, Weiss S, Heffner D. Desmoid fibromatosis of the sinonasal tract and nasopharynx. A clinicopathologic study of 25 cases. Cancer. 1996;78:2572–9.
65. Flucke U, Tops BB, van Diest PJ, Slootweg PJ. Desmoid-type fibromatosis of the head and neck region in the paediatric population: a clinicopathological and genetic study of seven cases. Histopathology. 2014;64:769–76.
66. Bhattacharya B, Dilworth HP, Iacobuzio-Donahue C, et al. Nuclear β-catenin expression distinguishes deep fibromatosis from other benign and malignant fibroblastic and myofibroblastic lesions. Am J Surg Pathol. 2005;29:653–9.
67. Carlson JW, Fletcher CDM. Immunohistochemistry for β-catenin in the differential diagnosis of spindle cell lesions: analysis of a series and review of the literature. Histopathology. 2007;51:509–14.
68. Le Guellec S, Soubeyran I, Rochaix P, et al. CTNNB1 mutation analysis is a useful tool for the diagnosis of desmoid tumors: a study of 260 desmoid tumors and 191 potential morphologic mimics. Mod Pathol. 2012;25:1551–8.
69. Alman BA, Li C, Pajerski ME, et al. Increased β-catenin protein and somatic APC mutations in

sporadic aggressive fibromatoses (desmoid tumors). Am J Pathol. 1997;151:329–34.

70. Kao YC, Lin PC, Yen SL, et al. Clinicopathological and genetic heterogeneity of the head and neck solitary fibrous tumours: a comparative histological, immunohistochemical and molecular study of 36 cases. Histopathology. 2016;68:492–501.
71. Smith SC, Gooding WE, Elkins M, et al. Solitary fibrous tumors of the head and neck: a multi-institutional clinicopathologic study. Am J Surg Pathol. 2017;41:1642–56.
72. Witkin GB, Rosai J. Solitary fibrous tumor of the upper respiratory tract. A report of six cases. Am J Surg Pathol. 1991;15:842–8.
73. Zukerberg LR, Rosenberg AE, Randolph G, et al. Solitary fibrous tumor of the nasal cavity and paranasal sinuses. Am J Surg Pathol. 1991;15:126–30.
74. Hicks DL, Moe KS. Nasal solitary fibrous tumor arising from the anterior cranial fossa. Skull Base. 2004;14:203–7.
75. Folpe AL, Fanburg-Smith JC, Billlings SD, et al. Most osteomalacia-associated mesenchymal tumors are a single histopathologic entity, the "phosphaturic mesenchymal tumor, mixed connective tissue variant": an analysis of 32 cases and a comprehensive review of the literature. Am J Surg Pathol. 2004;28:1–30.
76. Deep NL, Cain RB, McCullough AE, Hoxworth JM, Lal D. Sinonasal phosphaturic mesenchymal tumor: case report and systematic review. Allergy Rhinol (Providence). 2014;5:162–7.
77. Agaimy A, Michal M, Chiosea S, et al. Phosphaturic mesenchymal tumors: clinicopathologic, immunohistochemical and molecular analysis of 22 cases expanding their morphologic and immunophenotypic spectrum. Am J Surg Pathol. 2017;41:1371–80.
78. Lee JC, Jeng YM, Su SY, et al. Identification of a novel FN1-FGFR1 genetic fusion as a frequent event in phosphaturic mesenchymal tumour. J Pathol. 2015;235:539–45.
79. Lee JC, Su SY, Changou CA, et al. Characterization of FN1-FGFR1 and novel FN1-FGF1 fusion genes in a large series of phosphaturic mesenchymal tumors. Mod Pathol. 2016;29:1335–46.
80. Andrews T, Kountakis SE, Maillard AA. Myxomas of the head and neck. Am J Otolaryngol. 2000;21:184–9.
81. Heffner DK. Sinonasal myxomas and fibromyxomas in children. Ear Nose Throat J. 1993;72:365–8.
82. Yilmaz S, Edizer DT, Yağız C, Sar M, Cansız H. Maxillary sinus nonodontogenic myxoma extending into the sphenoid sinus and pterygopalatine fossa: case report. Ear Nose Throat J. 2011;90:E28–30.
83. Iatrou IA, Theologie-Lygidakis N, Leventis MD, Michail-Strantzia C. Sinonasal myxoma in an infant. J Craniofac Surg. 2010;21:1649–51.
84. Prasannan L, Warren L, Herzog CE, Lopez-Camarillo L, Frankel L, Goepfert H. Sinonasal myxoma: a pediatric case. J Pediatr Hematol Oncol. 2005;27:90–2.
85. Patel TD, Carniol ET, Vázquez A, Baredes S, Liu JK, Eloy JA. Sinonasal fibrosarcoma: analysis of the surveillance, epidemiology, and end results database. Int Forum Allergy Rhinol. 2016;6:201–5.
86. Plaza G, Ferrando J, Pinedo F. Sinonasal fibrosarcoma: a case report. Eur Arch Otorhinolaryngol. 2006;263:641–3.
87. Cai PQ, Wu YP, Li L, et al. CT and MRI of radiation-induced sarcomas of the head and neck following radiotherapy for nasopharyngeal carcinoma. Clin Radiol. 2013;68:683–9.
88. Wang CP, Chang YL, Ting LL, Yang TL, Ko JY, Lou PJ. Malignant fibrous histiocytoma of the sinonasal tract. Head Neck. 2009;31:85–93.
89. Rodrigo JP, Fernández JA, Suárez C, Gómez J, Llorente JL, Herrero A. Malignant fibrous histiocytoma of the nasal cavity and paranasal sinuses. Am J Rhinol. 2000;14:427–31.
90. Ko JY, Chen CL, Lui LT, Hsu MM. Radiation-induced malignant fibrous histiocytoma in patients with nasopharyngeal carcinoma. Arch Otolaryngol Head Neck Surg. 1996;122:535–8.
91. Iguchi Y, Takahashi H, Yao K, Nakayama M, Nagai H, Okamoto M. Malignant fibrous histiocytoma of the nasal cavity and paranasal sinuses: review of the last 30 years. Acta Otolaryngol Suppl. 2002;547:75–8.
92. Szablewski V, Neuville A, Terrier P, et al. Adult sinonasal soft tissue sarcoma: analysis of 48 cases from the French Sarcoma Group database. Laryngoscope. 2015;125:615–23.
93. Montgomery E, Goldblum JR, Fisher C. Leiomyosarcoma of the head and neck: a clinicopathological study. Histopathology. 2002;40:518–25.
94. Agaimy A, Semrau S, Koch M, Thompson LDR. Sinonasal leiomyosarcoma: clinicopathological analysis of nine cases with emphasis on common association with other malignancies and late distant metastasis. Head Neck Pathol. 2018;12:463–70.
95. Zahir ST, Sharahjin NS. Leiomyosarcoma of the maxilla in a 24-year-old man who initially presented with odontalgia, and suffered from tumour mismanagement. BMJ Case Rep. 2013. https://doi.org/10.1136/bcr-2013-200933.
96. Pinotti E, Sandini M, Famularo S, et al. Disseminated and late metastatic disease from nasal pit leiomyosarcoma after radical surgical resection. Case report of a singular presentation of a rare disease. Clin Sarcoma Res. 2017;7:12.
97. Callender TA, Weber RS, Janjan N, et al. Rhabdomyosarcoma of the nose and paranasal sinuses in adults and children. Otolaryngol Head Neck Surg. 1995;112:252–7.
98. Herrmann BW, Sotelo-Avila C, Eisenbeis JF. Pediatric sinonasal rhabdomyosarcoma: three cases and a review of the literature. Am J Otolaryngol. 2003;24:174–80.
99. Thompson LDR, Jo VY, Agaimy A, et al. Sinonasal tract alveolar rhabdomyosarcoma in adults: a clinicopathologic and immunophenotypic study of

fifty-two cases with emphasis on epithelial immunoreactivity. Head Neck Pathol. 2018;12:181–92.

100. Mosquera JM, Sboner A, Zhang L, et al. Recurrent NCOA2 gene rearrangements in congenital/infantile spindle cell rhabdomyosarcoma. Genes Chromosom Cancer. 2013;52:538–50.
101. Alaggio R, Zhang L, Sung YS, et al. A molecular study of pediatric spindle and sclerosing rhabdomyosarcoma: identification of novel and recurrent VGLL2-related fusions in infantile cases. Am J Surg Pathol. 2016;40:224–35.
102. Szuhai K, de Jong D, Leung WY, Fletcher CD, Hogendoorn PC. Transactivating mutation of the MYOD1 gene is a frequent event in adult spindle cell rhabdomyosarcoma. J Pathol. 2014;232:300–7.
103. Agaram NP, Chen CL, Zhang L, LaQuaglia MP, Wexler L, Antonescu CR. Recurrent MYOD1 mutations in pediatric and adult sclerosing and spindle cell rhabdomyosarcomas: evidence for a common pathogenesis. Genes Chromosom Cancer. 2014;53:779–87.
104. Franchi A. An update on sinonasal round cell undifferentiated tumors. Head Neck Pathol. 2016;10:75–84.
105. Bishop JA, Thompson LD, Cardesa A, et al. Rhabdomyoblastic differentiation in head and neck malignancies other than rhabdomyosarcoma. Head Neck Pathol. 2015;9:507–18.
106. Huang SC, Ghossein RA, Bishop JA, Zhang L, Chen TC, Huang HY, Antonescu CR. Novel PAX3-NCOA1 fusions in biphenotypic sinonasal sarcoma with focal rhabdomyoblastic differentiation. Am J Surg Pathol. 2016;40:51–9.
107. Thompson CF, Kim BJ, Lai C, et al. Sinonasal rhabdomyosarcoma: prognostic factors and treatment outcomes. Int Forum Allergy Rhinol. 2013;3:678–83.
108. Mouden K, Khmou M, Loughmari S, et al. Primary Kaposi's sarcoma of the nasal cavity: a case report and review of the literature. Clin Sarcoma Res. 2016;6:4.
109. Chen KH, Chen TD, Chen CW, Lee LY. Iatrogenic Kaposi's sarcoma in nasal cavity: a case report. World J Surg Oncol. 2014;12:172.
110. Venizelos I, Andreadis C, Tatsiou Z. Primary Kaposi's sarcoma of the nasal cavity not associated with AIDS. Eur Arch Otorhinolaryngol. 2008;265:717–20.
111. Wyatt ME, Finlayson CJ, Moore-Gillon V. Kaposi's sarcoma masquerading as pyogenic granuloma of the nasal mucosa. J Laryngol Otol. 1998;112:280–2.
112. Gnepp DR, Chandler W, Hyams V. Primary Kaposi's sarcoma of the head and neck. Ann Intern Med. 1984;100:107–14.
113. Stavord SD, Herdman RCD, Forster S, et al. Kaposi's sarcoma of the head and neck in patients with AIDS. J Laryngol Otol. 1989;103:379–82.
114. Lucente FE. Kaposi's sarcoma of the head and neck in patients with acquired immunodeficiency syndrome. Otolaryngol Head Neck Surg. 1994; 111:618.
115. Di Girolamo A, Giacomini PG, Coli A, et al. Epithelioid hemangioendothelioma arising in the nasal cavity. J Laryngol Otol. 2003;117:75–7.
116. Ogita S, Endo T, Nomura K, et al. Nasal cavity epithelioid hemangioendothelioma invading the anterior skull base. Surg Neurol Int. 2016;7:53.
117. Navalón-Ramon E, Pérez-Garrigues T, Meseguer-Garcia P, Pérez-Carbonell T. Epithelioid haemangioendothelioma of the nasal cavity in a woman. Acta Otorrinolaringol Esp. 2017;68:369–71.
118. Patnayak R, Jena A, Reddy MK, Chowhan AK, Rao LC, Rukhamangadha N. Epithelioid hemangioendothelioma of nasal cavity. J Lab Physicians. 2010;2:111–3.
119. Tseng CC, Tsay SH, Tsai TL, Shu CH. Epithelioid hemangioendothelioma of the nasal cavity. J Chin Med Assoc. 2005;68:45–8.
120. Naqvi J, Ordonez NG, Luna MA, Williams MD, Weber RS, El-Naggar AK. Epithelioid hemangioendothelioma of the head and neck: role of podoplanin in the differential diagnosis. Head Neck Pathol. 2008;2:25–30.
121. Errani C, Zhang L, Sung YS, et al. A novel WWTR1-CAMTA1 gene fusion is a consistent abnormality in epithelioid hemangioendothelioma of different anatomic sites. Genes Chromosomes Cancer. 2011;50:644–53.
122. Antonescu CR, Le Loarer F, Mosquera JM, et al. Novel YAP1-TFE3 fusion defines a distinct subset of epithelioid hemangioendothelioma. Genes Chromosomes Cancer. 2013;52:775–84.
123. Nelson BL, Thompson LD. Sinonasal tract angiosarcoma: a clinicopathologic and immunophenotypic study of 10 cases with a review of the literature. Head Neck Pathol. 2007;1:1–12.
124. Mannan AA, Singh MK, Bahadur S, Hatimota P, Sharma MC. Solitary malignant schwannoma of the nasal cavity and paranasal sinuses: report of two rare cases. Ear Nose Throat J. 2003;82:634–6.
125. Nagayama I, Nishimura T, Furukawa M. Malignant schwannoma arising in a paranasal sinus. J Laryngol Otol. 1993;107:146–8.
126. Heffner DK, Gnepp DR. Sinonasal fibrosarcomas, malignant schwannomas, and "Triton" tumors. A clinicopathologic study of 67 cases. Cancer. 1992;70:1089–101.
127. Fernández PL, Cardesa A, Bombí JA, Palacín A, Traserra J. Malignant sinonasal epithelioid schwannoma. Virchows Arch A Pathol Anat Histopathol. 1993;423:401–5.
128. Schaefer IM, Fletcher CD, Hornick JL. Loss of H3K27 trimethylation distinguishes malignant peripheral nerve sheath tumors from histologic mimics. Mod Pathol. 2016;29:4–13.
129. Kardon DE, Thompson LD. Sinonasal mucosal malignant melanoma: report of an unusual case mimicking schwannoma. Ann Diagn Pathol. 2000;4:303–7.
130. Lewis JT, Oliveira AM, Nascimento AG, et al. Low-grade sinonasal sarcoma with neural and myogenic

features: a clinicopathologic analysis of 28 cases. Am J Surg Pathol. 2012;36:517–25.
131. Jo VY, Mariño-Enríquez A, Fletcher CDM, Hornick JL. Expression of PAX3 distinguishes biphenotypic sinonasal sarcoma from histologic mimics. Am J Surg Pathol. 2018;42:1275–85.
132. Fritchie KJ, Jin L, Wang X, et al. Fusion gene profile of biphenotypic sinonasal sarcoma: an analysis of 44 cases. Histopathology. 2016;69:930–6.
133. Huang SC, Ghossein RA, Bishop JA, et al. Novel PAX3-NCOA1 fusions in biphenotypic sinonasal sarcoma with focal rhabdomyoblastic differentiation. Am J Surg Pathol. 2016;40:51–9.
134. Wong WJ, Lauria A, Hornick JL, Xiao S, Fletcher JA, Marino-Enriquez A. Alternate PAX3-FOXO1 oncogenic fusion in biphenotypic sinonasal sarcoma. Genes Chromosomes Cancer. 2016;55:25–9.
135. Wang X, Bledsoe KL, Graham RP, et al. Recurrent PAX3-MAML3 fusion in biphenotypic sinonasal sarcoma. Nat Genet. 2014;46:666–8.
136. Sturgis EM, Potter BO. Sarcomas of the head and neck region. Curr Opin Oncol. 2003;15:239–52.
137. Subramaniam MM, Shuen CS, Petersson F. Poorly differentiated synovial sarcoma of the sphenoid sinus: report of the first case and review of synovial sarcomas of the sinonasal tract. Histopathology. 2012;61:1232–7.
138. Kosemehmetoglu, Vrana JA, Folpe AL. TLE1 expression is not specific for synovial sarcoma: a whole section study of 163 soft tissue and bone neoplasms. Mod Pathol. 2009;22:872–8.
139. Knott PD, Gannon FH, Thompson LD. Mesenchymal chondrosarcoma of the sinonasal tract: a clinicopathological study of 13 cases with a review of the literature. Laryngoscope. 2003;113:783–90.
140. Guo L, Liu J, Sun X, Wang D. Sinonasal tract chondrosarcoma: 18-year experience at a single institution. Auris Nasus Larynx. 2014;41:290–3.
141. Fanburg-Smith JC, Auerbach A, Marwaha JS, Wang Z, Rushing EJ. Reappraisal of mesenchymal chondrosarcoma: novel morphologic observations of the hyaline cartilage and endochondral ossification and beta-catenin, Sox9, and osteocalcin immunostaining of 22 cases. Hum Pathol. 2010;41:653–62.
142. Cajaiba MM, Luo J, Goodman MA, Fuhrer KA, Rao UN. Sox9 expression is not limited to chondroid neoplasms: variable occurrence in other soft tissue and bone tumors with frequent expression by synovial sarcomas. Int J Surg Pathol. 2010;18:319–23.

Neuroectodermal and Melanocytic Tumors

Alessandro Franchi

Sinonasal Melanoma

Definition

Sinonasal melanoma (SM) is a malignant tumor derived from melanocytes of the nasal mucosa. There are no known precursor lesions, although an association with sinonasal mucosal melanosis has been reported [1, 2].

Clinical Features

SM is a rare tumor, representing <1% of all melanomas. However, considering only mucosal melanomas of the head and neck, the sinonasal tract is the most frequently affected anatomic site, followed by the oral cavity. The nasal cavities are more frequently involved than the paranasal sinuses (70–80% vs. 20–30%) [3]. Considering the subsites, in order of frequency, SM originates from the lateral wall of the nasal cavity (40%), the septum (25%), the maxillary sinus (20%), and the ethmoid sinus (10%).

SM typically affects adult patients, with a median age of approximately 60 years (range 40–90). The most common symptoms at presentation are epistaxis and nasal obstruction [4].

Pathologic Features

Grossly, most lesions are reported as polypoid masses, which are frequently brown or black. As with melanomas at other sites, the histologic appearance of SM is quite variable. Most tumors are large and ulcerated, and pagetoid spread or junctional activity cannot be always demonstrated. The surface epithelium often presents squamous metaplasia, while respiratory epithelium is seen in a minority of cases. Melanin pigment is detected in 30–60%, and it is located mainly within melanophages and less frequently in neoplastic cells, where the pigment is more finely granular. The tumor cells are markedly atypical and have an epithelioid, spindle, round, or pleomorphic morphology (Figs. 1, 2, 3, 4, and 5). The cytoplasm is eosinophilic, and the nucleus contains a large eosinophilic nucleolus. They are arranged in solid sheets and fascicles and often present a perithelio-matous arrangement or an alveolar pattern. Tumor giant cells presenting numerous irregular nuclei with prominent nucleoli are frequently identified. Atypical mitotic figures are numerous, and areas of necrosis are detected. An infiltrate of lymphocytes and plasma cells is often present. In some cases, areas of metaplastic bone formation or of osteocartilaginous differentiation have been reported [4, 5].

A. Franchi (✉)
Department of Translational Research and of New Technologies in Medicine and Surgery, University of Pisa, Pisa, Italy
e-mail: alessandro.franchi@unipi.it

A. Franchi (ed.), *Pathology of Sinonasal Tumors and Tumor-Like Lesions*,
https://doi.org/10.1007/978-3-030-29848-7_8

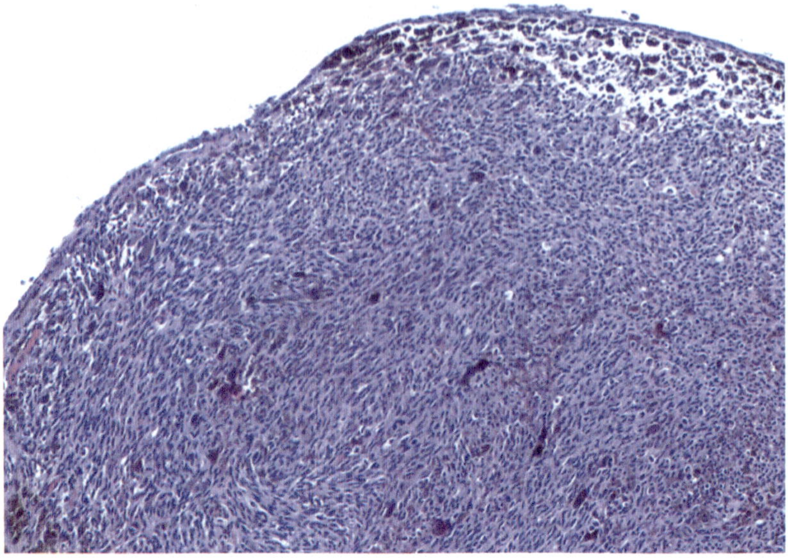

Fig. 1 Sinonasal melanoma. The tumor shows a predominant spindle cell morphology. Focal areas of melanin pigment formation are visible

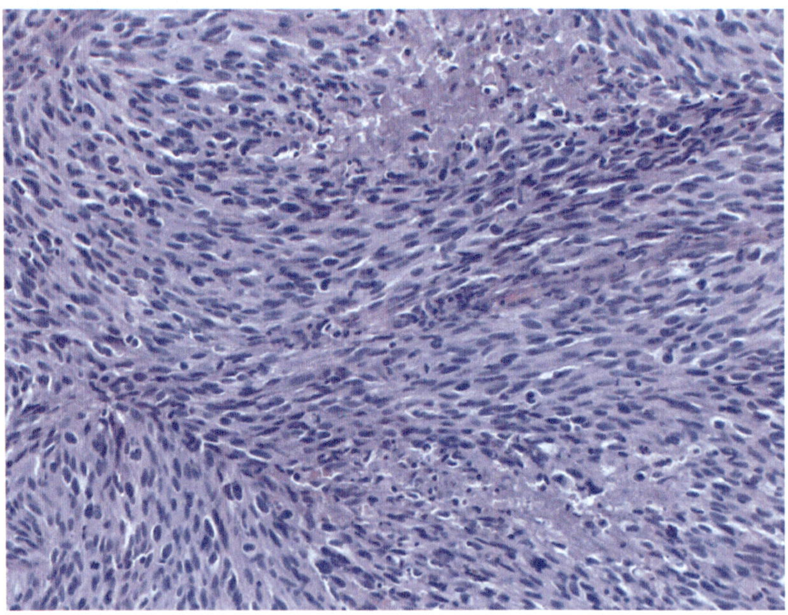

Fig. 2 This spindle cell melanoma shows a fascicular pattern and presents areas of necrosis. The differential diagnosis is mainly with spindle cell sarcomas and sarcomatous carcinoma

Immunohistochemical Profile

SM are variably positive for melanoma markers. S-100 protein, SOX10, and tyrosinase are more frequently positive than HMB-45 (Fig. 3), melan A, or microphthalmia transcription factor (MITF). Notably, SM is positive also for a number of other markers including NSE, CD117, CD99, synaptophysin, CD56, CD57 [4, 6], cytokeratins [7], and desmin [8].

Molecular Features

The molecular profile of SM differs from that of cutaneous melanoma and melanomas arising at other mucosal sites [9, 13, 14]. In particular, *KIT* and *BRAF* mutations are only rarely detected (4–22% of the cases), whereas *NRAS* mutations are relatively more frequent (15–30%) [9, 10, 13, 14]. *SF3B1* mutations have been documented in a minority of cases

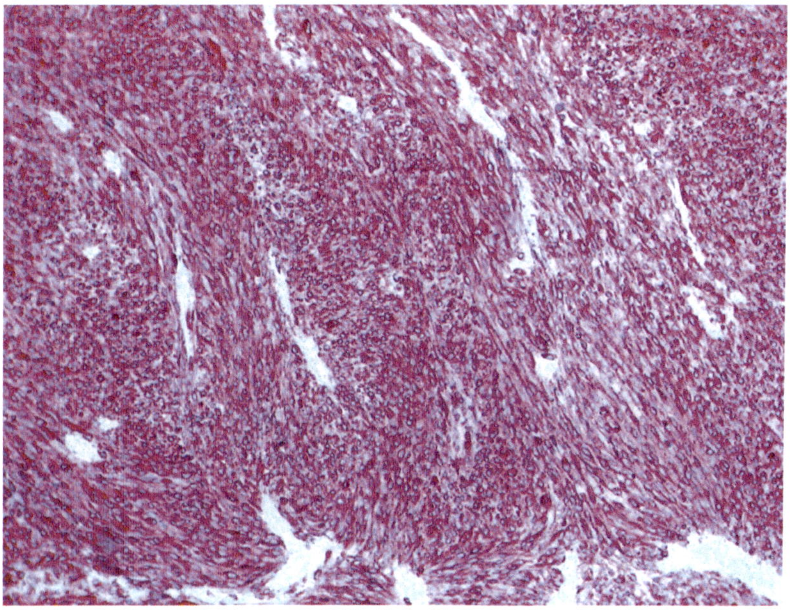

Fig. 3 The tumor is diffusely positive for HMB45

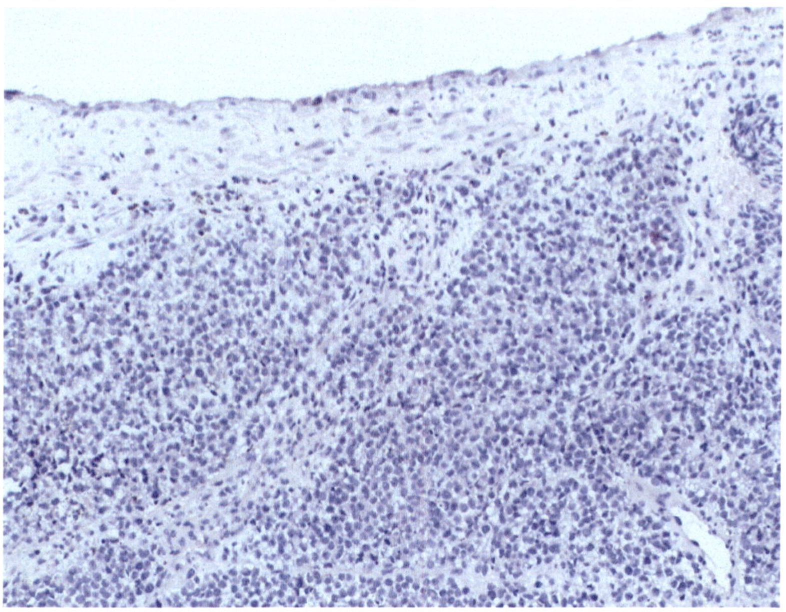

Fig. 4 Sinonasal melanoma with round cell morphology

[10–12]. These mutations are not mutually exclusive and may occur simultaneously [10]. *NRAS*, *KIT*, and *BRAF* mutations are more frequent in the United States and European sinonasal melanoma cases than in Asian cases [10]. There is no significant association between the mutation status of the tumors and survival outcomes [10, 13, 14].

In addition, loss of p16 expression appears to be a frequent event in this group of mucosal melanoma, occurring at higher frequency than cutaneous melanoma, and it is mainly related to deletion of 9p21 [14, 15]. No correlation between loss of p16 expression and the prognosis of patients affected by sinonasal melanoma has been demonstrated [15]. Other genetic

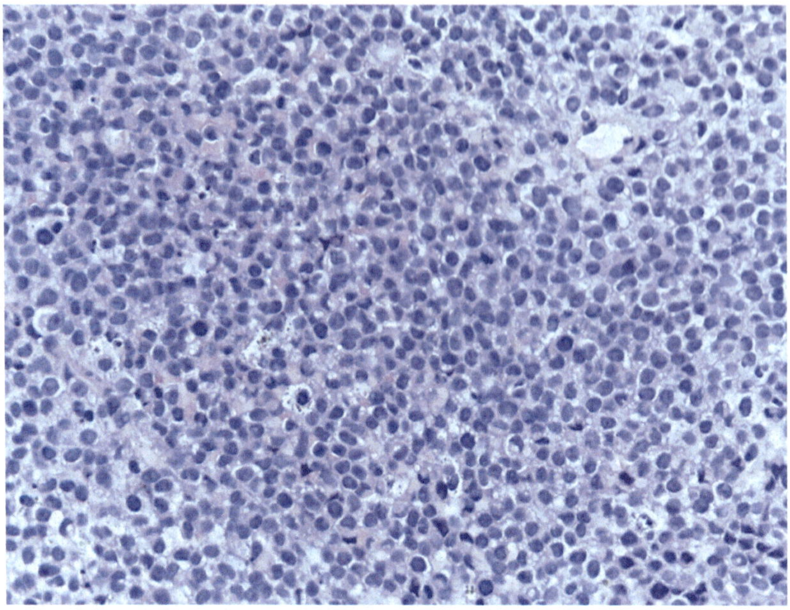

Fig. 5 In this sinonasal melanoma with round cell morphology, deposits of melanin pigment are present in the cytoplasm of few atypical cells

abnormalities include amplification of *RREB1*, loss of *MYB* and of *PTEN* [14]. This profile is partially similar to that of mucosal melanoma from other sites and to acral lentiginous melanoma, with the exception of gain at 11q13 (*CCND1*), which is not detected in SM.

Differential Diagnosis

The differential diagnosis of amelanotic SM is broad in relationship with the variable cytomorphology of these tumors. Epithelioid melanomas have to be mainly distinguished from various carcinoma types and from epithelioid malignant peripheral nerve sheath tumor, which is often S100 and SOX10 positive by immunohistochemistry. Undifferentiated round cell melanoma mimics quite closely several sinonasal small round cell tumors, including undifferentiated carcinomas, rhabdomyosarcoma, olfactory neuroblastoma, and lymphomas. Spindle cell melanoma may be mistaken for spindle cell sarcomas, particularly for malignant peripheral nerve sheath tumor [16]. Positivity for melanoma markers helps to rule out these entities.

Pigmented melanoma must be distinguished from sinonasal melanotic PEComa. This rare tumor shows an epithelioid morphology, production of melanin pigment, and expression of the melanocytic markers HMB45, melan A, tyrosinase, and MITF, but not of S100 or SOX10. In addition, PEComa is often positive for TFE3, while melanoma is not, whereas MUM1 is expressed by melanoma but not by PEComa. Finally, PEComas present *TFE3* gene translocations.

The presence of an intraepithelial component helps to exclude metastatic melanoma, but this scenario is seen in a minority of cases. However, the occurrence of metastatic melanoma in the sinonasal tract is a rare event, and it is usually part of widely disseminated disease.

Treatment and Prognosis

Complete surgical excision is accepted as the standard of care for treatment of patients with SM [17]. However, the anatomical complexity of the sinonasal region and the proximity to vital structures make radical resection virtually impossible in most cases. The use of postoperative radiation improves locoregional control, but does not improve survival [17].

At presentation, 10–20% of patients with SM have regional lymph node metastases, and approximately, 10% have distant metastases. During the course of disease, an additional 15–20% develops lymph node metastases, and 40–50% may develop distant metastases [18]. The lung, liver, and bone are the most frequent metastatic sites [4]. Locoregional failure quite often precedes the development of distant metastasis [4]. The 5-year overall survival ranges between 20 and 35% in the different series [4].

A number of pathologic and clinical parameters appears to be related to the clinical course. Tumor stage according to sinonasal AJCC staging system is an effective outcome predictor and should be the staging system of choice [4]. Paranasal sinus involvement indicates a poorer prognosis when compared to nasal cavity disease, and patients with multiple sinus involvement have the poorest prognosis [19].

Undifferentiated histology, >10 mitotic figures per 10 HPFs [4, 17], and presence of melanin pigment [17] are predictors of worse clinical outcome.

Tumor thickness greater than 7 mm was associated with a worse prognosis at 3 years in one study [20], but this parameter is often impossible to assess due to the fragmentation of the surgical material.

Olfactory Neuroblastoma

Definition

Olfactory neuroblastoma (ONB; synonyms: esthesioneuroblastoma, esthesioneuroepithelioma, esthesioneurocytoma) is a malignant tumor with neuroblastic differentiation typically derived from the olfactory membrane.

Clinical Features

ONB is an uncommon tumor that accounts for approximately 5% of all sinonasal malignancies. The incidence rate has been estimated at 0.4 cases/million inhabitants per year [21], and it has increased significantly over the period 1973–2006 [22], although these figures may reflect an improvement in the histopathological diagnosis. The peak age is in the fifth and sixth decades, but this tumor may also occur in the pediatric age [23]. Both sexes are equally involved.

The presenting symptoms are nonspecific and include nasal obstruction, rhinorrhea, and epistaxis. Anosmia and hyposmia are related to the involvement of the olfactory membrane. In rare instances, ONB may be associated with paraneoplastic syndromes that are determined either by tumor secretion of peptides and hormones or by immune cross-reactivity between tumor and normal host tissues [24]. Endocrinological paraneoplastic syndromes include syndrome of inappropriate ADH secretion (SIADH), ectopic ACTH syndrome, humoral hypercalcemia of malignancy, and hypertension due to catecholamine secretion by tumor cells. Neurological paraneoplastic syndromes described in ONB include opsoclonus–myoclonus–ataxia and cerebellar degeneration [24].

The site of origin of ONB is confined to the olfactory mucosa that lines the upper part of the nasal cavity. On rare occasions, ONB involves predominantly the superior aspect of the cribriform plate and grows as an intracranial mass [25, 26]. There are extremely rare cases of ONB that do not involve the olfactory membrane and have been termed "ectopic" ONBs. This diagnosis, however, requires the careful exclusion of all other sinonasal small round cell tumors that may mimic the appearance of ONB (see "Differential Diagnosis").

Pathologic Features

ONB presents usually as a unilateral, smooth, polypoid, or fungating mass of fleshy consistency and gray to pink or reddish color.

Histologically, ONB most often exhibits a lobular arrangement with well-defined nests of tumor cells separated by abundant edematous stroma (Fig. 6) or less frequently, it grows as solid sheets of cells with scanty but highly vascular stroma. The neoplastic population is typi-

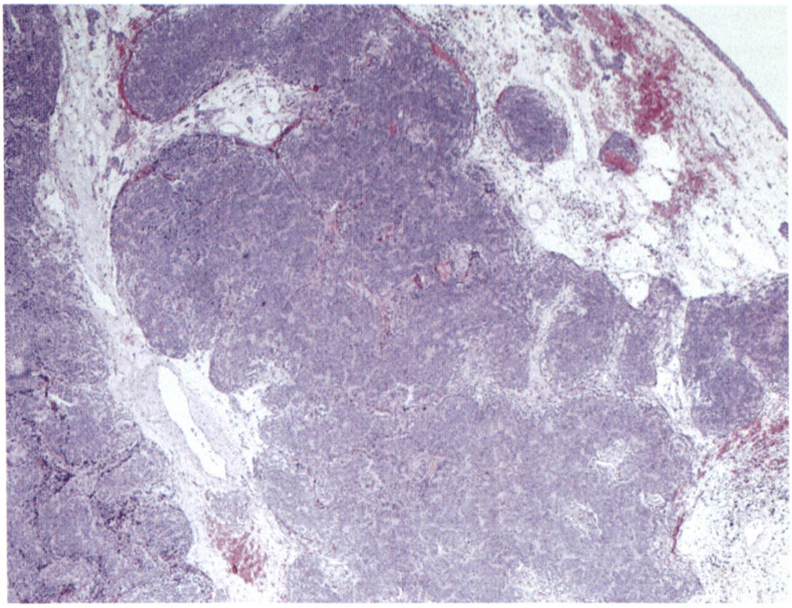

Fig. 6 At low power, most cases of olfactory neuroblastoma show a lobular arrangement with well-defined nests of tumor cells separated by abundant edematous stroma

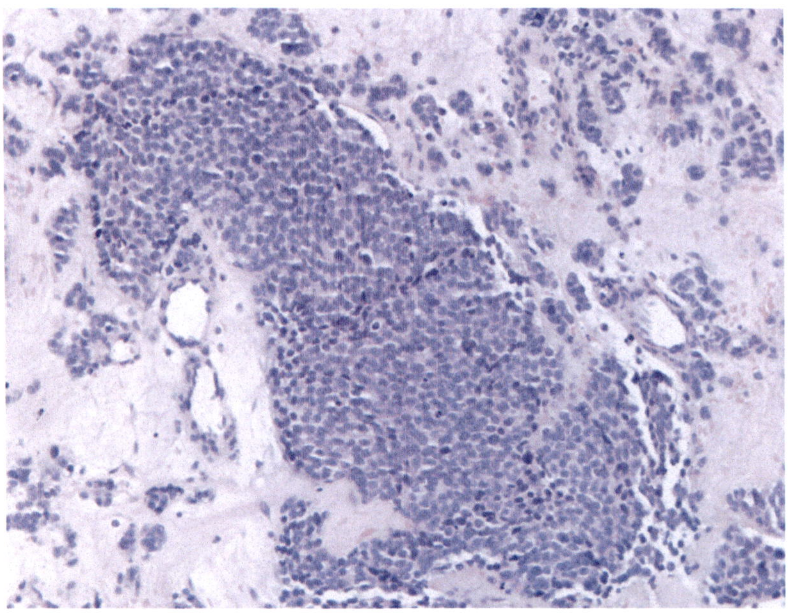

Fig. 7 The neoplastic population is typically uniform and consists of round cells, with round to oval nuclei with stippled chromatin, absent or small nucleoli, and minimal cytoplasm

cally uniform and consists of round cells, with round to oval nuclei with stippled chromatin, absent or small nucleoli, and minimal cytoplasm (Fig. 7). Neoplastic cells are separated by a neurofibrillary matrix formed by neuronal cell processes, in which axons may be better appreciated by conventional silver stains (Fig. 8). This neuropil is seen in about 85% of ONBs and is considered a useful diagnostic feature. Homer-Wright type of rosettes are also quite characteristic of ONB, but they are less commonly seen (Fig. 9). They form when the tumor cells surround the neurofibrillary matrix in collar-like arrangements. Even less frequent are true olfactory Flexner–Wintersteiner rosettes, in which the cells are arranged to form gland-like

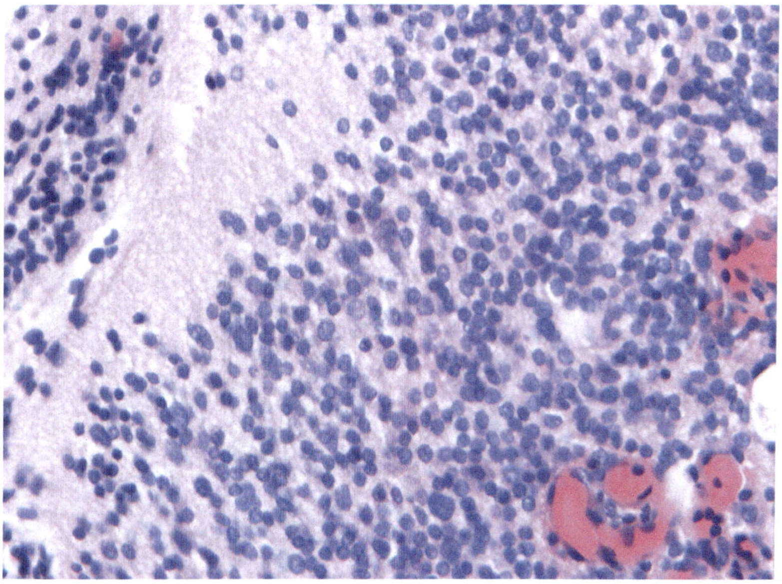

Fig. 8 Neoplastic cells are separated by a neurofibrillary matrix formed by neuronal cell processes

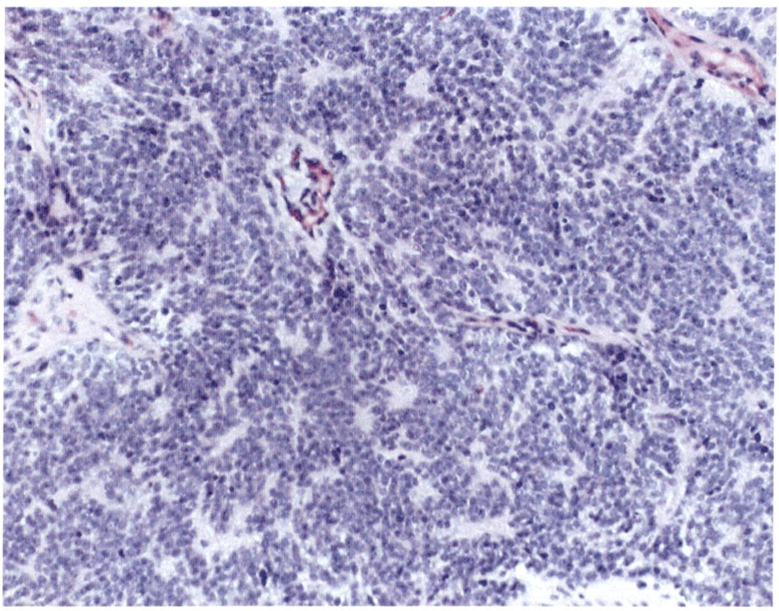

Fig. 9 Homer-Wright type of rosettes are frequently seen in olfactory neuroblastoma

structures with well-defined lumina (Fig. 10). These cuboidal or cylindrical cells generally have basally located nuclei and merge with the adjacent neoplastic neuroblasts without any intervening basal lamina. Perivascular pseudorosettes, formed by tumor cells arranged around capillaries are nonspecific. Presence of large ganglion-like cells is a rare finding (Fig. 11). Other uncommon features include stromal calcifications and melanin pigment deposition [27]. In rare instances, ONB may show a second neoplastic population with divergent differentiation, including myogenic [28] and epithelial elements [29].

As the differentiation of ON varies from tumor to tumor, a four-tiered grading scheme has been proposed by Hyams [30]. This system is based on the evaluation of several architectural and cyto-

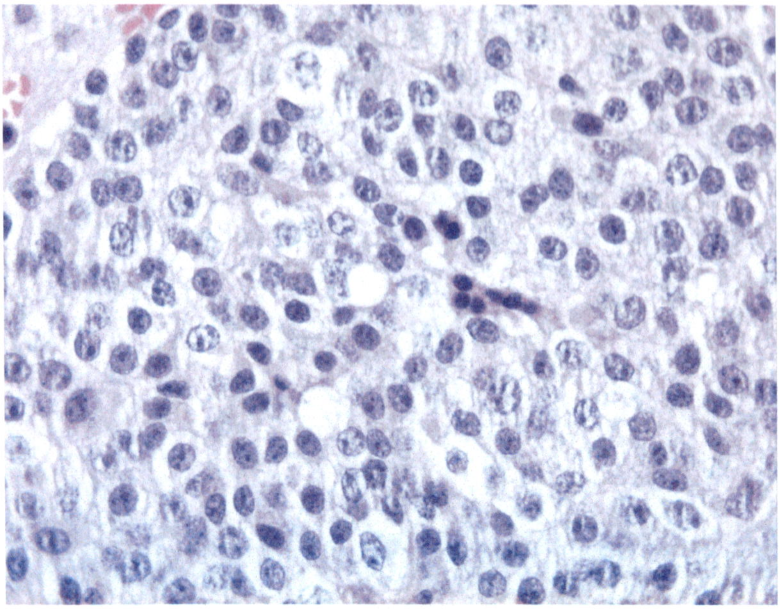

Fig. 10 In Flexner–Wintersteiner rosettes, neoplastic cells are arranged to form gland-like structures with well-defined lumina

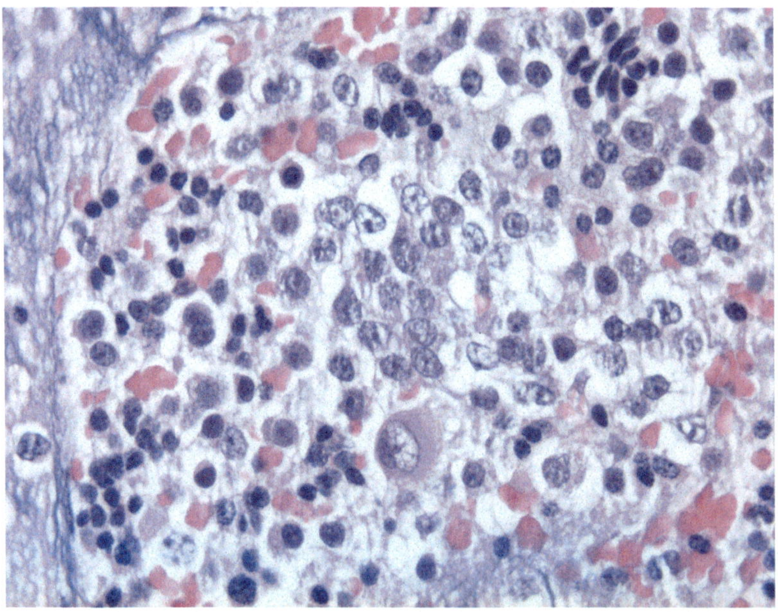

Fig. 11 Scattered large ganglion-like cells are rarely detected in olfactory neuroblastoma

logical parameters (Table 1). Lobular arrangement is present in all grades, although it is less pronounced in grades III and IV, similar to fibrillary matrix, which is prominent in grade I and absent in grade IV (Fig. 12). Nuclear pleomorphism, mitotic activity, and necrosis increase with grade (Fig. 13). Homer-Wright rosettes are a feature of grades I and II, whereas Flexner–Wintersteiner rosettes are present in grades III and IV. In a retrospective, population-based cohort study of patients affected by ON in the Surveillance, Epidemiology, and End Results (SEER) tumor registry, 48% had low-grade tumors (grade I–II) and 52% had a high-grade tumor (grade III–IV) [31]. Although the definite separation between grades is arbitrary and subjective, a number of studies have shown a good correlation with the clinical behavior of ONB [31].

Table 1 Hyams grading system for olfactory neuroblastoma

Histologic feature	Grade I	Grade II	Grade III	Grade IV
Lobular architecture	Present	Present	Attenuated	Usually absent, but may be retained
Fibrillary matrix	Present	Present	Attenuated	Absent
Homer-Wright rosettes	Present	Present	Absent	Absent
Flexner rosettes	Absent	Absent	Present	Absent
Nuclear pleomorphism	Absent	Moderate	Prominent	Marked
Mitotic activity	Absent	Present	Prominent	Brisk
Necrosis	Absent	Absent	Focal	Present

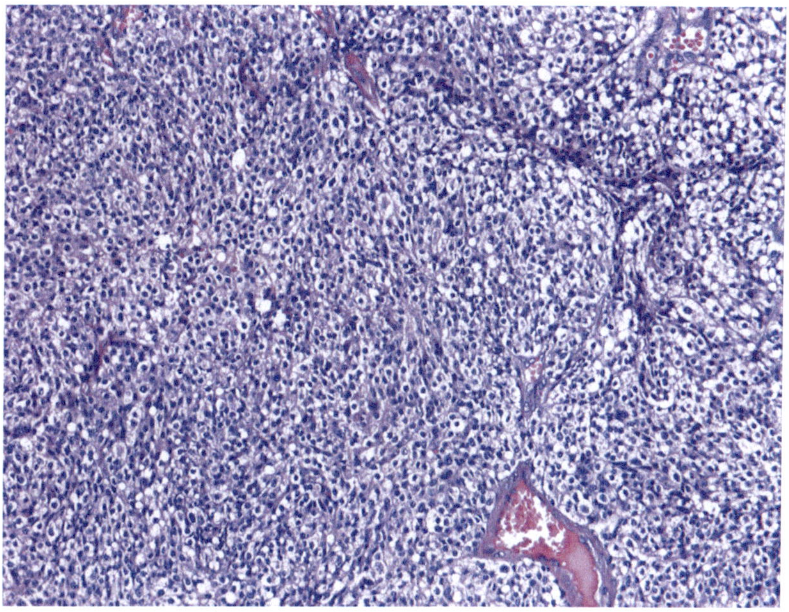

Fig. 12 High-grade olfactory neuroblastoma presents a solid architecture and cytologic atypia. This patient developed neck metastases 3 years after removal of the primary tumor

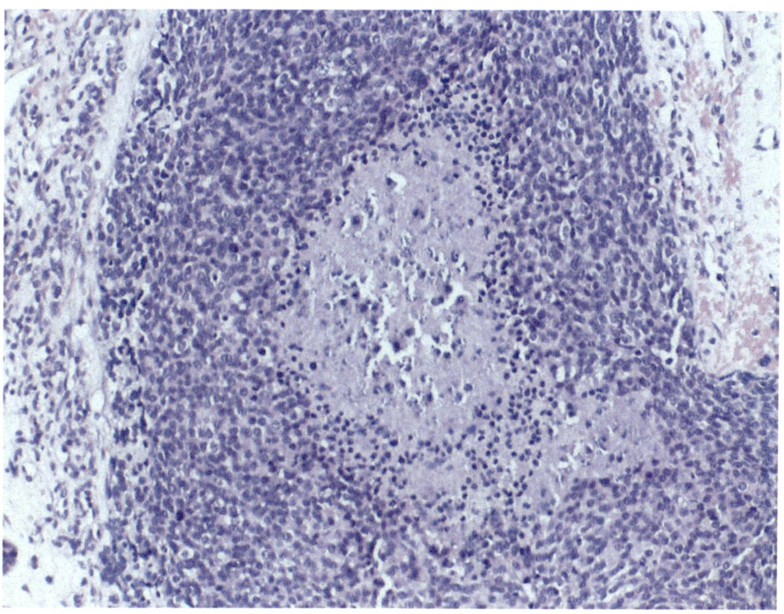

Fig. 13 Necrosis is a feature of high-grade olfactory neuroblastoma

Immunohistochemical Findings

ONB is typically positive for synaptophysin (Fig. 14a), chromogranin, CD56, neuron-specific enolase (NSE), beta-tubulin, and neurofilament protein [32, 33]. S-100 protein and GFAP are expressed by sustentacular cells present at the periphery of the neoplastic lobules (Fig. 14b). However, these cells are sparse or absent in high-grade lesions. Focal positivity for low molecular weight cytokeratins can also be seen in rare cases. Consistent staining for epithelial markers (EMA and cytokeratins) is present in the rare cases showing divergent epithelial differentiation. Calretinin positivity has recently been reported, but this marker does not seem to be entirely specific [34].

The neuroendocrine marker achaete-scute homolog 1 (ASH1) is expressed in ON, with increased positivity in high-grade tumor. However, this marker is of minimal diagnos-

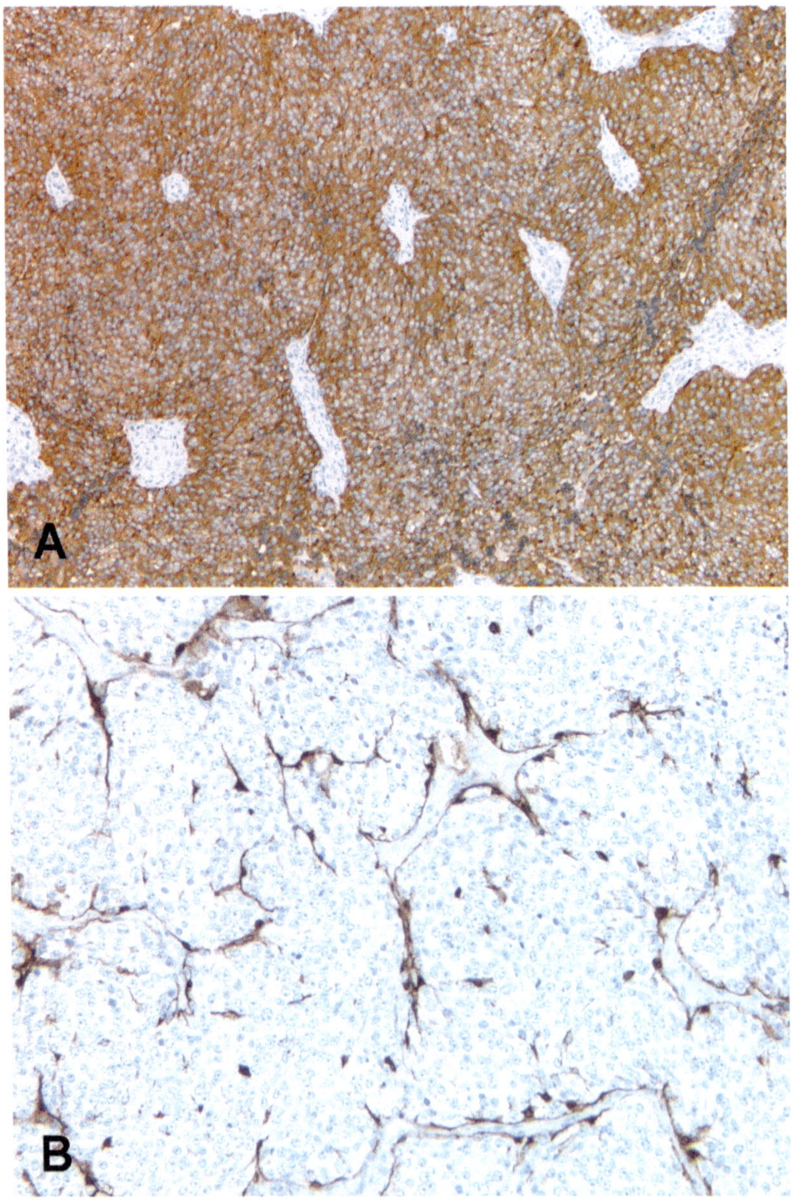

Fig. 14 Olfactory neuroblastoma is positive for synaptophysin (**a**). S100 highlights sustentacular cells (**b**)

tic utility, as it is expressed also in neuroendocrine carcinomas and sinonasal undifferentiated carcinoma [35]. Proliferative activity evaluated with Ki67 antibody varies widely between 0 and 50%. Negative markers include CD45, CD99, p63, FLI1, desmin, actin, and myogenin (with exception of cases showing divergent myogenic differentiation).

Ultrastructural Features

At the ultrastructural level, neoplastic cells present elongated neuritic processes containing microtubules, which form the fibrillary background seen histologically (Fig. 15). These processes are attenuated or absent in high-grade tumors. The nuclei are round and uniform, while the cytoplasm contains Golgi complexes, mitochondria, free polyribosomes, and dense core granules with diameters ranging from 150 to 350 nm [32, 36] (Fig. 16). Cells are closely packed and joined by occasional primitive and desmosome junctions [32]. Occasionally, synaptic junctions can be seen [36]. Sustentacular cells can be found at the periphery of tumor cell lobules and occasionally within them. They present elongated processes that encompass neoplastic nests and occasionally individual tumor cells. The cytoplasm is devoid of dense core granules and microtubules, and contains numerous intermediate filaments and small numbers of nonspecific organelles. They are covered by continuous basal lamina.

Molecular Features

There are only few genome-wide studies of ONB, and results are controversial, with reports indicating a high level of chromosomal instability and a greater frequency gain, while others have observed a low level of chromosomal instability and a greater frequency of losses [37]. By array comparative genomic hybridization, the most frequently reported changes included gains at 7q11.22-q21.11, 9p13.3, 13q, 20p/q, and Xp/q and losses at 2q31.1, 2q33.3, 2q37.1, 6q16.3, 6q21.33, 6q22.1, 22q11.23, 22q12.1, and Xp/q [38]. Genes relevant for ONB development appear to be located at 20q and 13q, and high-stage tumors show more alterations than low-stage ones [38]. Interestingly, recurrent focal amplifications included the receptor tyrosine kinase *FGFR3,* that could represent a novel therapeutic target [39].

Comprehensive genomic profiling showed some other clinically relevant recurrent altera-

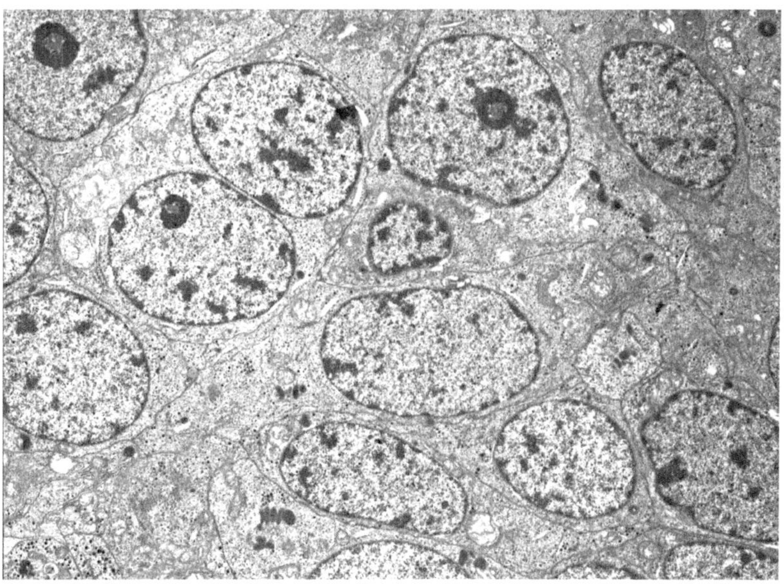

Fig. 15 Ultrastructurally, neoplastic cells of olfactory neuroblastoma are round to elongated, with round nucleus and cytoplasm containing Golgi complexes, mitochondria, free polyribosomes, and dense core granules

Fig. 16 Dense core neurosecretory granules are present in the cell processes

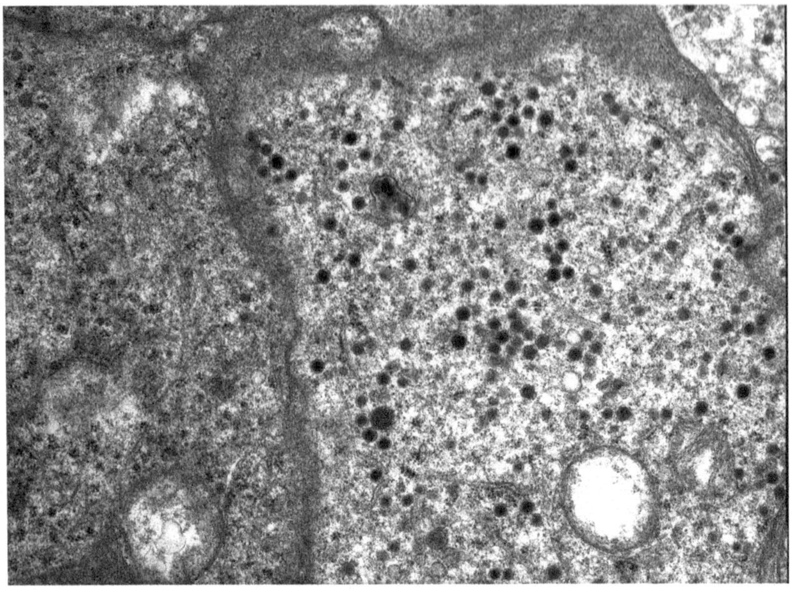

tions, including amplification of tyrosine kinases encoded on chromosome 5q and mutations affecting genes in the mTOR/PI3K pathway [40].

Other genes involved with lower frequency are *TP53*, *PIK3CA*, *NF1*, *CDKN2A*, and *CDKN2C* [40]. However, *TP53* mutations appear to be a late event in ONB progression and probably are not involved in the initial phases of tumorigenesis [32, 41, 42].

Differential Diagnosis

ON is frequently misdiagnosed with other sinonasal tumors, including neuroendocrine carcinoma, pituitary adenoma, melanoma, lymphoma, sinonasal undifferentiated carcinoma, alveolar rhabdomyosarcoma, and Ewing's sarcoma [43].

The distinction between ON and neuroendocrine carcinoma is clinically relevant because ON usually shows a less aggressive clinical behavior than neuroendocrine carcinoma [44–46]. Careful histologic evaluation, with search of the characteristic features of ON, including the lobular architecture and the neurofibrillary background, integrated with imaging information on the site of the tumor, is the prerequisite for a correct diagnosis. However, in small biopsy specimen and moderately/poorly differentiated lesions, a panel of immunohistochemical markers helps in the distinction. Absence of significant cytokeratin positivity in ON is a useful feature; in addition, the punctate cytoplasmic cytokeratin positivity of neuroendocrine carcinoma is not a feature of ON [45]. Positivity for p63 and p40 is also useful to separate poorly differentiated squamous cell carcinoma and NUT carcinoma from ON. Teratocarcinosarcoma may be entered in the differential diagnosis of ON for the presence of areas with round cell morphology and neural immunophenotype, which may closely resemble the histological appearance of ON. However, epithelial and mesenchymal elements can be recognized with a thorough sampling of the lesion.

Round cell melanoma can be distinguished from ON, which can seldom present melanin pigment depositions, based on the diffuse positivity for S100, HMB45, MART1, and SOX10. Rhabdomyosarcoma, particularly the alveolar variant, may be included in the differential diagnosis for its architectural features and for the expression of neuroendocrine markers, but it can be separated based on the positivity for desmin and myogenin. However, the presence of heterologous myogenic differentiation in rare cases of ON should also be taken into account. Finally, sinonasal lymphomas and plasmacytoma may be difficult to separate from ON on pure morphological grounds in small biopsies, but their immunoprofiles do not overlap, and therefore the differential diagnosis is usually straightforward.

Treatment and Prognosis

A combination of surgery and radiotherapy is considered the optimal approach to the treatment of ONB [47–49]. Even in advanced stage cases, an endoscopic approach can provide a resection with negative margins, with survival outcomes equivalent to or better than open resections [50]. Patients with aggressive and locoregional advanced disease may benefit from induction chemotherapy. A better response has been observed in high Hyams grade [51].

ON is characterized by slow onset of symptoms and excellent 5-year survival rates but with a propensity for delayed locoregional recurrence that warrants long-term follow-up. In a meta-analysis of the literature, the 5-year overall survival for ONB was 45% [47], although most larger series reported a survival of about 60–85% [23, 31, 52, 53].

Local recurrence occurs with a frequency of approximately 30%, while regional spread is observed in 15–20% and distant metastases in less than 10% of patients [54]. Distant metastases mainly involve the bone, lung, brain, and spine [47, 54]. However, the risk for lymph node and distant spread remains high even after 5 years, and long-term follow-up is recommended. Neck recurrence tends to be associated with poorer survival because neck recurrence often portends subsequent development of distant metastases [53].

The clinical staging system of ON was first introduced by Kadish et al. in 1976, and it is still in use [55]. Tumors limited to the nasal cavity only are in stage A, involvement of the paranasal sinuses is a feature of tumors in stage B, and stage C is used for tumors with extension outside the paranasal sinuses. A revision by Morita et al. introduced a stage D to include tumors with cervical node metastasis and distant metastasis [56].

Approximately 15%–20% of the cases are in stage A, 20–50% in stage B, 5–35% in stage C, and 5–35% in stage D [23, 31, 45, 52]. This staging system shows a good correlation with the clinical behavior, and the 5-year survival is 75–90% for Stage A, 65–70% for Stage B, 40–47% for Stage C, and 15–35% for stage D [23, 31, 45, 52, 53].

Considering histopathological parameters, there is accumulating evidence that Hyams grading system is a good predictor of prognosis, with high-grade tumors showing a significantly worst clinical behavior than low-grade ones [51, 52, 56]. In addition, in a recent study, a Ki67-index ≥20% was associated with an increased risk of recurrence and poorer outcomes [46].

Ewing Sarcoma

Definition

Ewing sarcoma (ES; synonym: peripheral neuroectodermal tumor) is a round cell malignancy with variable neuroectodermal differentiation. It is characterized by recurrent translocations involving the *EWSR1* gene on chromosome 22 and a member of the ETS family of transcription factors.

Clinical Features

ES of the head and neck region is extremely rare, comprising 4% of all cases of Ewing's sarcoma [57], and ES of the sinonasal tract represent only <10% of these cases [58]. Sinonasal ES occurs over a wide age range, although most patients are in the pediatric age or young adults [59]. Presenting symptoms are nasal obstruction and/or epistaxis [59]. The tumor involves the nasal cavity and/or one or more sinuses, most often the maxillary and the ethmoid sinuses [59]. *Dural*, brain, or orbital invasion is present in about one-third of the cases.

Pathologic Features

Histologically, the lesion consists of a uniform population of round to oval cells, with scant clear or eosinophilic cytoplasm, organized in solid sheets, nests, and cords (Fig. 17). Pseudorosette formation can be present in tumors showing neuroectodermal differentiation. Microscopic evidence of bone invasion is observed in most cases [59]. Mitotic activity is variable, but generally low, and foci of necrosis can be present. Cases showing cellular heterogeneity and nuclear pleomorphism are classified as atypical ES.

Rare examples of ES may show prominent epithelial differentiation associated with diffuse cytokeratin expression [60]. These tumor variants present a prominently nested growth, with tumor lobules composed of basaloid cells with peripheral palisading, separated by fibrotic bands. Focal squamous differentiation and intraepithelial growth can also be present [60].

Immunohistochemical Findings

ES is diffusely and intensely positive for CD99 with a membrane or cytoplasmic pattern. Nuclear positivity for FLI1 is observed in the majority of cases. Neural markers, including synaptophysin, NSE, S100, and chromogranin, are also frequently positive. Focal positivity for cytokeratins can be present in conventional ES, while the adamantinoma-like variant presents diffuse positivity for cytokeratins and p40 [60]. Myogenic, melanoma, and hematolymphoid markers are negative, as it is NUT1.

Molecular Features

The majority of ES (90–95%) presents the t(11;22) reciprocal translocation involving the *EWSR1* and *FLI-1* genes. Less frequently, the *EWSR1* gene is fused with another member of the ETS family, such as *ERG* or *ETV1*, or exceptionally with a non-ETS partner gene.

Differential Diagnosis

The distinction of sinonasal ES from other round cell malignancies may be challenging, especially in small biopsy material, and the differential diagnosis includes several non-epithelial and epithelial malignancies (Table 2). Alveolar rhabdomyosarcoma can be ruled out

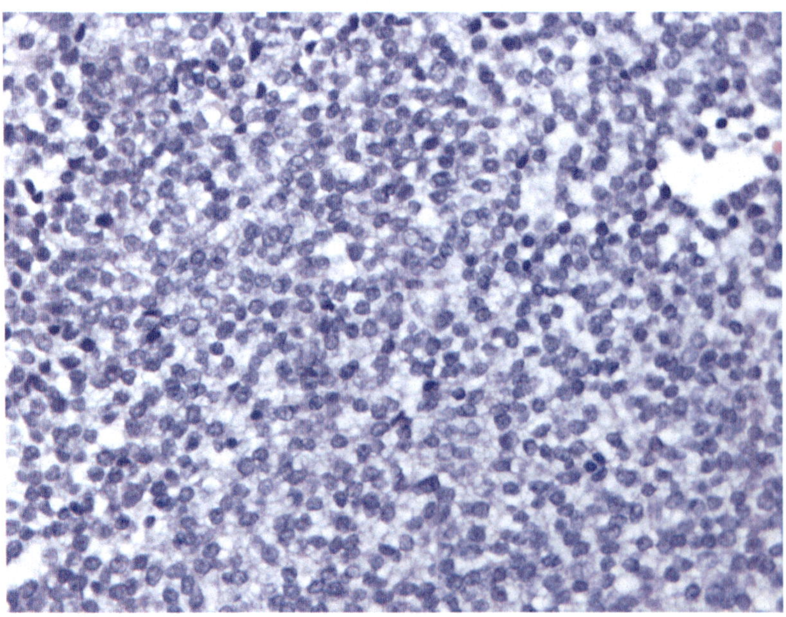

Fig. 17 Ewing sarcoma. The tumor consists of a uniform population of round cells

Table 2 Summary of the diagnostic features of sinonasal "round cell" sarcomas

	Histologic features	Immunohistochemical markers	Diagnostic gene fusion(s)
Rhabdomyosarcoma	Loose myxoid areas, subepithelial cellular areas, solid, alveolar	Myogenin, desmin, actin	*PAX3* or *PAX7-FOXO1* (alveolar rhabdomyosarcoma)
Ewing sarcoma	Solid, pseudorosettes	CD99, variable expression of neuroectodermal markers and cytokeratins	*EWSR1-FLI1* or other ETS family members
Desmoplastic small round cell tumor	Solid areas separated by desmoplastic stroma	Cytokeratins, desmin, WT1, neuron-specific enolase, CD99	*EWSR1-WT1*
Synovial sarcoma (poorly differentiated)	Solid, prominent vascular channels	Cytokeratins, EMA, TLE1	*SS18-SSX1* or *SSX2*
Mesenchymal chondrosarcoma	Biphasic, small cells, and islands of cartilage	SOX9	*HEY1-NCOA2*
Small cell osteosarcoma	Solid, osteoid deposition	SATB2	Not determined

for its positivity for myogenin and desmin, while round cell melanoma stains for S100 and melanoma markers. Mesenchymal chondrosarcoma is easily separated from ES if areas of cartilage matrix formation are present in the biopsy material. Otherwise, this differential diagnosis may be challenging, also for the CD99 positivity often seen in mesenchymal chondrosarcoma. Immunostaining for SOX9 or search for the *HEY1-NCOA2* fusion helps to recognize this entity. Cases of ES with nesting pattern may be difficult to separate from olfactory neuroblastoma, a tumor that occurs also in the same age group. In addition, both tumor types are positive for neural markers. However, in olfactory neuroblastoma, CD99 is not expressed, and S100 expression is limited to sustentacular cells. In equivocal cases, search for *EWSR1* rearrangement, which is not present in olfactory neuroblastoma, is useful.

Adamantinoma-like ES is almost indistinguishable from poorly differentiated carcinomas and myoepithelioma, also for the strong and diffuse positivity for cytokeratins and p40 and for S100 protein and synaptophysin. CD99 immunostaining is not entirely specific, and therefore search for the *EWSR1* gene rearrangement is necessary. However, it should be kept in mind that the use of FISH analysis with *EWSR1* probes, while helpful to rule out a poorly differentiated carcinoma, is not useful in excluding other possibilities such as myoepithelial carcinoma [60].

Treatment and Prognosis

There are only few cases of sinonasal ES with molecular confirmation and clinical information with follow-up data reported in the literature [59]. Most cases have been treated with chemotherapy and radiotherapy, and the prognosis seems to be better than more typical extremity bone and soft tissue tumors [59].

References

1. Cove H. Melanosis, melanocytic hyperplasia, and primary malignant melanoma of the nasal cavity. Cancer. 1979;44:1424–33.
2. Hofbauer GF, Böni R, Simmen D, Mihic D, Nestle FO, Burg G, Dummer R. Histological, immunological and molecular features of a nasal mucosa primary melanoma associated with nasal melanosis. Melanoma Res. 2002;12:77–82.
3. Clifton N, Harrison L, Bradley PJ, Jones NS. Malignant melanoma of nasal cavity and paranasal sinuses: report of 24 patients and literature review. J Laryngol Otol. 2011;125:479–85.
4. Thompson LD, Wieneke JA, Miettinen M. Sinonasal tract and nasopharyngeal melanomas: a clinicopathologic study of 115 cases with a proposed staging system. Am J Surg Pathol. 2003;27:594–611.
5. Takeshita H, Miwa T, Furukawa M. Osteocartilaginous differentiation of mucosal melanoma in the sinonasal cavity. Ann Otol Rhinol Laryngol. 2002;111:1112–5.
6. Lee H, Torres FX, McLean SA, Chen R, Lee MW. Immunophenotypic heterogeneity of primary sinonasal melanoma with aberrant expression of neuroendocrine markers and calponin. Appl Immunohistochem Mol Morphol. 2011;19:48–53.

7. Safadi RA, Bader DH, Abdullah NY, Sughhayer MA. Immunohistochemical expression of keratins 6, 7, 8, 14, 16, 18, 19, and MNF-116 pancytokeratin in primary and metastatic melanoma of the head and neck. Oral Surg Oral Med Oral Pathol Oral Radiol. 2016;121:510–9.
8. Smith SM, Schmitt AC, Carrau RL, Iwenofu OH. Primary sinonasal mucosal melanoma with aberrant diffuse and strong desmin reactivity: a potential diagnostic pitfall! Head Neck Pathol. 2015;9:165–71.
9. Zebary A, Jangard M, Omholt K, Ragnarsson-Olding B, Hansson J. KIT, NRAS and BRAF mutations in sinonasal mucosal melanoma: a study of 56 cases. Br J Cancer. 2013;109:559–64.
10. Wroblewska JP, Mull J, Wu CL, et al. SF3B1, NRAS, KIT, and BRAF mutation; CD117 and cMYC expression; and tumoral pigmentation in Sinonasal melanomas: an analysis with newly found molecular alterations and some population-based molecular differences. Am J Surg Pathol. 2019;43:168–77.
11. Cosgarea I, Ugurel S, Sucker A, et al. Targeted next generation sequencing of mucosal melanomas identifies frequent NF1 and RAS mutations. Oncotarget. 2017;8:40683–92.
12. Hintzsche JD, Gorden NT, Amato CM, et al. Whole-exome sequencing identifies recurrent SF3B1 R625 mutation and comutation of NF1 and KIT in mucosal melanoma. Melanoma Res. 2017;27:189–99.
13. Amit M, Tam S, Abdelmeguid AS, et al. Mutation status among patients with sinonasal mucosal melanoma and its impact on survival. Br J Cancer. 2017;116:1564–71.
14. Turri-Zanoni M, Medicina D, Lombardi D, et al. Sinonasal mucosal melanoma: molecular profile and therapeutic implications from a series of 32 cases. Head Neck. 2012;35(8):1066–77.
15. Franchi A, Alos L, Gale N, et al. Expression of p16 in sinonasal malignant melanoma. Virchows Arch. 2006;449:667–72.
16. Kardon DE, Thompson LD. Sinonasal mucosal malignant melanoma: report of an unusual case mimicking schwannoma. Ann Diagn Pathol. 2000;4:303–7.
17. Moreno MA, Roberts DB, Kupferman ME, et al. Mucosal melanoma of the nose and paranasal sinuses, a contemporary experience from the M. D. Anderson Cancer Center. Cancer. 2010;116:2215–23.
18. Prasad ML. Update on pigmented lesions of the sinonasal tract. Head Neck Pathol. 2007;1:50–4.
19. Khan MN, Kanumuri VV, Raikundalia MD, et al. Sinonasal melanoma: survival and prognostic implications based on site of involvement. Int Forum Allergy Rhinol. 2014;4:151–5.
20. Trapp TK, Fu YS, Calcaterra TC. Melanoma of the nasal and paranasal sinus mucosa. Arch Otolaryngol Head Neck Surg. 1987;113:1086–9.
21. Theilgaard SA, Buchwald C, Ingeholm P, et al. Esthesioneuroblastoma: a Danish demographic study of 40 patients registered between 1978 and 2000. Acta Otolaryngol. 2003;123:433–9.
22. Turner JH, Reh DD. Incidence and survival in patients with sinonasal cancer: a historical analysis of population based data. Head Neck. 2012;34:877–85.
23. Jethanamest D, Morris LG, Sikora AG, Kutler DI. Esthesioneuroblastoma: a population-based analysis of survival and prognostic factors. Arch Otolaryngol Head Neck Surg. 2007;133:276–80.
24. Kunc M, Gabrych A, Czapiewski P, Sworczak K. Paraneoplastic syndromes in olfactory neuroblastoma. Contemp Oncol (Pozn). 2015;19:6–16.
25. Ng HK, Poon WS, Poon CY, South JR. Intracranial olfactory neuroblastoma mimicking carcinoma: report of two cases. Histopathology. 1988;12:393–403.
26. Banerjee AK, Sharma BS, Vashista RK, Kak VK. Intracranial olfactory neuroblastoma: evidence for olfactory epithelial origin. J Clin Pathol. 1992;45:299–302.
27. Curtis JL, Rubinstein LJ. Pigmented olfactory neuroblastoma: a new example of melanotic neuroepithelial neoplasm. Cancer. 1982;49:2136–43.
28. Bishop JA, Thompson LD, Cardesa A, et al. Rhabdomyoblastic differentiation in head and neck malignancies other than rhabdomyosarcoma. Head Neck Pathol. 2015;9:507–18.
29. Meyer C, Hamersley ERS, Manosalva RE, Torske K, McIntyre N, Mitchell A. Olfactory neuroblastoma with divergent differentiation: an unusual histologic finding in a rare tumor. Head Neck Pathol. 2017;11:531–6.
30. Hyams VJ, Batsakis JG, Michaels L. Tumors of the upper respiratory tract and ear. Armed forces Institute of Pathology Fascicles, 2nd series. Washington: American Registry of Pathology Press; 1988.
31. Tajudeen BA, Arshi A, Suh JD, St John M, Wang MB. Importance of tumor grade in esthesioneuroblastoma survival. A population-based analysis. JAMA Otolaryngol Head Neck Surg. 2014;140:1124–9.
32. Hirose T, Scheithauer BW, Lopes MB, Gerber HA, Altermatt HJ, Harner SG, VandenBerg SR. Olfactory neuroblastoma. An immunohistochemical, ultrastructural, and flow cytometric study. Cancer. 1995;76:4–19.
33. Frierson HF Jr, Ross GW, Mills SE, Frankfurter A. Olfactory neuroblastoma. Additional immunohistochemical characterization. Am J Clin Pathol. 1990;94:547–53.
34. Wooff JC, Weinreb I, Perez-Ordonez B, Magee JF, Bullock MJ. Calretinin staining facilitates differentiation of olfactory neuroblastoma from other small round blue cell tumors in the sinonasal tract. Am J Surg Pathol. 2011;35:1786–93.
35. Taggart MW, Hanna EY, Gidley P, Weber RS, Bell D. Achaete-scute homolog 1 expression closely correlates with endocrine phenotype and degree of differentiation in sinonasal neuroendocrine tumors. Ann Diagn Pathol. 2015;19:154–6.
36. Min KW. Usefulness of electron microscopy in the diagnosis of "small" round cell tumors of the sinonasal region. Ultrastruct Pathol. 1995;19:347–63.

37. López-Hernández A, Vivanco B, Franchi A, et al. Genetic profiling of poorly differentiated sinonasal tumours. Sci Rep. 2018;8:3998.
38. Guled M, Myllykangas S, Frierson HF Jr, et al. Array comparative genomic hybridization analysis of olfactory neuroblastoma. Mod Pathol. 2008;21:770–8.
39. Lazo de la Vega L, McHugh JB, Cani AK, et al. Comprehensive molecular profiling of olfactory neuroblastoma identifies potentially targetable FGFR3 amplifications. Mol Cancer Res. 2017;15:1551–7.
40. Gay LM, Kim S, Fedorchak K, et al. Comprehensive genomic profiling of esthesioneuroblastoma reveals additional treatment options. Oncologist. 2017;22:834–42.
41. Papadaki H, Kounelis S, Kapadia SB, Bakker A, Swalsky PA, Finkelstein SD. Relationship of p53 gene alterations with tumor progression and recurrence in olfactory neuroblastoma. Am J Surg Pathol. 1996;20:715–21.
42. Weiss GJ, Liang WS, Izatt T, et al. Paired tumor and normal whole genome sequencing of metastatic olfactory neuroblastoma. PLoS One. 2012;7:e37029.
43. Cohen ZR, Marmor E, Fuller GN, DeMonte F. Misdiagnosis of olfactory neuroblastoma. Neurosurg Focus. 2002;12:e3.
44. Franchi A, Palomba A, Cardesa A. Current diagnostic strategies for undifferentiated tumours of the nasal cavities and paranasal sinuses. Histopathology. 2011;59:1034–45.
45. Thompson LD. Olfactory neuroblastoma. Head Neck Pathol. 2009;3:252–9.
46. Turri-Zanoni M, Maragliano R, Battaglia P, et al. The clinicopathological spectrum of olfactory neuroblastoma and sinonasal neuroendocrine neoplasms: refinements in diagnostic criteria and impact of multimodal treatments on survival. Oral Oncol. 2017;74:21.
47. Dulguerov P, Allal AS, Calcaterra TC. Esthesioneuroblastoma: a meta-analysis and review. Lancet Oncol. 2001;2:683–90.
48. Platek ME, Merzianu M, Mashtare TL, et al. Improved survival following surgery and radiation therapy for olfactory neuroblastoma: analysis of the SEER database. Radiat Oncol. 2011;6:41.
49. Yin ZZ, Gao L, Luo JW, et al. Long-term outcomes of patients with esthesioneuroblastomas: a cohort from a single institution. Oral Oncol. 2016;53:48–53.
50. Harvey RJ, Nalavenkata S, Sacks R, et al. Survival outcomes for stage-matched endoscopic and open resection of olfactory neuroblastoma. Head Neck. 2017;39:2425–32.
51. Su SY, Bell D, Ferrarotto R, et al. Outcomes for olfactory neuroblastoma treated with induction chemotherapy. Head Neck. 2017;39:1671–9.
52. Bell D, Saade R, Roberts D, Ow TJ, Kupferman M, Demonte F, et al. Prognostic utility of Hyams histological grading and Kadish-Morita staging systems for esthesioneuroblastoma outcomes. Head Neck Pathol. 2015;9:51–9.
53. Banuchi VE, Dooley L, Lee NY, et al. Patterns of regional and distant metastasis in esthesioneuroblastoma. Laryngoscope. 2016;126:1556–61.
54. Eden BV, Debo RF, Larner JM, et al. Esthesioneuroblastoma. Long term outcome and patterns of failure. The University of Virginia experience. Cancer. 1994;73:2556–62.
55. Kadish S, Goodman M, Wang CC. Olfactory neuroblastoma. A clinical analysis of 17 cases. Cancer. 1976;37:1571–6.
56. Morita A, Ebersold MJ, Olsen KD, Foote RL, Lewis JE, Quast LM. Esthesioneuroblastoma: prognosis and management. Neurosurgery. 1993;32:706-15.
57. Cotterill SJ, Ahrens S, Paulussen M, Jurgens HF, Voute PA, Gadner H, Craft AW. Prognostic factors in Ewing's tumor of bone: analysis of 975 patients from the European Intergroup Cooperative Ewing's Sarcoma study group. J Clin Oncol. 2000;18:3108–14.
58. Allam A, El-Husseiny G, Khafaga Y, et al. Ewing's sarcoma of the head and neck: a retrospective analysis of 24 cases. Sarcoma. 1999;3:11–5.
59. Hafezi S, Seethala RR, Stelow EB, et al. Ewing's family of tumors of the sinonasal tract and maxillary bone. Head Neck Pathol. 2011;5:8–16.
60. Bishop JA, Alaggio R, Zhang L, Seethala RR, Antonescu CR. Adamantinoma-like Ewing family tumors of the head and neck: a pitfall in the differential diagnosis of basaloid and myoepithelial carcinomas. Am J Surg Pathol. 2015;39:1267–74.

Hematolymphoid Tumors

Alessandro Franchi

Sinonasal hematolymphoid tumors represent up to 17% of all sinonasal malignancies, and in some series, they represent the second most common sinonasal malignancy after squamous cell carcinoma. B- and T-cell non-Hodgkin lymphomas are by far the most frequent entities in this group of tumors, followed by extramedullary plasmacytoma. Classical and nodular lymphocyte-predominant Hodgkin lymphomas do not typically involve the sinonasal tract. Examples of Rosai-Dorfman disease, myeloid sarcoma, and histiocytic sarcoma have also been reported.

Lymphomas

Definition

Sinonasal lymphomas are malignant tumors with phenotypic features of B or T cells with variable differentiation. Diffuse large B-cell lymphoma (DLBCL) and natural killer/T-cell (NK/T-cell) lymphoma (previously known as lethal midline granuloma or angiocentric lymphoma) are the most commonly encountered types at this anatomic site.

Clinical Features

Overall, sinonasal lymphomas represent approximately 1% of all lymphomas and 6–14% of all sinonasal malignancies [1–3].

There are significant differences in the geographic distribution of sinonasal lymphoma types, as DLBCL is the most common in Europe and the Unites States, whereas extranodal natural killer/T-cell (NK/T-cell) lymphoma, nasal type, is more frequent in Asia and South America [4]. DLBCL tends to affect an older population than NKTL (mean age 68 years and 52 years, respectively) [4], and there is a slight male predominance for both types. Symptoms at the onset are nonspecific and include nasal obstruction, ocular disturbances, rhinorrhea, and epistaxis. General symptoms, including fever, lymphadenopathy, pruritus, night sweats, and malaise, are present in 10–40% of patients and are more frequently reported in patients affected by NKTL [4, 5]. Sinonasal DLBCL may occur in HIV-positive patients [6].

The most common location for DLBCL is the maxillary sinus, followed by the nasal cavity and ethmoid sinus, whereas NKTL affects more frequently the nasal cavities or the nasal cavities and paranasal sinuses and only rarely involves the sinuses alone [6].

A. Franchi (✉)
Department of Translational Research and of New Technologies in Medicine and Surgery, University of Pisa, Pisa, Italy
e-mail: alessandro.franchi@unipi.it

A. Franchi (ed.), *Pathology of Sinonasal Tumors and Tumor-Like Lesions*,
https://doi.org/10.1007/978-3-030-29848-7_9

Pathologic Features

In DLBCL the sinonasal mucosa is occupied by a diffuse growth of large atypical B lymphoid cells. Morphologically centroblastic, immunoblastic, and anaplastic variants can be recognized (Fig. 1). In the centroblastic variant, neoplastic cells present vesicular nuclei with two to four peripherally located nucleoli and scant cytoplasm, while in the immunoblastic variant, they show a single, centrally located nucleolus and more abundant basophilic cytoplasm. The anaplastic variant is characterized by large bizarre and pleomorphic nuclei that resemble those of Reed–Sternberg cells. Apoptotic bodies and mitotic figures are easily identified.

In NKTL the infiltrate is more polymorphic, containing varying proportions of admixed reactive lymphocytes, plasma cells, and histiocytes, and it is typically angiocentric and angiodestructive (Fig. 2). The size of neoplastic is variable, the nuclei have an irregular contour and present inconspicuous nucleoli, and the cytoplasm is scanty and often pale to clear. Initially, neoplastic cells may be interspersed within the reactive infiltrate, but with time they tend to coalesce to diffuse sheets and cause mucosal ulceration and destruction of blood vessels. Apoptotic bodies and areas of geographic, coagulative necrosis are easily identified. Pseudoepitheliomatous hyperplasia of the covering epithelium may occur and destruction of the mucosal glands.

Several other B-cell lymphoma types may involve the nasal cavities and paranasal sinuses (Table 1), including *Burkitt's lymphoma, B-lymphoblastic leukemia/lymphoma, and plasmablastic lymphoma* among the aggressive types and *marginal zone B-cell lymphoma, chronic lymphocytic leukemia/small lymphocytic lymphoma, and follicular lymphoma* among the low-grade types [7]. Among T-cell lymphomas, involvement of the sinonasal tract is reported for *adult T-cell leukemia/lymphoma, anaplastic large cell lymphoma, peripheral T-cell lymphoma NOS (not otherwise specified),* and *T-lymphoblastic leukemia/lymphoma* [7]. The latter has to be distinguished from the so-called indolent T-lymphoblastic proliferation, that has been described also in the upper aerodigestive and sinonasal tract and pursue a benign course [8]. The cytological and immunophenotypic features are similar, but the indolent T-lymphoblastic proliferation does not show involvement of the surface and glandular epithelium.

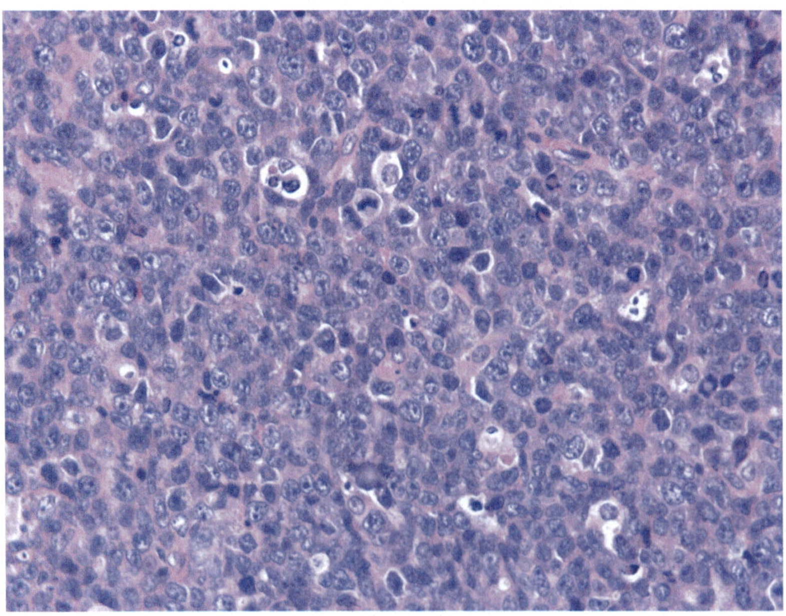

Fig. 1 Diffuse large B-cell lymphoma of the nasal cavity. The tumor consists of large atypical cells. Atypical mitotic figures and apoptotic bodies are present

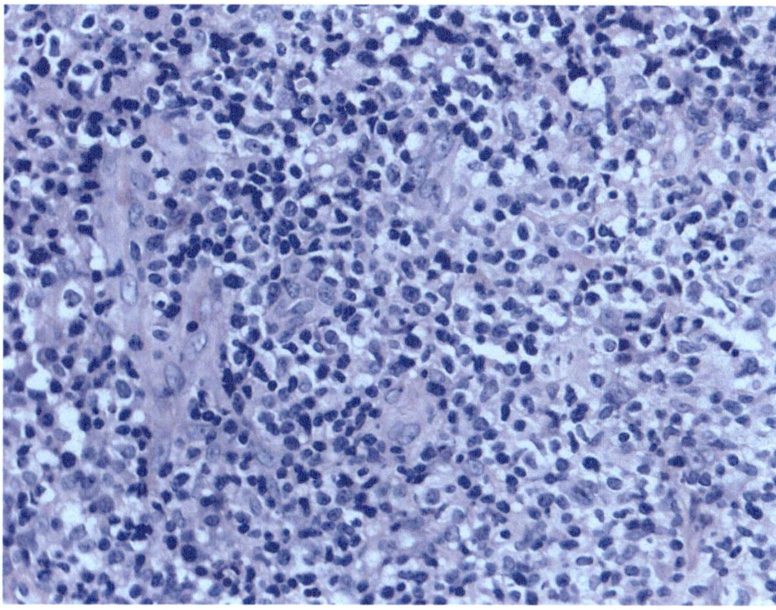

Fig. 2 In NK-T cell lymphoma the infiltrate is polymorphic containing varying proportions of admixed reactive lymphocytes, plasma cells, and histiocytes. Vessels with prominent endothelial lining are present

Immunohistochemical Features

DLBCL is positive for pan B-cell markers including CD19, CD20, CD22, and CD79a. EBV markers are negative, except for rare cases arising in HIV-positive patients [6]. Rare examples of sinonasal ALK-positive DLBCL have been reported [9].

In NKTL, neoplastic cells are positive for CD2, cytoplasmic CD3 (CD3 epsilon), and CD56 and often positive for granzyme B, TIA-1, and perforin (Fig. 3). Other T-cell markers are usually negative, including CD4, CD5, CD8, and CD3 surface antigen. NK/T-cell lymphoma is almost always associated with EBV positivity (EBER-1) (Fig. 3). Sinonasal lymphomas demonstrating CD3epsilon+, CD56-, cytotoxic molecule+, and EBV+ are also included within the NK/T category.

Molecular Features

DLBCL can be divided in two main molecular subgroups, the germinal center B-cell like (GCB), and the post-germinal center or activate B-cell like (ABC). The Hans algorithm can be used to distinguish the two subtypes using an immunohistochemical approach [10]. Cases can be assigned to the GCB group if CD10 alone is positive or if both bcl-6 and CD10 are positive, while if bcl-6 is positive and CD10 is negative, then the expression of MUM1 determines the group: if MUM1 is negative, then the case is assigned to the GCB group; if MUM1 is positive, then the case is assigned to the non-GCB group (Hans CP). CD10, BCL6, and MUM1 are considered positive if >30% of neoplastic cells are stained. The molecular landscape varies according to the cell of origin subtype.

In NKTL the most common alteration is deletion of 6q, which is found in approximately 40–50% of cases and determines the loss of putative tumor suppressor genes such as *FOXO3*, *AIM1*, and *PRDN1* [11].

Differential Diagnosis

Lymphomas must be separated from other sinonasal non-hematopoietic round cell malignancies, including melanoma, carcinomas, sarcomas, and olfactory neuroblastoma. An appropriate panel of immunohistochemical markers helps in these differentials. The distinction between sinonasal DLBCL cell lymphoma and NKTL is based on

Table 1 Summary of the salient diagnostic features of sinonasal hematolymphoid malignancies

	Median age	Geographic distribution	Histologic features	Immunophenotype	Molecular features
Diffuse large B-cell lymphoma	V/VI decades	Western countries	Rather uniform population of large pleomorphic cells infiltrating the mucosa and the underlying bone	CD45, CD19, CD20, CD22, CD79a, high Ki67 proliferative index (>50%)	EBV negative (rare cases EBER+)
Burkitt lymphoma	Children and young adults	Endemic variant limited to equatorial Africa and Papua New Guinea; sporadic variant is seen worldwide	Medium-sized atypical lymphocytes with a high nuclear to cytoplasmic ratio, nuclei with finely clumped chromatin, and multiple basophilic nucleoli; apoptotic bodies; scattered tingible body macrophages impart a "starry sky" appearance	CD19, CD20, CD10, bcl-6, PAX5; bcl-2 negative; Ki67 proliferative index nearly 100%	*MYC* rearrangements
B-lymphoblastic leukemia/lymphoma	Children	Worldwide	Medium-sized atypical lymphoid cells with frequent admixed mitotic figures and apoptotic bodies, and occasional tingible body macrophages	TdT and/or CD34, CD10, PAX5; CD20 variably expressed	Frequent cytogenetic abnormalities that define specific entities
Plasmablastic lymphoma	IV decade in HIV-related cases; VIII decade in sporadic cases	Worldwide	Variable appearance with tumors composed of cells with immunoblastic features and others composed of cells with plasmacytic differentiation	CD138, CD38, MUM-1; light chain restriction; CD45, CD20, and PAX5 usually negative	*MYC* translocation in 50% of cases; EBV positive in 65%–70%
Chronic lymphocytic leukemia/small lymphocytic lymphoma	VII decade	Worldwide	Small lymphocytes with scant cytoplasm condensed chromatin and inconspicuous nucleoli	CD20, CD23, CD5; cyclin D1 not expressed	No specific markers
Follicular lymphoma	VI decade	More frequent in western Europe and the United States	Closely packed follicles that are not polarized, lack tingible body macrophages, and are composed of a mixture of centrocytes and larger centroblasts	CD19, CD20, CD22, bcl2, bcl6, CD10	t(14;18)(q23;q21)
MALT lymphoma	Mainly adults, but pediatric cases also reported	Worldwide	Mixture of small and medium-sized lymphocytes with scattered immunoblasts and diffuse plasma cell differentiation; residual secondary follicles	CD20, CD79a; CD10 negative; kappa and lambda clonal expression; CD21, CD23, CD35 highlight expanded meshworks of follicular dendritic cells in colonized follicles	Various chromosomal translocations
Extramedullary plasmacytoma	VI decade	Worldwide	Diffuse mucosal infiltration of neoplastic plasma cells	CD38, CD138, MUM1; kappa and lambda light chains	Rare cases EBV positive

Nasal natural killer/T-cell lymphoma	V–VI decades	Asia, Mexico, Central and South America	Angiocentric/angiodestructive pleomorphic neoplastic infiltrate, composed of small, medium-sized, large-sized, or anaplastic cells; Admixture of inflammatory cells (histiocytes, lymphocytes, granulocytes); necrosis	CD2, cytoplasmic CD3 (CD3ε), and CD56; often positive for granzyme B, TIA-1, and perforin	EBV positive
Adult T-cell leukemia/lymphoma	Adults	Japan, Caribbean basin, parts of Central Africa	Large pleomorphic cells with indented and often elongated nuclei and moderately abundant eosinophilic cytoplasm	CD2, CD3, CD5, CD25, and often CD4	Associated with human T-lymphotropic virus-1 (HTLV-1)
Anaplastic large cell lymphoma	Adults	Worldwide	Large cells with eccentric irregular nuclei ("hallmark cells"), but a variable number of small cells may be present, together with an abundant inflammatory background composed of histiocytes or neutrophils that may obscure the tumor cells	CD30, CD25, and most are positive for CD43 and EMA; variable expression of T-cell markers; CD15 negative	*ALK* translocations
T-lymphoblastic leukemia/lymphoma	Adolescents, adults	Worldwide	Round cells with high nuclear to cytoplasm ratio, round to oval to irregularly shaped nuclei with dispersed chromatin and usually inconspicuous nucleoli	CD3 and CD7 with concurrent expression of one or more markers of immaturity including CD34, TdT, CD99, CD10; possible expression of CD56	Various chromosomal aberrations
Myeloid sarcoma	VI decade	Worldwide	Diffuse mucosal infiltration of primitive myeloid cells	Chloroacetate esterase, myeloperoxidase, lysozyme, CD33, CD34, CD68 (KP1), CD117	Various chromosomal aberrations
Histiocytic sarcoma	Wide age range, but most cases occur in adults	Worldwide	Infiltrate of large and pleomorphic neoplastic cells; accompanying inflammatory infiltrate, most often of neutrophils or lymphocytes	CD45, CD45RO, CD4, CD68, lysozyme, CD31	*BRAF* V600E mutation reported

the differences in their histopathological features and immunohistochemical markers (Table 1). Typically, NKTL shows an angiocentric infiltrate, marked necrosis, and a polymorphous infiltrate which are not features of DLBCL.

NKTL has to be distinguished from inflammatory nonneoplastic conditions, including fungi and bacterial infections with marked inflammation and necrosis and Wegener's granulomatosis, for its clinical presentation and the features of the inflammatory infiltrate. The presence of cellular atypia and numerous mitotic figures is helpful to rule out nonneoplastic infiltrates. In small biopsies, search for EBV may help in the differential diagnosis between NKTL and Wegener's granulomatosis or nonspecific rhinitis [12]. However, EBV positivity in lymphoid cells in the sinonasal mucosa

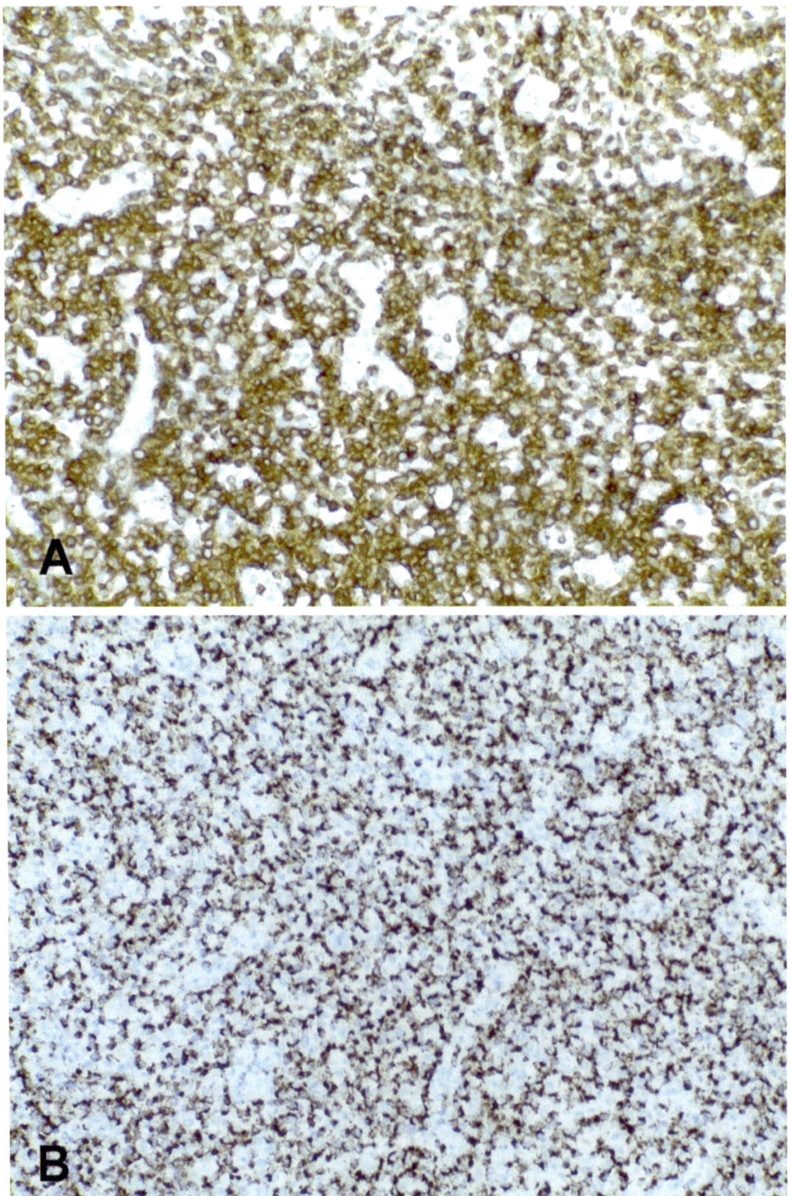

Fig. 3 NK-T cell lymphoma with positivity for CD3 epsilon (**a**), granzyme B (**b**), and EBV (EBER) (**c**)

Fig. 3 (continued)

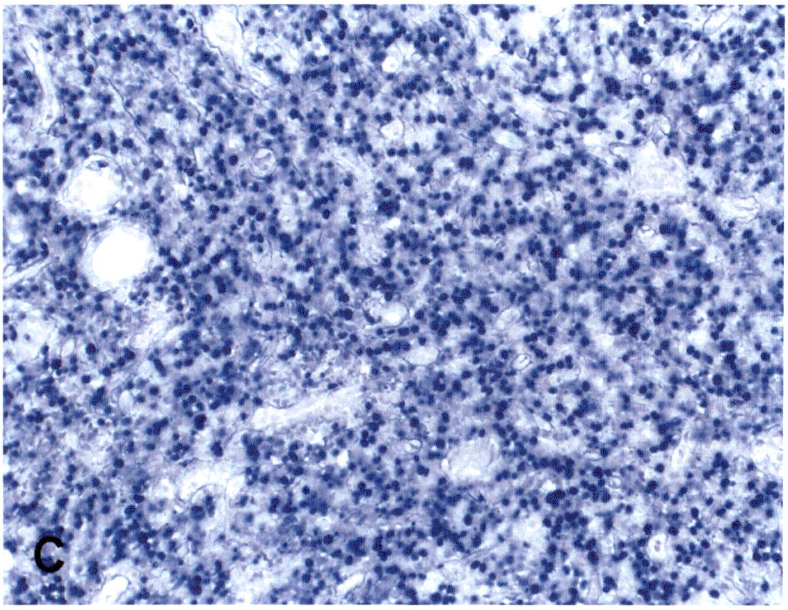

should not be interpreted "per se" as evidence as nasal NKTL, especially in pediatric patients, because in rare instances EBV-positive lymphocytes can be present in reactive infiltrates of small lymphocytes, which are in addition of B lineage [13].

Treatment and Prognosis

Treatment for sinonasal DLBCL and NKTL depends on the stage at diagnosis and histologic subtype. For NKTL, combined radiotherapy and chemotherapy are preferred for localized disease and when patients are healthy enough to tolerate the treatment, while for advanced stages, chemotherapy alone is typically used [4]. For DLBCL in early stage, chemotherapy followed by radiotherapy is the preferred treatment, whereas patients in advanced stages are treated with the CHOP chemotherapeutic regimen plus rituximab (R-CHOP) [4, 14].

The 5-year survival rate is better for DLBCL (60–70%) than NKTL (approximately 30%) [4, 15], but this difference is lost when general B symptoms, such as fever, lymphadenopathy, pruritus, night sweats, general malaise, and weight loss, are present [4].

Extraosseous Plasmacytoma

Definition

Sinonasal extramedullary plasmacytoma (SEP) is a localized monoclonal plasma cell neoplasm. The diagnosis of SEP requires the exclusion of systemic disease.

Clinical Features

The mucosa sites of the upper respiratory tract are the most frequently affected sites by extra osseous plasmacytoma (80%), and SED represents from 35 to 55% of all cases [16–18]. The mean age at diagnosis is 55–60 years, and there is a significant male prevalence (M:F = 3:1) [18]. The most common anatomic site is the nasal cavity and septum (approximately one-third of the cases), and the most common presenting symptom is nasal obstruction (30% of cases) [16].

Pathological Features

SEP appears more often as a polypoid, soft, often bleeding lesion. Histologically, there is diffuse infiltration of the mucosa by neoplastic plasma cells that can vary in appearance from well-differentiated and indistinguishable from normal plasma cells (Fig. 4) to less mature plasmablastic or anaplastic morphologies (Fig. 5). Well-differentiated SEP shows a proliferation of relatively uniform small plasma cells with abundant cytoplasm and eccentrically located nuclei with the characteristic "clockface" chromatin. By contrast, in less differentiated SEP, neoplastic cells are larger, with increased nuclear to cytoplasmic ratio, nuclei with finely dispersed chromatin, and prominent nucleoli. The anaplastic variant is characterized by neoplastic cells of large size showing pleomorphic nuclei or multinucleation, and it may be difficult to recognize it as a plasma cell neoplasm. In well-differentiated SEP, neoplastic plasma cells can contain cytoplasmic inclusions composed of immunoglobulin: "grapelike" cytoplasmic inclusions characterize the so-called "Mott cells," while plasma cells with one large cytoplasmic inclusion are termed "Russel bodies," and cytoplasmic inclusions that overlie the nucleus are designated "Dutcher bodies." However, these inclusions can be seen also in nonneoplastic plasma cells.

Immunohistochemical Features

Neoplastic plasma cells express CD79a, CD38, CD138, and MUM1, but may aberrantly co-

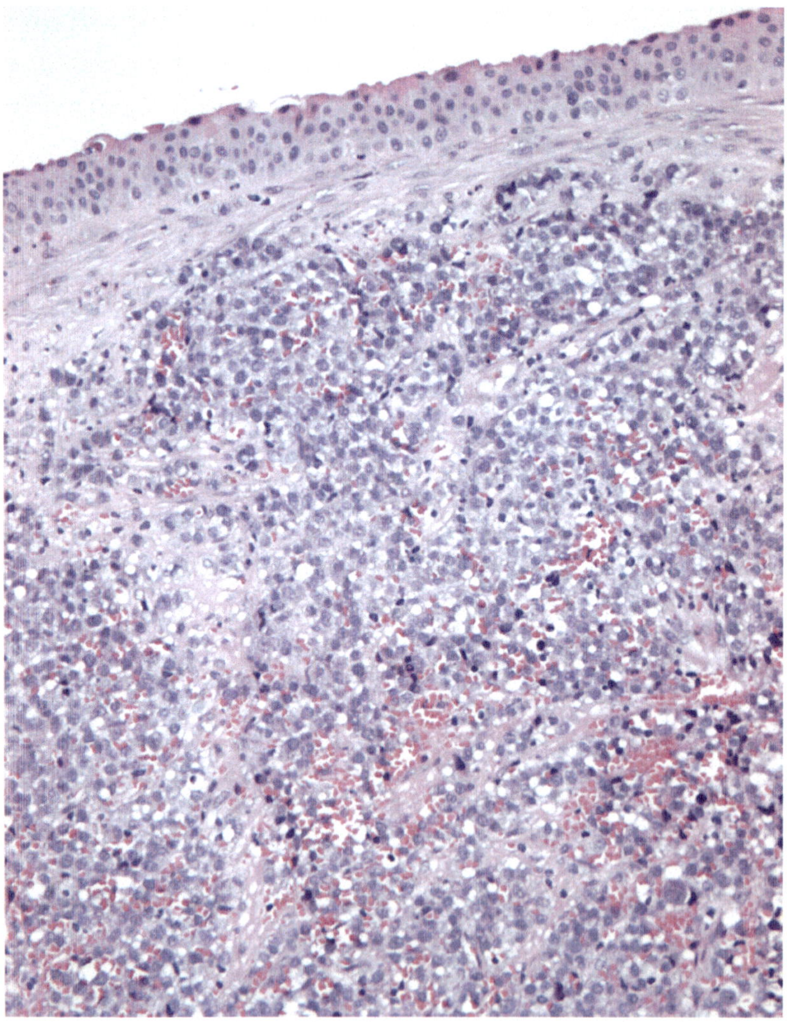

Fig. 4 Plasmacytoma of the nasal cavity. The tumor presents as an infiltrate of uniform medium-sized cells of the mucosa

express also CD56, CD117, CD20, CD52, and CD10 (Fig. 6a). Plasmacytoma typically presents immunoglobulin light chain restriction, which can be demonstrated by immunohistochemical staining with light chain antibodies (Fig. 6b) or by in situ hybridization for light chain mRNA.

Differential Diagnosis

Lymphomas with prominent plasmacytic differentiation, such as extranodal marginal zone lymphoma, must be excluded. Diffuse expression of B-cell markers, such as CD19, CD20, CD79a, and CD22, and positivity for CD45, which is

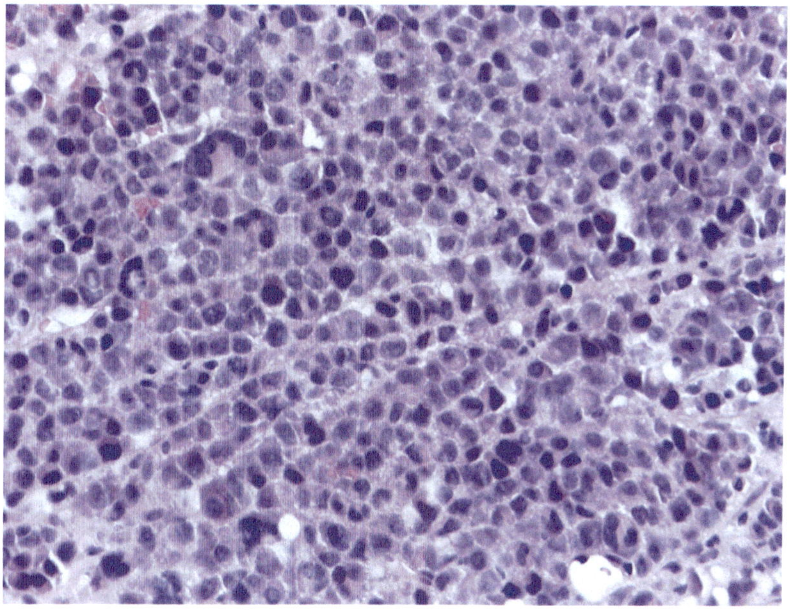

Fig. 5 The infiltrate consists of atypical elements with plasma cell features

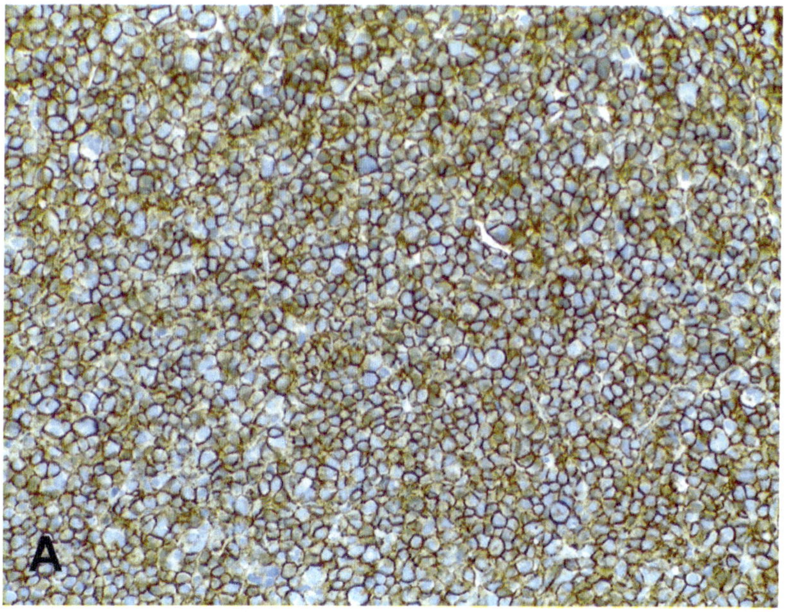

Fig. 6 The tumor is positive for CD138 (**a**) and presents monoclonal restriction of the expression of lambda light chain (**b**)

Fig. 6 (continued)

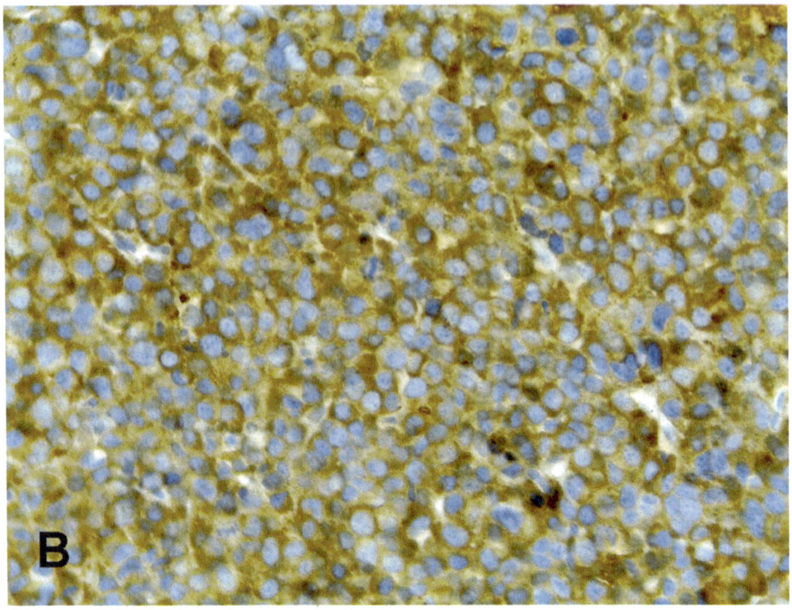

usually absent or weakly positive in neoplastic plasma cells, supports the diagnosis of marginal zone lymphoma.

Plasmablastic lymphoma, a high-grade lymphoma associated with HIV characterized by a "blastic" morphology, can also be considered in the differential diagnosis. Plasmablastic lymphoma frequently shows extranodal occurrence of the upper aerodigestive tract with a predilection for the oral cavity and is positive for plasma cell markers such as CD38 and CD138 and for in situ hybridization for EBER, which in turn is negative in SEP.

Treatment and Prognosis

Similar to other head and neck sites, SEP has a favorable outcome, with an estimated 10-year survival of 80–85% [16, 18]. Patients receiving a combination of radiotherapy and surgery show the best outcomes [16]. Approximately 10% of SEPs progress to multiple myeloma, with the majority of these patients (75.0%) receiving radiotherapy alone as their treatment modality [16].

Other Sinonasal Hematolymphoid Disorders

Rosai-Dorfman disease (synonym: *sinus histiocytosis with massive lymphadenopathy*) is a rare nonneoplastic histiocytic proliferative disorder that most commonly affects children and young adults with massive painless cervical lymphadenopathy, fever, and leukocytosis [19]. Extranodal sinonasal involvement occurs in 11% of cases [20], usually in association with other sites and only rarely as the only localization [21]. Concomitant nodal involvement is present in 30–50% of patients, while localization at other extranodal sites is detected in up to 65% of patients. The mean age presentation is 40 years, and there is no gender predilection. Clinical presentation depends on the predominant localization (anterior or posterior nasal cavity) [21]. Histologically, the nasal mucosa is occupied by a proliferation of large histiocytes, with vesicular nuclei containing distinct nucleoli and abundant pale-to-eosinophilic cytoplasm. The histiocytic cells may contain intact erythrocytes, lymphocytes, and plasma cells (emperipolesis). The groups of histiocytes are separated by chronic inflammatory cells, mainly small lymphocytes and plasma cells. Immunohistochemically, the histiocytic cells are strongly reactive for S-100 protein, the histiocytic markers CD68 and CD163, whereas CD1a and langerin are negative, thus excluding Langerhans cell histiocytosis.

The disease is considered benign, and patients have been treated mainly with endoscopic surgery for symptomatic control, although there is no consensus on treatment guidelines. Radiotherapy, chemotherapy, or steroid therapy have also been employed with variable results [22]. Based on the review of Chen et al., the clinical course of sinonasal Rosai-Dorfman disease is self-limiting in only 0.7% of patients, while approximately half of the patients have a persistent or progressive course and 5% die from the disease [22]. In general, factors associated with death include: multisystem dissemination; involvement of vital organs such as the liver, pancreas, kidneys, lower respiratory tract, and heart; and immunological disorders or anemia. In sinonasal cases, no recurrence has been observed if the initial treatment consisted of complete resection of the mass [22].

Myeloid sarcoma (synonyms: granulocytic sarcoma, chloroma, extramedullary myeloid tumor) is a localized tumor of myeloid blasts occurring at an anatomical site other than the bone marrow, which can rarely arise in the sinonasal tract [23–25]. It may develop prior to, concurrently with, or following the presentation of acute myeloid leukemia. The mucosa is infiltrated by diffuse sheets of primitive myeloid cells with high nuclear to cytoplasmic ratio, and the histologic appearance may mimic that of lymphoma or other poorly differentiated malignant neoplasms of the sinonasal tract (Fig. 7). The diagnosis can be confirmed using a panel of immunohistochemical staining including chloroacetate esterase, myeloperoxidase (Fig. 8), lysozyme, CD68, and CD43, while CD34, CD117, CD99, TdT, and CD33 are variably expressed [26, 27].

Histiocytic sarcoma is a rare malignant neoplasm of cells showing morphologic and immunophenotypic features of mature tissue histiocytes that can occasionally involve the nasal cavity [28, 29]. Neoplastic cells are large and pleomorphic, with abundant eosinophilic cytoplasm, well-defined cell borders, ovoid to irregular nuclei with large nucleoli. There is usually an accompanying inflammatory infiltrate, most often of neutrophils or lymphocytes. Neoplastic cells are positive for

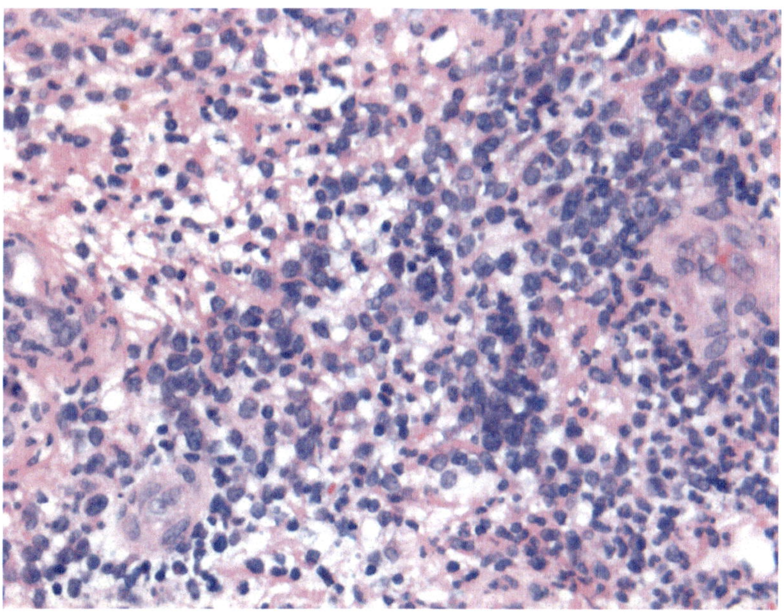

Fig. 7 Myeloid sarcoma. The nasal mucosa is infiltrated by primitive myeloid cells with high nuclear to cytoplasmic ratio, with a histologic appearance that mimics that of lymphoma

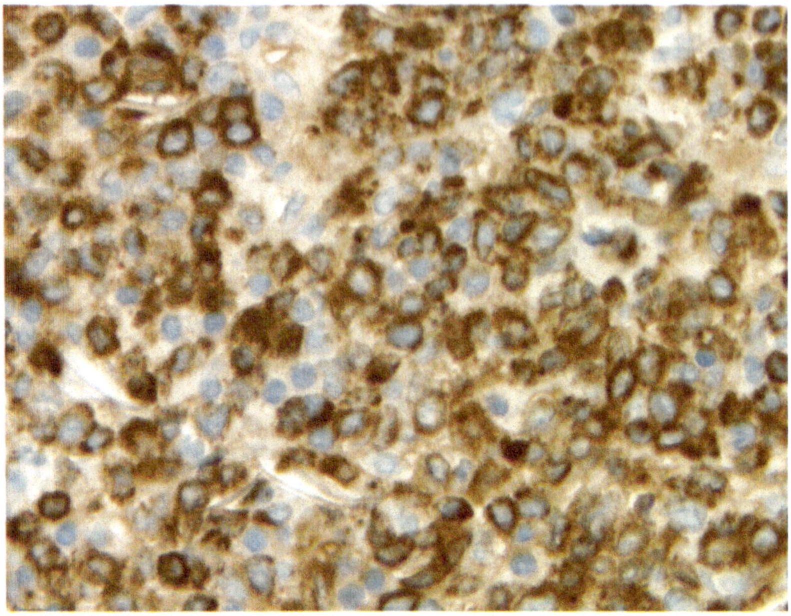

Fig. 8 Tumor cells are positive for myeloperoxidase

the histiocytic markers CD163, CD68, and lysozyme, while CD1a is negative and S100 only focally and weakly positive. CD45, CD45RO, and CD4 (cytoplasmic) are also usually positive.

References

1. Kapadia SB, Barnes L, Deutsch M. Non-Hodgkin's lymphoma of the nose and paranasal sinuses: a study of 17 cases. Head Neck Surg. 1981;3:490–9.
2. Abbondanzo SL, Wenig BM. Non-Hodgkin's lymphoma of the sinonasal tract. A clinicopathologic and immunophenotypic study of 120 cases. Cancer. 1995;75:1281–91.
3. Harbo G, Grau C, Bundgaard T, et al. Cancer of the nasal cavity and paranasal sinuses. A clinicopathological study of 277 patients. Acta Oncol. 1997;36:45–50.
4. Dubal PM, Dutta R, Vazquez A, Patel TD, Baredes S, Eloy JA. A comparative population-based analysis of sinonasal diffuse large B-cell and extranodal NK/T--cell lymphomas. Laryngoscope. 2015;125:1077–83.
5. Kim GE, Koom WS, Yang W-I, et al. Clinical relevance of three subtypes of primary sinonasal lymphoma characterized by immunophenotypic analysis. Head Neck. 2004;26:584–93.
6. Cuadra-Garcia I, Proulx GM, Wu CL, et al. Sinonasal lymphoma: a clinicopathologic analysis of 58 cases from the Massachusetts General Hospital. Am J Surg Pathol. 1999;23:1356–69.
7. Crane GM, Duffield AS. Hematolymphoid lesions of the sinonasal tract. Semin Diagn Pathol. 2016;33:71–80.
8. Ohgami RS, Arber DA, Zehnder JL, et al. Indolent T-lymphoblastic proliferation (iT-LBP): a review of clinical and pathologic features and distinction from malignant T-lymphoblastic lymphoma. Adv Anat Pathol. 2013;20:137–40.
9. Beltran B, Castillo J, Salas R, et al. ALK-positive diffuse large B-cell lymphoma: report of four cases and review of the literature. J Hematol Oncol. 2009;2:11.
10. Hans CP, Weisenburger DD, Greiner TC, et al. Confirmation of the molecular classification of diffuse large B-cell lymphoma by immunohistochemistry using a tissue microarray. Blood. 2004;103:275–82.
11. Huang Y, De Reyniès A, de Leval L, et al. Gene expression profiling identifies emerging oncogenic pathways operating in extranodal NK/T-cell lymphoma, nasal type. Blood. 2010;115:1226–37.
12. Dictor M, Cervin A, Kalm O, Rambech E. Sinonasal T-cell lymphoma in the differential diagnosis of lethal midline granuloma using in situ hybridization for Epstein-Barr virus RNA. Mod Pathol. 1996;9:7–14.
13. Ha SY, An J, Park S. Detection of Epstein–Barr virus-infected lymphoid cells in nasal mucosa or nasopharynx: appearances can be deceptive. Virchows Arch. 2013;462:391–7.
14. Sehn LH, Donaldson J, Chhanabhai M, et al. Introduction of combined CHOP plus rituximab therapy dramatically improved outcome of diffuse large B cell lymphoma in British Columbia. J Clin Oncol. 2005;23:5027–33.
15. Kanumuri VV, Khan MN, Vazquez A, et al. Diffuse large B-cell lymphoma of the sinonasal tract: analy-

sis of survival in 852 cases. Am J Otolaryngol. 2014;35:154–8.
16. D'Aguillo C, Soni RS, Gordhan C, et al. Sinonasal extramedullary plasmacytoma: a systemic review of 175 patients. Int Forum Allergy Rhinol. 2014;4:156–63.
17. Vento SI, Vähämurto P, Silventoinen K, et al. Clinical findings in 25 patients with sinonasal or nasopharyngeal extramedullary plasmacytoma in a four-decade single-Centre series. Acta Otolaryngol. 2017;137:975–80.
18. Patel TD, Vázquez A, Choudhary MM, Kam D, Baredes S, Eloy JA. Sinonasal extramedullary plasmacytoma: a population-based incidence and survival analysis. Int Forum Allergy Rhinol. 2015;5:862–9.
19. Rosai J, Dorfman RF. Sinus histiocytosis with massive lymphadenopathy. A newly recognized benign clinicopathological entity. Arch Pathol. 1969;87:63–70.
20. Foucar E, Rosai J, Dorfman R. Sinus histiocytosis with massive lymphadenopathy (Rosai-Dorfman disease): review of the entity. Semin Diagn Pathol. 1990;7:19–73.
21. Duan HG, Zheng CQ, Wang DH, Ding GQ, Luo JQ, Zang CP, Yu C. Extranodal sinonasal Rosai-Dorfman disease: a clinical study of 10 cases. Eur Arch Otorhinolaryngol. 2015;272:2313–8.
22. Chen HH, Zhou SH, Wang SQ, et al. Factors associated with recurrence and therapeutic strategies for sinonasal Rosai-Dorfman disease. Head Neck. 2012;34:1504–13.
23. Prades JM, Alaani A, Mosnier JF, Dumollard JM, Martin C. Granulocytic sarcoma of the nasal cavity. Rhinology. 2002;40:159–61.
24. Gorman M, Ahmed KA, Pallera A, Samant S. Granulocytic sarcoma of the nasal cavity: a case report. Ear Nose Throat J. 2009;88:1210–2.
25. Gupta AJ, Mandal S, Gupta R, Khurana N, Gulati A. Myeloid sarcoma presenting as nasal and orbital mass: an initial manifestation of an acute myeloid Leukaemia. J Clin Diagn Res. 2017;11:ED24–6.
26. Roth MJ, Medeiros LJ, Elenitoba-Johnson K, Kuchnio M, Jaffe ES, Stetler-Stevenson M. Extramedullary myeloid cell tumors. An immunohistochemical study of 29 cases using routinely fixed and processed paraffin-embedded tissue sections. Arch Pathol Lab Med. 1995;119:790–8.
27. Menasce LP, Banerjee SS, Beckett E, Harris M. Extra-medullary myeloid tumour (granulocytic sarcoma) is often misdiagnosed: a study of 26 cases. Histopathology. 1999;34:391–8.
28. Pileri SA, Grogan TM, Harris NL, et al. Tumours of histiocytes and accessory dendritic cells: an immunohistochemical approach to classification from the International Lymphoma Study Group based on 61 cases. Histopathology. 2002;41:1–29.
29. Hornick JL, Jaffe ES, Fletcher CD. Extranodal histiocytic sarcoma: clinicopathologic analysis of 14 cases of a rare epithelioid malignancy. Am J Surg Pathol. 2004;28:1133–44.

Germ Cell Tumors

Alessandro Franchi

Dermoid Cyst

Definition

Nasal dermoid cyst (NDC; synonym: dermoid sinus cyst) is a developmental lesion composed of elements from the ectoderm and mesoderm. By contrast to teratomas, it contains no endodermal elements.

Clinical Features

NDCs are relatively common lesions, as they represent 1–3% of all dermoids and 3.5–12.5% of dermoids arising in the head and neck region [1–3]. They are the commonest midline congenital nasal lesions accounting for 60% of midline nasal masses in children [2]. However, cases occurring in adulthood have been reported [2]. Craniofacial congenital anomalies can be associated with NDC [4]. NDC typically arises in the midline, involving the subcutaneous tissue of the nasal bridge. Intracranial extension has been reported with variable frequency (20% in average) [3], and it is more frequent in patients with other craniofacial abnormalities. NDC arising in the paranasal sinuses are exceptional [5].

Pathologic Findings

NDC is lined by mature keratinizing squamous epithelium supported by variably dense fibrovascular connective tissue. Skin appendages can be identified within the wall of the cyst. Abundant keratin debris are present within the lumen, and a chronic inflammatory infiltrate is often noted within the connective tissue of the wall.

Differential Diagnosis

Clinically, NDC should be distinguished from encephalocele that occurs at the same site. Histologically, epidermal inclusion cysts may resemble NDCs, but they do not contain adnexa. Mature teratomas have a more complex structure and contain endodermal elements.

Treatment and Prognosis

NDC is a benign lesion, which is treated by complete surgical excision. Transnasal endoscopic excision is performed if the cyst is located within the nasal cavity and there is minimal or no cutaneous involvement [3, 6]. The same approach can be

A. Franchi (✉)
Department of Translational Research and of New Technologies in Medicine and Surgery, University of Pisa, Pisa, Italy
e-mail: alessandro.franchi@unipi.it

A. Franchi (ed.), *Pathology of Sinonasal Tumors and Tumor-Like Lesions*,
https://doi.org/10.1007/978-3-030-29848-7_10

used even if preoperative radiologic studies show extension to the anterior cranial fossa [3]. When the NDC extends to the falx cerebri, a frontal craniotomy may be required [3]. If dermal remnants remain unresected, the NDC may recur locally.

Mature Teratoma

Definition

Sinonasal mature teratoma (SMT) is a benign germ cell tumor that shows similar histologic features to the counterparts arising in the gonads and at other extragonadic sites. It is composed of a variety of mature tissues that are foreign to the site of occurrence and are derived from two or three germ cell layers.

Clinical Features

SMTs are very rare. The reported cases have occurred almost exclusively in neonates and infants, who presented with facial deformity, nasal obstruction, and nasal mass [7–11]. SMTs can be associated with other congenital anomalies [12]. The nasal septum and the maxillary sinus are the most commonly affected sites.

Pathologic Features

SMTs may be cystic or solid. Microscopically, they are composed of variable admixtures of the skin with appendages, adipose tissue, smooth muscle, skeletal muscle, cartilage, bone, glial tissue, primitive and mature glandular epithelium, respiratory epithelium, and gastrointestinal epithelium. Malignant transformation in invasive squamous cell carcinoma has been described in a benign teratoma of the maxilla of a 13-month-old boy [13].

Differential Diagnosis

Nasal glial heterotopia, meningocele, and dermoid cyst can be separate from SMT because they lack the variegated histological appearance of mature teratoma. Teratocarcinosarcoma may present mature elements that resemble a mature teratoma, but presents also clear histologic malignant features that allow its distinction.

Treatment and Prognosis

The treatment is surgical, and intranasal teratomas have been successfully resected endoscopically [7, 10].

Yolk Sac Tumor

Definition

Yolk sac tumor (YST; synonym: endodermal sinus tumor) is a malignant germ cell tumor which is histologically undistinguishable from YST of the gonads.

Clinical Features

YST is an extremely rare malignant tumor in the sinonasal tract, with only few examples reported in the literature. It affects mainly children, but cases arising in adult patients have also been reported [14–19]. Presenting symptoms are nonspecific and include headache, nasal obstruction, rhinorrhea, and epistaxis.

Pathologic Features

YST is characterized by multiple histologic patterns, frequently encountered in the same tumor. The most common are the reticular (microcystic) and endodermal, but macrocystic, solid, alveolar-glandular, and polyvesicular vitelline patterns are also described. Cuboidal and cylindrical neoplastic cells have a primitive appearance, with clear, glycogen-rich cytoplasm, and hyperchromatic irregular nuclei with prominent nucleoli. Mitotic figures are usually numerous. A characteristic feature of YST is the presence of Schiller–Duval bodies, which consist of round or elongated papillae with a fibrovascular core, which occupy spaces lined by cuboidal cells. PAS-positive diastase-resistant intracellular hyaline bodies are another common histologic feature of YST, usually associated with the reticular or solid patterns.

In adult patients, YST has developed in combination with carcinomas, including non-keratinizing squamous cell carcinoma [14], undifferentiated carcinoma [17], and SMARCB1 deficient carcinoma [20]. This scenario raises the possibility that, at least in adult patients, YST may represent a divergent "dedifferentiation" of other malignancies. Foci of choriocarcinoma have also been observed in sinonasal YST [15]. A yolk cell component has been documented in a case of sinonasal teratocarcinosarcoma [21].

Immunohistochemistry

Considering that YST may occur in association with carcinomas, immunohistochemical panels should aim to characterize the different components. YST is positive for low molecular weight cytokeratins, α-fetoprotein, and SALL4. Glypican-3 is positive not only in YST but also in choriocarcinoma and metastatic hepatocellular carcinoma and may be expressed in immature teratoma [22]. Human chorionic gonadotropin-positive syncytiotrophoblasts are detected in areas of associated choriocarcinoma.

Differential Diagnosis

The differential diagnosis is broad and depends on the predominant pattern. Tumors with solid growth have to be distinguished from various carcinoma types, including non-keratinizing squamous cell carcinoma, basaloid squamous cell carcinoma, and sinonasal undifferentiated carcinoma. Tumors with cystic and microcystic architecture may be confused mainly with non-intestinal-type adenocarcinomas. Immunostaining for α-fetoprotein helps in the distinction.

Treatment and Prognosis

In general, the prognosis of sinonasal YST is poor, both for the tendency to local recurrence and the high incidence of metastasis to lung, liver, regional lymph nodes, and bone at the time of presentation. Surgical excision is the treatment of choice for patients with localized tumors, and induction or adjuvant chemotherapy can be considered in the treatment of advanced disease [17]. Radiotherapy may be used in surgically inaccessible regions [17]. YST produces α-fetoprotein, which, although not specific, can be used as a marker to monitor residual and metastatic disease.

Choriocarcinoma

Definition

Choriocarcinoma is a malignant tumor composed of an admixture of syncytiotrophoblast, cytotrophoblast, and intermediate trophoblast.

Clinical Features

It is an extremely rare tumor in the sinonasal tract. One reported case involved the maxillary antrum, and another one affected the nasal cavity, the ethmoid, and sphenoid sinuses [23]. Both patients were males in the fifth decade of life, presented with nasal obstruction and epistaxis, and had elevated serum levels of human chorionic gonadotropin.

Pathologic Features

Grossly, the tumor is friable, necrotic, and hemorrhagic. Histologically, it consists of a population of smaller mononuclear, round to polygonal cells with clear cytoplasm, ovoid nuclei with prominent nucleoli resembling cytotrophoblast or intermediate trophoblast, admixed with multinucleated syncytiotrophoblastic cells with abundant eosinophilic cytoplasm and multiple large nuclei with prominent nucleoli.

Immunohistochemistry

Syncytiotrophoblastic cells are positive for β-HCG. Cytokeratins and CD10 are positive in all choriocarcinoma cells, while CK5/6, p63,S-100 protein, α-fetoprotein, OCT4, and renal cell carcinoma marker are negative.

Differential Diagnosis

The differential diagnosis includes poorly differentiated carcinomas and adenocarcinomas, and sinonasal melanoma. In addition, a choriocarcinoma component may be encountered in sinonasal yolk sac tumor. Finally, metastatic gestational and nongestational choriocarcinoma must be ruled out before establishing a diagnosis of primary sinonasal choriocarcinoma [24–26].

Treatment and Prognosis

Contrary to gestational choriocarcinoma that shows an extreme sensitivity for chemotherapy, extragonadal tumors are usually unresponsive to surgical and chemotherapeutic treatment and present a poor prognosis [23].

References

1. Hughes GB, Sharpino G, Hunt W, Tucker HM. Management of the congenital midline nasal mass—a review. Head Neck Surg. 1980;2:222–33.
2. Rohrich RJ, Lowe JB, Schwartz MR. The role of open rhinoplasty in the management of nasal dermoid cysts. Plast Reconstr Surg. 1999;104:2163–70.
3. Hanikeri M, Waterhouse N, Kirkpatrick N, Peterson D, Macleod I. The management of midline transcranial nasal dermoid sinus cysts. Br J Plast Surg. 2005;58:1043–50.
4. Wardinsky TD, Pagon RA, Kropp RJ, Hayden PW, Clarren SK. Nasal dermoid sinus cysts: association with intracranial extension and multiple malformations. Cleft Palate Craniofac J. 1991;28:87–95.
5. Torske KR, Benson GS, Warnock G. Dermoid cyst of the maxillary sinus. Ann Diagn Pathol. 2001;5:172–6.
6. Zapata S, Kearns DB. Nasal dermoids. Curr Opin Otolaryngol Head Neck Surg. 2006;14:406–11.
7. Yeo WX, Tan KK. Diagnosis and surgical management of congenital intranasal teratoma in a newborn: a rare case report. Case Rep Otolaryngol. 2018;2018:1403912.
8. Cukurova I, Gumussoy M, Yaz A, Bayol U, Yigitbasi OG. A benign teratoma presenting as an obstruction of the nasal cavity: a case report. J Med Case Rep. 2012;6:147.
9. Ibekwe TS, Kokong DD, Ngwu BA, Akinyemi OA, Nwaorgu OG, Akang EE. Nasal septal teratoma in a child. World J Surg Oncol. 2007;5:58.
10. Huth ME, Heimgartner S, Schnyder I, Caversaccio MD. Teratoma of the nasal septum in a neonate: an endoscopic approach. J Pediatr Surg. 2008;43:2102–5.
11. Streetharan SS, Prepageran N. Benign teratoma of nasal cavity. Med J Malaysia. 2004;59:678–9.
12. Kamyar K, Seedebrahim T, Nazanin H. A rare case of large nasal teratoma associated with congenital heart anomalies in a neonate. Iran J Pediatr. 2013;23:120–1.
13. Kuhn JJ, Schoem SR, Warnock GR. Squamous cell carcinoma arising in a benign teratoma of the maxilla. Otolaryngol Head Neck Surg. 1996;114:447–52.
14. Manivel C, Wick MR, Dehner LP. Transitional (cylindric) cell carcinoma with endodermal sinus tumor-like features of the nasopharynx and paranasal sinuses. Clinicopathologic and immunohistochemical study of two cases. Arch Pathol Lab Med. 1986;110:198–202.
15. Filho BC, McHugh JB, Carrau RL, Kassam AB. Yolk sac tumor in the nasal cavity. Am J Otolaryngol. 2008;29:250–4.
16. Gangopadhyay K, McArthur PD, Martin JM, Saleem M. Endodermal sinus tumor of the maxillary sinus: a case report. Ear Nose Throat J. 1999;78:376–2.
17. Mishra A, El-Naggar AK, Demonte F, Hanna EY. Endodermal sinus tumor of the paranasal sinuses. Head Neck. 2008;30:539–43.
18. Westerveld GJ, Quak JJ, Bresters D, Zwaan CM, van der Valk P, Leemans CR. Endodermal sinus tumor of the maxillary sinus. Otolaryngol Head Neck Surg. 2001;124:691–2.
19. Chuang HC, Kang CJ, Lee LY. Sinonasal pure yolk sac tumor: a case report and literature review. Fetal Pediatr Pathol. 2014;33:127–34.
20. Zamecnik M, Rychnovsky J, Syrovatka J. Sinonasal SMARCB1 (INI1) deficient carcinoma with yolk sac tumor differentiation: report of a case and comparison with INI1 expression in gonadal germ cell tumors. Int J Surg Pathol. 2018;26:245–9.

21. Thomas J, Adegboyega P, Iloabachie K, Mooring JW, Lian T. Sinonasal teratocarcinosarcoma with yolk sac elements: a neoplasm of somatic or germ cell origin? Ann Diagn Pathol. 2011;15:135–9.
22. Rabban JT, Zaloudek CJ. A practical approach to immunohistochemical diagnosis of ovarian germ cell tumors and sex cord-stromal tumors. Histopathology. 2013;62:71–88.
23. Bell DM, Porras G, Tortoledo ME, Luna MA. Primary sinonasal choriocarcinoma. Ann Diagn Pathol. 2009;13:96–100.
24. Salimi R. Metastatic choriocarcinoma of the nasal mucosa. J Surg Oncol. 1977;9:301–5.
25. Mukherjee DK. Choriocarcinoma of the nose. Ann Otol Rhinol Laryngol. 1978;87:257–9.
26. Tangtrakul S, Linasmita V, Wilailak S, Srisupandit S, Bullangpoti S, Ayudhya NI. An HIV-infected woman with choriocarcinoma presenting with a nasal mass. Gynecol Oncol. 1998;68:304–6.

Metastatic Tumors

Alessandro Franchi

Definition

Sinonasal metastases are malignant tumors deriving from noncontiguous anatomic sites, thus excluding direct extension from an adjacent structure and also localization of leukemia/lymphoma. They occur through hematogenous spread, possibly through the venous Batson route along the prevertebral venous plexus [1].

The most frequently involved anatomic sites are the maxillary (33%), sphenoid (22%), ethmoid (14%), and frontal (9%) sinuses [4–6]. Multiple sinuses are involved in approximately 20% of the cases, while in 10–15% the metastases are limited to the nasal cavity [7]. The most frequent primary sites of origin of the tumors are the kidney (40%), lung (9%), breast (8%), thyroid (8%), prostate (7%), and others (28%).

Clinical Features

Sinonasal metastases are rare. Usually they present in patients with a known history of a primary, and only occasionally they are the first manifestation of a clinically occult malignancy [2, 3]. In most cases, metastatic disease involves only one paranasal sinus or one site in the nasal cavity. The clinical presentation is similar to that of primary sinonasal tumors, and symptoms are nonspecific. They include recurrent epistaxis, which is more common in metastases from renal and thyroid carcinomas, nasal obstruction, headache, and facial pain. Visual disturbances, exophthalmos, and palpebral ptosis are also common symptoms.

Pathologic Features

The histopathologic features of metastatic tumors to the sinonasal tract reproduce more often the histological features of the primary tumors, which may facilitate their recognition.

Among the several variants of renal cell carcinoma, the clear cell type is the most frequent, while other types are very rarely seen [8–10]. Clear-cell renal carcinoma presents with polygonal tumor cells with optically clear cytoplasm arranged in acinar, alveolar, or solid pattern, with a rich network of capillary and sinusoidal vascular structures. There are often associated hemorrhage and necrosis which are visible on both gross and microscopic examination.

Thyroid carcinomas are usually of the papillary and follicular types [11, 12] and may show clear cell morphology [13].

Rare examples of colorectal adenocarcinoma metastatic to the sinonasal tract have been

A. Franchi (✉)
Department of Translational Research and of New Technologies in Medicine and Surgery, University of Pisa, Pisa, Italy
e-mail: alessandro.franchi@unipi.it

A. Franchi (ed.), *Pathology of Sinonasal Tumors and Tumor-Like Lesions*,
https://doi.org/10.1007/978-3-030-29848-7_11

reported, occurring mainly as a late manifestation of the disease [14, 15].

Hepatocellular carcinoma may metastasize to the sinonasal region both as presenting sign or in the advanced stages of the disease [16–18]. Neoplastic cells are large and polygonal, with eosinophilic cytoplasm, and are arranged in nests and thick trabeculae. The presence of bile production is a helpful histological sign for the diagnosis.

Breast carcinoma is among the most common tumors to metastasize to the head and neck, but involvement of the sinonasal tract is exceptional [19]. Histologically, it shows features of ductal or lobular histological types, but a mucinous component may be present as well, thus requiring careful distinction from a primary adenocarcinoma [19].

Differential Diagnosis

Metastatic clear cell carcinoma of the kidney has to be distinguished mainly from primary sinonasal renal cell-like adenocarcinoma. An immunohistochemical panel including vimentin and RCC, that are usually positive in clear cell renal carcinoma and negative in renal cell-like adenocarcinoma, and CK7, which is positive in only a minority of conventional clear cell RCC but always positive in sinonasal renal cell-like adenocarcinoma [20], helps in the distinction.

Metastatic small and large cell neuroendocrine carcinomas, mainly originating from the lung, have to be distinguished from their primary sinonasal counterparts. The histological and immunohistochemical profile is similar, including positivity for cytokeratins, neuroendocrine markers, and TTF1, and therefore the distinction must rely on the correlation with clinical data [21].

Metastatic thyroid carcinomas have to be differentiated from primary sinonasal low-grade tubulopapillary adenocarcinomas. Positivity for TTF-1 and thyroglobulin helps in the distinction.

Metastatic intestinal adenocarcinomas require precise distinction from primary intestinal-type adenocarcinoma, because of the different treatment modalities and prognosis [22]. The histopathologic aspect is completely overlapping, as it is the immunohistochemical profile, with both primary and secondary tumors being positive for cytokeratin 20 and CDX2, as well as for other markers of intestinal differentiation, although positivity for cytokeratin 7 speaks more in favor of a primary adenocarcinoma [23]. However, secondary tumors usually develop in patients with a history of colorectal adenocarcinoma, and thus clinical data are essential for the correct diagnosis In addition, while sinonasal intestinal-type adenocarcinoma originates in most cases from the upper nasal cavities and ethmoid sinuses, metastatic deposits tend to involve other sites, like the maxillary sinus.

The diagnosis of metastatic hepatocellular carcinoma may be suggested by the identification of bile production by neoplastic cells and is supported by the positivity for Hepar-1, glypican-3, and arginase.

The distinction of metastatic breast carcinoma from a primary sinonasal carcinoma is supported by the positivity for breast markers, including GATA-3 and mammaglobin, while GCDFP-15 is less frequently positive [19].

Metastatic prostatic adenocarcinoma is often poorly differentiated, and therefore distinction from sinonasal adenocarcinomas is supported by immunohistochemical positivity with antibodies to prostatic-specific antigen and prostatic acid phosphatase, while prostatic adenocarcinoma is usually negative for EMA and cytokeratin 7.

Treatment and Prognosis

The prognosis of patients with sinonasal metastases is poor, and treatment usually aims at palliation, trying to avoid a relevant morbidity. Minimally invasive endoscopic surgical treatments and palliative radiotherapy may prolong survival and provide a rapid improvement of symptoms and quality of life. Medical treatments are also employed, for example, in metastatic breast carcinoma, but still with a palliative aim, though associated with high rates of clinical improvement of local symptoms [24, 25].

Preoperative embolization and endoscopic resection followed by proton beam radiation is the treatment algorithm for resectable metastases from renal cell carcinoma [10].

References

1. Batson OV. The function of the vertebral veins and their role in the spread of metastasis. Ann Surg. 1988;112:138–49.
2. Fyrmpas G, Adeniyi A, Baer S. Occult renal cell carcinoma manifesting with epistaxis in a woman: a case report. J Med Case Rep. 2011;5:79.
3. Lee HM, Kang HJ, Lee SH. Metastatic renal cell carcinoma presenting as epistaxis. Eur Arch Otorhinolaryngol. 2005;262:69–71.
4. Prescher A, Brors D. Metastases to the paranasal sinuses: case report and review of the literature. Laryngorhinootologie. 2001;80:583–94.
5. McClatchey KD, Lloyd RV, Schaldenbrand JD. Metastatic carcinoma to the sphenoid sinus. Case report and review of the literature. Arch Otorhinolaryngol. 1985;241:219–24.
6. López F, Devaney KO, Hanna EY, Rinaldo A, Ferlito A. Metastases to nasal cavity and paranasal sinuses. Head Neck. 2016;38:1847–54.
7. Barnes L. Metastases to the head and neck: an overview. Head Neck Pathol. 2009;3:217–24.
8. Remenschneider AK, Sadow PM, Lin DT, Gray ST. Metastatic renal cell carcinoma to the sinonasal cavity: a case series. J Neurol Surg Rep. 2013;74:67–72.
9. Terada T. Renal cell carcinoma metastatic to the nasal cavity. Int J Clin Exp Pathol. 2012;5:588–91.
10. Bastier PL, Dunion D, de Bonnecaze G, Serrano E, de Gabory L. Renal cell carcinoma metastatic to the sinonasal cavity: a review and report of 8 cases. Ear Nose Throat J. 2018;97:E6–E12.
11. Altman KW, Mirza N, Philippe L. Metastatic follicular thyroid carcinoma to the paranasal sinuses: a case report and review. J Laryngol Otol. 1997;111:647–51.
12. Freeman JL, Gershon A, Liavaag PG, Walfish PG. Papillary thyroid carcinoma metastasizing to the sphenoid-ethmoid sinuses and skull base. Thyroid. 1996;6:59–61.
13. Altinay S, Taşkin Ü, Aydin S, Oktay MF, Özen A, Ergül N. Metastatic follicular thyroid carcinoma masquerading as olfactory neuroblastoma: with skull-base, cranium, paranasal sinus, lung, and diffuse bone metastases. J Craniofac Surg. 2015;26:e3–6.
14. Conill C, Vargas M, Valduvieco I, Fernandez PL, Cardesa A, Capurro S. Metastasis to the nasal cavity from primary rectal adenocarcinoma. Clin Transl Oncol. 2009;11:117–9.
15. Tanaka K. A case of metastases to the paranasal sinus from rectal mucinous adenocarcinoma. Int J Clin Oncol. 2006;11:64–5.
16. Mohammed H, Sheikh R, Rahman W, Sheta S, Dogan Z. Undiagnosed hepatocellular carcinoma presenting as nasal metastases. Case Rep Otolaryngol. 2015;2015:856134.
17. Hashim H, Rahmat K, Abdul Aziz YF, Chandran PA. Metastatic hepatocellular carcinoma presenting as a sphenoid sinus mass and meningeal carcinomatosis. Ear Nose Throat J. 2014;93:E20–3.
18. Lee TH, Rangan V, Khallafi H. A case of sphenoid sinus metastasis in hepatocellular carcinoma. Hepatology. 2016;63:2050–3.
19. Gondim DD, Chernock R, El-Mofty S, Lewis JS Jr. The great mimicker: metastatic breast carcinoma to the head and neck with emphasis on unusual clinical and pathologic features. Head Neck Pathol. 2017;11:306–13.
20. Storck K, Moh'd Hadi U, Simpson R, Ramer M, Brandwein-Gensler M. Sinonasal renal cell-like adenocarcinoma: a report on four patients. Head Neck Pathol. 2008;2:75–80.
21. Kaufmann O, Dietel M. Expression of thyroid transcription factor-1 in pulmonary and extrapulmonary small cell carcinomas and other neuroendocrine carcinomas of various primary sites. Histopathology. 2000;36:415–20.
22. Conill C, Vargas M, Valduvieco I, Fernández PL, Cardesa A, Capurro S. Metastasis to the nasal cavity from primary rectal adenocarcinoma. Clin Transl Oncol. 2009;11:117–9.
23. Resto VA, Krane JF, Faquin WC, Lin DT. Immunohistochemical distinction of intestinal-type sinonasal adenocarcinoma from metastatic adenocarcinoma of intestinal origin. Ann Otol Rhinol Laryngol. 2006;115:59–64.
24. Weng B, Wang Q, Lin S, Lu Y. Nasal cavity metastasis of breast cancer: a case report and review of the literature. Int J Clin Exp Pathol. 2014;7:7028–33.
25. Pittoni P, Di Lascio S, Conti-Beltraminelli M, et al. Paranasal sinus metastasis of breast cancer. BMJ Case Rep. 2014;2014:bcr2014205171.

Index

A. Franchi (ed.), *Pathology of Sinonasal Tumors and tumor-like lesions*,
https://doi.org/10.1007/978-3-030-29848-7

The manufacturer's authorised representative in the EU is Springer Nature Customer Service Centre GmbH, Europaplatz 3, 69115 Heidelberg, Germany. If you have any concerns regarding our products, please contact ProductSafety@springernature.com

Printed and bound by CPI Group (UK) Ltd, Croydon, CR0 4YY
27/07/2026
02177354-0001